Contents

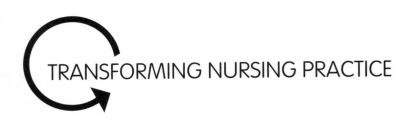

TRANSFORMING NURSING PRACTICE

Transforming Nursing Practice is a series tailor made for pre-registration students nurses. Each book in the series is:

 Affordable

 Full of active learning features

 Mapped to the NMC Standards of proficiency for registered nurses

 Focused on applying theory to practice

Each book addresses a core topic and they have been carefully developed to be simple to use, quick to read and written in clear language.

An invaluable series of books that explicitly relates to the NMC standards. Each book covers a different topic that students need to explore in order to develop into a qualified nurse... I would recommend this series to all Pre-Registered nursing students whatever their field or year of study.

LINDA ROBSON,
Senior Lecturer at Edge Hill University

Many titles in the series are on our recommended reading list and for good reason - the content is up to date and easy to read. These are the books that actually get used beyond training and into your nursing career.

EMMA LYDON,
Adult Student Nursing

ABOUT THE SERIES EDITORS

DR MOOI STANDING is an Independent Nursing Consultant (UK and International) and is responsible for the core knowledge, adult nursing and personal and professional learning skills titles. She is an experienced NMC Quality Assurance Reviewer of educational programmes and a Professional Regulator Panellist on the NMC Practice Committee. Mooi is also Board member of Special Olympics Malaysia, enabling people with intellectual disabilities to participate in sports and athletics nationally and internationally.

DR SANDRA WALKER is a Clinical Academic in Mental Health working between Southern Health Trust and the University of Southampton and responsible for the mental health nursing titles. She is a Qualified Mental Health Nurse with a wide range of clinical experience spanning more than 25 years.

Nursing Adults with Long Term Conditions

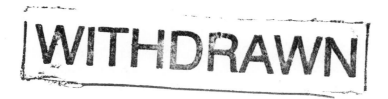

Sara Miller McCune founded SAGE Publishing in 1965 to support the dissemination of usable knowledge and educate a global community. SAGE publishes more than 1000 journals and over 800 new books each year, spanning a wide range of subject areas. Our growing selection of library products includes archives, data, case studies and video. SAGE remains majority owned by our founder and after her lifetime will become owned by a charitable trust that secures the company's continued independence.

Los Angeles | London | New Delhi | Singapore | Washington DC | Melbourne

3rd Edition

Nursing Adults with Long Term Conditions

Jane Nicol &
Lorna Hollowood

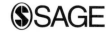

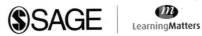

Learning Matters
An imprint of SAGE Publications Ltd
1 Oliver's Yard
55 City Road
London EC1Y 1SP

SAGE Publications Inc.
2455 Teller Road
Thousand Oaks, California 91320

SAGE Publications India Pvt Ltd
B 1/I 1 Mohan Cooperative Industrial Area
Mathura Road
New Delhi 110 044

SAGE Publications Asia-Pacific Pte Ltd
33 Pekin Street #02–01
Far East Square
Singapore 048763

Editor: Donna Goddard
Development editor: Richenda Milton-Daws
Senior project editor: Chris Marke
Project management: Deer Park Productions
Marketing manager: George Kimble
Cover design: Wendy Scott
Typeset by: C&M Digitals (P) Ltd, Chennai, India
Printed in the UK

Library of Congress Control Number: 2019931376

British Library Cataloguing in Publication data

A catalogue record for this book is available from
the British Library

ISBN 978-1-5264-5919-0
ISBN 978-1-5264-5920-6 (pbk)

At SAGE we take sustainability seriously. Most of our products are printed in the UK using responsibly sourced
papers and boards. When we print overseas we ensure sustainable papers are used as measured by the
Egmont grading system. We undertake an annual audit to monitor our sustainability.

BESTSELLING TEXTBOOKS

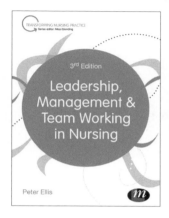

3rd Edition

Leadership, Management & Team Working in Nursing

Peter Ellis

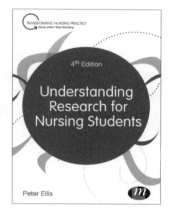

4th Edition

Understanding Research for Nursing Students

Peter Ellis

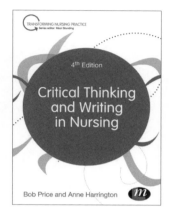

4th Edition

Critical Thinking and Writing in Nursing

Bob Price and Anne Harrington

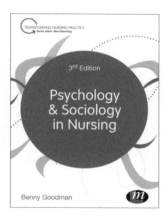

3rd Edition

Psychology & Sociology in Nursing

Benny Goodman

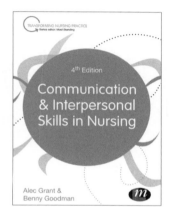

4th Edition

Communication & Interpersonal Skills in Nursing

Alec Grant & Benny Goodman

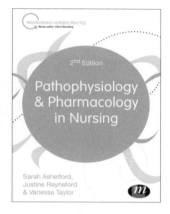

2nd Edition

Pathophysiology & Pharmacology in Nursing

Sarah Ashelford, Justine Raynsford & Vanessa Taylor

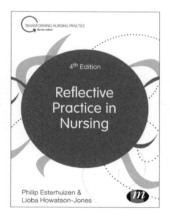

4th Edition

Reflective Practice in Nursing

Philip Esterhuizen & Lioba Howatson-Jones

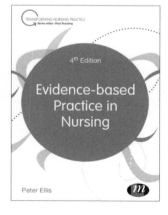

4th Edition

Evidence-based Practice in Nursing

Peter Ellis

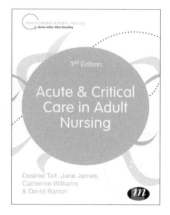

3rd Edition

Acute & Critical Care in Adult Nursing

Desiree Tait, Jane James, Catherine Williams & David Barton

You can find a full list of textbooks in the
Transforming Nursing Practice series at

https://uk.sagepub.com

This book is dedicated to:
Neil Anderson

About the authors

Jane Nicol is a Registered General Nurse and Lecturer in the School of Nursing at the University of Birmingham. During her career she has worked across a range of clinical settings in both primary and secondary care, enabling her to develop a broad knowledge and skill base. She currently teaches pre-registration nursing students at the University of Birmingham. Jane's specialist areas of teaching are the care and management of people living with long term conditions and palliative and end-of-life care. She is a published author in both these areas. Jane's contribution to student learning has been recognised nationally, she has been shortlisted for both Nursing Times and Student Nursing Times Awards.

Lorna Hollowood is a Registered Adult Nurse and Lecturer in the School of Nursing at the University of Birmingham. Lorna has a clinical background in District Nursing and palliative care. She teaches on a variety of modules with a focus on public health, long term conditions and contributes to palliative and end-of-life care teaching across the programme. She maintains her clinical activity through assessing and supporting the care home sector in the provision of end-of-life care.

Acknowledgements

The publishers and author would like to thank the following for their very helpful feedback during the writing of this book:

Maggie Roberts, Health Lecturer and Pathway Leader for Primary Care, and Chair of the Community Practice Learning Team, at the University of Nottingham;

Paul Macreth, Senior Lecturer and Course Leader for District Nursing, at Leeds Metropolitan University.

They would also like to thank Pilgrim Projects Ltd and the Patient Voices website (www.patientvoices.org.uk) for Bill's story and the accompanying word cloud (Figure 2.1) in the case study on page 31. The word cloud was created at www.wordle.net.

Introduction

About this book

People living with long term conditions (LTCs) are often experts in their own condition, living with and managing it on a day-to-day basis. Therefore, nurses and other healthcare professionals caring for, and working with, people living with LTCs have to possess the knowledge, skills and attributes that will foster partnership working, encourage self-management and support those whose condition requires more active care and management. The aim of this book is to provide an overview of the key aspects of the care and management of LTCs and to relate these to clinical practice. While the chapters in this book are presented sequentially, it is recognised that aspects of the care and management of a person living with an LTC, such as health promotion and symptom management, feature throughout their journey, from diagnosis through to palliative and end-of-life care. This book is aimed at pre-registration students, with the topics covered applied across the lifespan. It is aimed at supporting the development of knowledge and skills required to work with people living with long term conditions, both physical and mental health. In addition to pre-registration students, this book may be of relevance to qualified health and social care professionals keen to develop their knowledge of supporting people living with long term conditions.

A note on terminology

Given that the underlying premise of the care and management of long term conditions is based on self-care and self-management, the term 'person/individual' has been used, but when the context demands, the term 'patient' has been used.

Book structure

The chapters in this book are written sequentially and are designed to take you on the journey a person with an LTC travels from diagnosis through to palliative care. However, the book can be read by dipping in and out of chapters, though it is recommended that Chapter 1 is read first. Chapter 1 provides an overview of LTCs, their impact across the lifespan, and the importance of planning for transition of care from child to adult services. Models of care delivery and the impact that LTCs have on individuals, both physically and psychologically, are explored.

In Chapter 2, the focus is on developing and maintaining an effective nurse–patient relationship with both the person living with an LTC and their carer. The role that emotional intelligence and resilience have in the care and management of LTCs is examined. The importance of effective communication is reviewed with some useful communication strategies outlined and related to LTCs. Chapter 3 uses an exploration of the determinants of health and public health to set the context of health promotion in LTCs demonstrating the multifactorial nature of health and health promotion. The importance of health promotion in LTCs is explained and applied to practice; health promotion models are outlined and their relevance to LTCs discussed. Strategies for health promotion such as motivational interviewing are examined and related to people living with an LTC. Chapter 4 focuses on the importance of promoting self-management for people living with an LTC. The importance of self-efficacy and patient activation enabling people living with an LTC to self-manage is explored. By examining the skills and knowledge necessary to become successful self-managers, and by applying them to clinical scenarios, self-efficacy and patient activation of people living with LTCs can be increased. In Chapter 5, quality of life and symptom management in long term conditions are addressed, highlighting the areas of a person's life that influence and affect their quality of life. Effective symptom management is discussed using a framework such as the nursing process to support care. In Chapter 6, the emphasis is on case management. The roles and responsibilities of case managers are reflected upon, explored and related to case scenarios. Strategies to support complex care, such as care pathways and effective discharge planning, emphasise the need for collaborative working in the care and management of people living with an LTC.

Chapter 7 is the final chapter and introduces palliative care as a key part of the care and management of people with LTCs. The concept of 'bad news' is discussed, and the importance of effective communication skills when breaking 'bad news' are emphasised and reflected upon. Specific strategies, including assessment frameworks, that can be used to support person-centred palliative and end-of-life care are examined and related to clinical practice.

Requirements from the NMC standards

Evidence-based nursing requires the nurse to have knowledge and skills, which are outlined in detail in the document Standards of Proficiency for Registered Nurses (NMC, 2018). These standards are used by educational institutions when planning professional courses. They are grouped into seven 'Platforms', as shown in the box.

Standards of proficiency for registered nurses (NMC, 2018)

- Platform 1: Being an accountable professional

Registered nurses act in the best interests of people, putting them first and providing nursing care that is person-centred, safe and compassionate. They act professionally at all times and use their knowledge and experience to make evidence-based decisions about care. They communicate care effectively, are role models for others and are accountable for their actions. Registered nurses continually reflect on their practice and keep abreast of new and emerging developments in nursing, health and care.

- Platform 2: Promoting health and preventing ill health

Registered nurses play a key role in improving and maintaining the mental, physical and behavioural health and well-being of people, families, communities and populations. They support and enable people at all stages of life and in all care settings to make informed choices about how to manage health challenges in order to maximise their quality of life and improve health outcomes. They are actively involved in the prevention of and protection against disease and ill health, and engage in public health, community development and global health agendas, and in the reduction of health inequalities.

- Platform 3: Assessing needs and planning care

Registered nurses prioritise the needs of people when assessing and reviewing their mental, physical, cognitive, behavioural, social and spiritual needs. They use information obtained during assessments to identify the priorities and requirements for person-centred and evidence-based nursing interventions and support. They work in partnership with people to develop person-centred care plans that take into account their circumstances, characteristics and preferences.

- Platform 4: Providing and evaluating care

Registered nurses take the lead in providing evidence-based, compassionate and safe nursing interventions. They ensure that the care they provide and delegate is person-centred and of a consistently high standard. They support people of all ages in a range of care settings. They work in partnership with people, families and carers to evaluate whether care is effective and the goals of care have been met in line with their wishes, preferences and desired outcomes.

- Platform 5: Leading and managing nursing care and working in teams

Registered nurses provide leadership by acting as a role model for best practice in the delivery of nursing care. They are responsible for managing nursing care and are accountable for the appropriate delegation and supervision of care provided by others in the team including lay carers. They play an active and equal role in the interdisciplinary team, collaborating and communicating effectively with a range of colleagues.

- Platform 6: Improving safety and quality of care

Registered nurses make a key contribution to the continuous monitoring and quality improvement of care and treatment in order to enhance health outcome and people's experience of nursing and related care. They assess risks to safety or experience and take appropriate action to manage those, putting the best interests, needs and preferences of people first.

(Continued)

(Continued)

- Platform 7: Coordinating care

Registered nurses play a leadership role in coordinating and managing the complex nursing and integrated care needs of people at any stage of their lives, across a range of organisations and settings. They contribute to the processes of organisational change through an awareness of local and national policies.

This book draws from these Standards and presents the relevant ones at the beginning of each chapter.

Learning features

Throughout this book you will be presented with a range of learning activities that will help you to understand what you are reading. A series of case studies have been included to support the integration of theory and practice. These activities will encourage you to undertake some further independent study and to think more critically about the topics being discussed. Some of the activities will ask you to reflect on your previous clinical experience; reflection allows you to develop your understanding of yourself and your nursing practice, and to identify how things can be improved. Where relevant, sample answers are provided at the end of each chapter; it is hoped that these activities will encourage you to become increasingly self-directed in your learning. It may be appropriate for you to consider completing these activities, and including these in your personal and professional development portfolio.

There is a Glossary to explain some of the terms used at the end of the book. Glossary terms are in bold on the first instance that they appear.

Chapter 1

Long term conditions across the lifespan

(Continued)

Annexe B:

Part 1: Procedures for assessing people's needs for person-centred care

1   Use evidence based, best practice approaches to take a history, observe, recognise and accurately assess people of all ages:

    1.1   mental health and wellbeing status

    1.2   physical health and wellbeing

Chapter aims

After reading this chapter, you will be able to:

- describe the difference between an LTC and an acute condition;
- discuss the incidence of LTCs and their impact on healthcare provision;
- understand how the care and management of people living with a long term condition are organised;
- reflect on the physical and psychological impacts of living with LTCs;
- recognise the importance of appropriate care during the transition from child to adult services.

Introduction

When I was looking after it I could cope better, I checked her blood levels, made sure her insulin was given properly, but now I'm supposed to let go, trust her to manage and it's terrifying.

(Mother of a 15-year-old girl living with type 1 diabetes)

The amount of times I was going to give up (smoking), after every big birthday, and now the doctor says this is it, it'll only get worse, I can't run around with the grandkids without getting out of breath, I feel old before I'm ready . . . I know I've got to stop but I don't know how.

(54-year-old male diagnosed with COPD)

There's a sense of hopelessness as everyday things I took for granted become more difficult. You have to adjust your goal posts. I focus on tomorrow now, not so much about what I won't be able to control in the future.

(62-year-old female diagnosed with motor neurone disease six months ago)

Diagnosis of a long term condition (LTC) can occur at all stages across the lifespan, resulting in different implications for the person, their future and for those caring for them. For a child and their family, a diagnosis of asthma will mean a lifetime of adjustment and self-management of their condition. For a person diagnosed with type 1 diabetes, it may mean making lifestyle choices that they do not want to make, or living with the consequences. For a person learning to live with the long term complications of a condition, this could mean a long process of readjustment and finding new ways of doing things. Not only will their immediate concerns be different, the impact that their condition has on their day-to-day life will vary across the person's life. This will result in a range of needs having to be met, with the impact being felt physically, emotionally, socially and psychologically. In order for you to effectively support people living with LTCs, their family and carers, it is important to have an understanding of what LTCs are, their incidence across the lifespan and the frameworks used to guide their care and management. In order to do this, this chapter will develop your knowledge and understanding about LTCs, including transition of care from child to adult services and the importance of recognising the physical and psychological impact of living with LTCs.

Activity 1.1   Critical thinking

The Department of Health (DH) defines an LTC as: *a condition that cannot, at present, be cured but is controlled by medication and/or other treatment/therapies* (DH, 2012).

Using the above quote as a starting point, take some time to answer these questions.

- How many LTCs can you list?
- What is the difference between an acute condition and an LTC? Can you answer in terms of onset, duration, treatment and outcome?

A brief outline answer is given at the end of the chapter.

Activity 1.1 has drawn your attention to the complex nature of LTCs, their care, management and prognosis. Over time, it is likely that the symptoms of the condition become worse and there is a gradual, or sometimes sudden, deterioration in the health and well-being of the person living with the condition.

The incidence and impact of LTCs globally and in the UK

Globally, 70 per cent of deaths are attributable to LTCs, totalling over 40 million deaths a year. Cardiovascular disease, cancers, respiratory diseases and diabetes account for 80 per cent of all of these deaths and between them they share the following risk factors: tobacco use, physical inactivity, harmful alcohol use and unhealthy diets (WHO, 2017). This highlights and emphasises the fact that the majority of LTCs are exacerbated by lifestyle choices.

Living with an LTC can have a profound effect on a person's quality of life. Over 40 percent of people living with one LTC and over 80 per cent of people living with three or more report chronic pain (DH, 2012). However, the impact of LTCs can be felt beyond the person and their family. Globally, the rise in LTCs and the associated health costs in low-income countries can reduce household incomes; this in turn forces people into poverty and prevents economic development (WHO, 2013).

Since the National Health Service was founded in 1948, both life expectancy and the incidence of LTCs have increased. The Office for National Statistics (ONS) states that today, the life expectancy for men in the UK is 79.2 years and for women 82.9 years (ONS, 2017a). In addition, figures identify that the population of the UK is getting older, with the number of people over the age of 85 doubling in 25 years, equating to 5 per cent of the population (ONS, 2017b). These developments have led to an increase in the incidence and prevalence of LTCs, especially some cancers – e.g., prostate, chronic kidney disease and diabetes (DH, 2012).

The Department for Health (DH) estimates that the number of people living with LTCs will remain relatively stable over the next ten years, but that the number of people living with multiple LTCs will rise from 1.9 million (in 2008) to 2.9 million in 2018 (DH, 2012). Figures from the DH (2012) estimate that approximately 10 per cent of children under the age of 10 are living with one or more LTC, and of these, 2 per cent are living with a mental health LTC and 4 per cent are living with asthma. By the age of 60, 40 per cent of people have one or more LTCs, rising to 70 per cent in the over 80s (DH, 2012).

The most common LTCs are diabetes, mental health problems, hypertension, asthma, musculoskeletal problems and heart disease (DH, 2012). In the UK, people living with LTCs are the most intensive users of health and social care services; currently, 70 per cent of the health budget is spent on the 30 per cent of the population living with LTCs (George and Martin, 2016). Therefore, to promote well-being and to reduce pressures on health and social care services, the care and management for people with LTCs should focus on delaying the progression of LTCs through effective self-management. Combating LTCs, both in the UK and globally, requires change on many levels, from supporting a person to make a change in their lifestyle to promoting public health policies that promote the prevention of LTCs.

Case study: Frazer

Frazer was diagnosed with type 1 diabetes when he was 8 years old. As a child, Frazer was supported in managing his condition by his parents. However, as he grew up and became a young person, he did not manage his diabetes well. He started to smoke and drink heavily; this made it harder for him to maintain his blood glucose levels below 7.8mmol/l and throughout his early adulthood his blood glucose levels were consistently raised.

Frazer lives with his partner Claire and their 11-year-old daughter Fiona. Claire works full time for a local whisky distillery. Frazer works part time as an office administrator and takes care of his daughter after school. Frazer stopped smoking five years ago; however, he continues to drink alcohol on a daily basis, despite being asked to stop by family and healthcare professionals.

Frazer is now 47 years old and was diagnosed with diabetic **polyneuropathy** in his late 30s; this means that he has reduced nerve sensation in his feet. He has had both great toes amputated as a result of this; in addition, he has had longstanding problems with foot ulcers and recurrent infections. Most recently, Frazer has received negative pressure wound therapy as an inpatient to try to prevent amputation of his lower leg.

Activity 1.2   Critical thinking

Read the case study above about Frazer and then answer the following questions.

- Over the course of his disease progression, what health and social care services would Frazer and his family access? Can you identify these services within the clinical area that you work in and do you know how to refer to them?
- What impact will Frazer's LTC have on his family?

A brief outline answer is given at the end of the chapter.

Activity 1.2 emphasises the impact that caring and managing LTCs has not only for health and social care services, but for the family of the person living with the condition. Over the course of their life, people living with LTCs will have contact with many health and social care professionals. Their care may be delivered in a **primary**, **secondary** or **tertiary** care setting. However, public policy (NHS, Scotland, 2010; Department of Health, Social Services and Public Safety (DHSSPS), 2012; NHS England, 2017; Wales Audit Office, 2014) emphasises the importance of health promotion and self-management in LTCs with out-of-hospital care playing a larger part in overall NHS services. This is reflected in Activity 1.2 where it can be seen that the majority of Frazer's care and management is provided in primary care. In all of these documents there is a clear emphasis on the importance of working with the person to provide patient-centred care and promote empowerment, self-care and management. As an LTC progresses, professionals are expected to deliver effective care and case management, and prepare for palliative care requirements.

Quality Outcomes Framework

The Quality Outcomes Framework (QOF) is a voluntary, annual incentive programme that pays GP surgeries for achievement in three domains: clinical, public health and additional services. Within the QOF the clinical domain there is a focus on the successful management of LTCs through the use of specific indicators (see Table 1.1).

Conditions listed on the QOF (listed alphabetically)	Examples of QOF indicators (listed alphabetically)
• Asthma • Atrial fibrillation • Cancer • Chronic kidney disease (CKD) • Chronic obstructive pulmonary disease • Coronary heart disease • Dementia • Depression • Diabetes mellitus • Epilepsy • Heart failure • Hypertension • Hypothyroid • Learning disability • Mental health • Obesity • Palliative care • Smoking • Stroke and transient ischaemic attack (TIA)	• Achieving target blood pressure – e.g., maintaining a blood pressure of 150/90 for people with hypertension • Achieving target cholesterol level • Confirming diagnosis with objective measures – e.g., echocardiogram confirming heart failure • Condition-specific reviews – e.g., retinal screening for people with diabetes • Influenza immunisation – e.g., for those with COPD • Maintaining an accurate register of each condition – applicable to all LTCs • Measuring blood pressure • Measuring cholesterol • Offering smoking cessation advice • Other condition-specific outcomes – e.g., lifestyle advice for people with cardiovascular disease • Recording a person's smoking status • Specific therapy – e.g., lithium therapy for psychotic disorders • Taking condition-specific blood tests – e.g., thyroid function tests for those with hypothyroid

Table 1.1 Quality Outcome Framework LTCs and examples of performance indicators (NHS Digital, 2017)

As you can see from Table 1.1, the QOF framework focuses on those LTCs with the greatest prevalence in the UK and incorporates areas of care such as health promotion, medication management and review to maximise efficacy. The aim of this is to improve patient prognosis, reduce disease burden and improve quality of life. You can find the latest advice on the QOF framework at **www.bma.org.uk/qofguidance**.

Models of care to support people living with one or more LTCs

Within the UK, the theoretical frameworks that can be used to organise services and care in the management of LTCs focus on increasing the level of control and input a person living with an LTC has in relation to how services are delivered and in managing their condition. The House of Care model is a whole-system approach that signifies a change from the traditional 'medical model' that was used to manage LTCs. NHS England (2013) believe the model puts the individual living with LTCs at the centre of care and takes into account their own skills and expertise in effective management. The holistic model provides person-centered care by building a 'house' consisting of four components (see Figure 1.1): commissioning; engaged, informed individuals and carers; organisational and clinical processes; and health and care professionals working in partnership. These four interdependent components encourage individuals to self-manage the condition with the support of structured services working in partnership around them. It is about a whole-system approach that places the person living with the LTC at the heart of the delivery of care (Coulter et al., 2013).

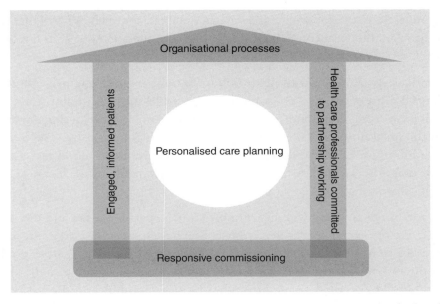

Figure 1.1   The House of Care model (Coulter, Roberts and Dixon, King's Fund, 2013, reproduced with permission)

Activity 1.3   Decision-making

Read the following case scenarios and consider how application of different components of the House of Care framework can be implemented to support the individuals.

For Linda, consider the right wall of the 'house' – professionals committed to partnership working.

Q1 Which members of the multidisciplinary team (MDT) could help Linda?

Q2 What are the potential barriers to these teams working effectively in partnership?

For Peter, consider the left wall of the 'house' – engaged informed patients.

Q1 What may help Peter be prepared for consultations with healthcare professionals?

Q2 What sources of emotional and psychological support could he access?

For Temi, consider the roof of the 'house' – organisational processes.

Q1 How can organisations involved in Temi's care keep an up-to-date record of her condition?

Linda

Linda is 78 years old; she lives alone in a one-bedroomed bungalow that she rents from the local council. Linda has one son, aged 53, who visits her twice a week.

Linda was diagnosed with heart failure in her 60s when she presented to her GP with occasional chest pain and breathlessness. Initially, Linda put this down to anxiety about her job; she was working in the catering department at the local hospital. Following a series of investigations, physical examination, EEG and BNP (brain natriuretic peptide) blood test, Linda was diagnosed with heart failure and was prescribed a diuretic, an ACE inhibitor and a beta blocker.

Linda has been living with heart failure for the past ten years and has tried to make some changes in her lifestyle. She has changed her diet, but still smokes (ten a day) and is reluctant to take much exercise; she does not like going out on her own as she is anxious that she may become unwell. This has led Linda to become isolated from her local community and she has recently begun to feel that she is a burden on her son.

Peter

Peter is 55 years old, married to Sarah (53) and they have three children (25, 22 and 18). Their oldest child (a son) lives and works abroad in France; their middle child (a daughter) works in a local estate agent and their youngest child (another daughter) has just started at university studying to be a primary school teacher. Both daughters still live at home. Peter works as a freelance graphic designer; Sarah is a librarian at the local library.

Peter was diagnosed with Alzheimer's disease about a year ago. Initially, his GP diagnosed depression and he was started on antidepressants; however, Peter's symptoms became worse: coming home from an appointment, he became lost and had to phone Sarah as he couldn't remember how to get home. Following this incident, Peter and Sarah went to see his GP again, and it was then that he was referred on for a neurology outpatient appointment. At this appointment the Mini Mental State Exam was used, alongside taking Peter and Sarah's history and a physical examination, and a provisional diagnosis of Alzheimer's was made.

Following his diagnosis, Peter was commenced on donepezil (Aricept), which he found improved his memory and his ability to find the right words. He has been able to carry on working, though he focuses on online consultancy (Sarah helps with the computer side of things) and works closer to home. Sarah has reduced the hours she works so that she can drive Peter to his appointments as he still struggles with directions.

Temi

Temi is 17 years old and has sickle cell disease. She was screened at birth through a heel prick test, screening suggested sickle cell disease and this was confirmed through a second blood test. Throughout her life Temi has experienced sickle cell crises; during these crises she suffers severe pain, typically in her pelvis and legs, usually lasting up to six days. Temi is currently studying for her A levels and is determined not to let sickle cell prevent her from doing what she wants. Her ambition is to go to university to study medicine, and work as a paediatrician with children who have sickle cell disease. As a young adult, she is better able to identify triggers, dehydration and stress, and manage these to reduce crises occurring. Temi has had one hospital admission in the past 12 months for a sickle cell crisis; she has been able to self-manage the other three crises she has had through taking analgesia, keeping hydrated and rest.

A brief outline answer is given at the end of the chapter.

The impact of living with an LTC

As the quotations at the start of this chapter indicate, a diagnosis of an LTC can have a negative impact on the person and their family. Such a diagnosis is generally seen as being 'bad news' – that is to say, news that implies the loss of something. The loss can relate to physical ability, loss of mobility and the ability to do things for yourself due to motor neurone disease, something/someone that an individual values, altered body image – e.g., following mastectomy – which affects the way in which a person sees themselves, or loss of position or role in the family. The diagnosis of an LTC is usually given by a member of the medical profession. However, as a member of the healthcare team involved in that person's care, it is important that you are aware of the information a person has the right to know at the time of their diagnosis. The General Medical Council in their *Good Medical Practice* guide (2013) states that a person has the right to know: their diagnosis, likely progression, treatment options, the outcome of treatment, side effects of any treatment and the cost of the treatment options where relevant. During this initial consultation it is unlikely that the person will hear all that is being said and will leave with questions to ask. Adler et al. (1989) recognise the impact of physical and psychological noise on communication: physical noise could include the environment that the interaction is taking place in and sensory impairment, and psychological noise could be the distractions, fears and preconceptions, of both the patient and the nurse, that are brought to the situation.

Case study: Anisa

Following the birth of her son Aroon, six months ago, Anisa (age 28) has been feeling tired and has been experiencing muscular aches and pains. Initially, she put these down to being a 'new mum'; however, she was persuaded to see her general practitioner (GP) by her husband Kaldeep. She has been undergoing a series of investigations and she is attending an appointment with her consultant to find out the results of the investigations. Both Kaldeep and Aroon have come along to the appointment with Anisa.

You are on placement in the outpatient department, and the consultant has asked that your mentor sits in on Anisa's consultation – you go in with her. It is during this consultation that Anisa is given her diagnosis of relapsing remitting multiple sclerosis (RRMS).

Activity 1.4   Critical thinking

Read Anisa's case study above and answer the following questions. You may want to discuss your thoughts with a fellow student and compare notes.

- What physical and psychological noise may impact on Anisa and Kaldeep's ability to take on board information?
- What could you do to minimise the impact of these?

A brief outline answer is given at the end of the chapter.

Activity 1.4 demonstrates the need for ongoing communication for people diagnosed with LTCs and their family. You should provide relevant information in an appropriate format and recap as necessary to ensure that the information has been understood by the person and their family. The impact of living with LTCs goes beyond the point of diagnosis and stays with the person and their family as their condition progresses. It is important, therefore, to remember that 'noise' may be present at other times during a person's health journey. People living with LTCs will feel the impact of their diagnosis in all areas of their life – physically, psychologically and socially. The remainder of this section will discuss the physical and psychological impact of living with LTCs. The social impact will be discussed in Chapter 3 in relation to **determinants of health** and public health.

The physical impact of living with an LTC

Many of the physical effects of living with LTCs are condition-specific. As there is not scope in this section to outline the altered pathology and the signs and symptoms of all LTCs, it will outline the altered physiology and the main signs and symptoms of the following LTCs: asthma, chronic heart failure, motor neurone disease, prostate cancer and dementia. Information on the altered physiology and the signs and symptoms of cardiovascular disease, depression and type 2 diabetes can be found in Activity 5.1 in Chapter 5.

Asthma

Asthma is an inflammatory lung condition where the airways in the lungs are hyperresponsive to a range of irritants. Asthma can be described as being intrinsic, where no specific irritant can be found, or extrinsic, where an identifiable irritant is present. Such irritants include smoke, pollen, household allergens (e.g., dust mites), medication (e.g., non-steroidal anti-inflammatory drugs) and infection (e.g., upper respiratory tract). When exposed to an irritant, the muscle in the airways contracts and the membranes shrink, resulting in a narrowing of the airways. As the airway narrows, the flow of air to the lungs is disrupted, resulting in an 'asthma attack' when the person experiences wheeze, chest tightness, shortness of breath and coughing (CKS, 2018). As well as narrowing of the airways, the irritants cause inflammation of the membranes and excessive production of mucus (Lorig et al., 2006). This inflammatory response is reversible;

however, if it is not managed correctly, it can lead to complication such as respiratory failure, **status asthmaticus** and irreversible damage of the airways. Asthma can also lead to fatigue, resulting in time off work or school (CKS, 2018).

Chronic heart failure

Chronic heart failure (CHF) can be associated with previous myocardial infarction or other cardiovascular conditions, e.g., hypertension. It can be caused by either high or low cardiac output. High cardiac output is where the heart is working at a normal or increased rate but the requirements of the body are more than the heart can supply – e.g., anaemia, hyperthyroidism. Low cardiac output is caused by a reduction in the function of the heart and is due to the following (Simon et al., 2014):

- increased pre-loading of the heart – e.g., fluid overload or mitral regurgitation;
- failure of the pumping mechanism of the heart – e.g., ischaemic heart disease;
- inadequate heart rate – e.g., use of beta blockers;
- arrhythmia, e.g., atrial fibrillation;
- excessive overloading, e.g., hypertension.

When discussing CHF, it is common to use the terms 'right heart failure' and 'left heart failure', resulting in differing signs and symptoms due to the nature of the heart failure. Right heart failure is usually associated with congestion of the veins throughout the person's body, while left heart failure is usually associated with congestion of the pulmonary veins (CKS, 2017a). In right heart failure a person can experience the following: ankle oedema, abdominal discomfort due to liver distension, fatigue, nausea and anorexia. People with left heart failure can experience the following: shortness of breath (on exertion) and **orthopnea**, fatigue, reduced exercise tolerance and nocturnal cough (Simon et al., 2014; CKS, 2017a).

Motor neurone disease

Motor neurone disease (MND) is a progressive neurodegenerative disease, which results in muscle weakness, reduced mobility, dysphagia, and speech and breathing difficulties with no curative treatment or remission; 50 per cent of patients die within three years of their first symptom and many die within a year of diagnosis (Wood-Allum, 2014; NICE, 2016a). People presenting with the disease may experience muscle weakness, wasting, cramps and limb stiffness. For others, it may be speech and swallowing problems, and, more rarely, difficulties with breathing. The disease is progressive and will result in increased muscle weakness in arms and legs, problems swallowing and communicating, and respiratory weakness that ultimately leads to death (NICE, 2016a). It is a rare disease currently affecting 1 in 100,000 people. It can often take a long time to diagnose, meaning that people do not receive a definitive diagnosis until up to 18 months after experiencing initial symptoms. Care for people with MND is complex and multifaceted, and requires specialist palliative care and clinical skills.

Prostate cancer

Prostate cancer is the most common cancer in men: more than 47,000 men are diagnosed with prostate cancer each year (Cancer Research UK, 2015). The prostate gland is found only in men; it lies just beneath the bladder and is normally the size of a walnut and is divided into two lobes. The urethra runs through the middle of the prostate: the main function of the prostate is to produce fluid that enriches and protects sperm. The growth and function of the prostate gland depends on the production of testosterone, a hormone produced in the testes. Prostate cancer develops due to the formation of abnormal cells in the prostate gland. These cells cause the prostate to increase in size: as prostate cancer is a slow-growing cancer, in the early stages of the disease there may be no symptoms. Symptoms of local prostate cancer include urinary retention and haematuria; frequency of micturition and urgency can be present. As the cancer spreads, the person may experience symptoms such as weight loss, bone pain and fatigue (Simon et al., 2014).

Dementia

Dementia is a **syndrome** that occurs due to damage to a person's brain, resulting in many problems, such as memory loss, although their level of consciousness is not affected (Simon et al., 2014). Most of these syndromes progress gradually over a period of years; a person's ability to manage their activities of daily living (ADL) independently is affected by their declining memory and cognitive ability.

The symptoms of dementia occur in three areas (CKS, 2017b).

1. Cognitive dysfunction – this results in a person experiencing many problems – e.g., language (both speech and written), memory and orientation to time, place and person.
2. Psychiatric and behavioural problems – these include personality changes, reduced emotional control (emotionally labile) and agitation.
3. Difficulties with ADLs – areas that are affected include driving, personal care and shopping.

The incidence of dementia in the population increases with age; conventionally, a person developing dementia under the age of 65 is classed as having early or young-onset dementia. The most common causes of dementia are listed below (CKS, 2017b).

- Alzheimer's disease accounts for approximately 50 per cent of all cases of dementia. It is caused by degenerative changes in the cerebral cortex, resulting in pathological changes to the structure and chemistry of a person's brain. The cortex of the brain atrophies, and amyloid (fibrous protein) plaques form on and around the neurones. Neurones affected by this have reduced production of acetylcholine (a neurotransmitter involved in learning, memory and mood). Initially, a person experiences memory lapses – e.g., forgetting names and places. As the disease progresses, symptoms such as problems with language and mood changes (depression and agitation) occur.

- Vascular dementia accounts for about 25 per cent of dementia cases and is sometimes called vascular cognitive impairment. Damage to the brain is as a result of cerebrovascular disease, including cerebrovascular accident (CVA), small undetected CVAs (multi-infarct) or ongoing changes in the small cerebral blood vessels (subcortical dementia). In this type of dementia, each cerebrovascular event causes an increase in the person's symptoms; these include personality changes, some focal neurological deficit and apathy.

Management of dementia includes providing the person and their carer with strategies to manage their memory loss, social and carer support, and management of presenting symptoms – e.g., agitation, sleep disturbance (Simon et al., 2014).

Activity 1.5   Evidence-based practice and research

To develop your understanding of the pathophysiology of LTCs further, briefly outline the altered physiology and the main signs and symptoms of:

- depression;
- type 2 diabetes;
- venous leg ulcers.

Some useful resources:

- your preferred applied anatomy and physiology text books;
- **http://cks.nice.org.uk/#?char=A** – this is a useful website for healthcare professionals working in primary care, and provides evidence-based information on managing common conditions seen in primary care;
- **www.nhs.uk/pages/home.aspx** – this comprehensive website contains information on many health conditions.

A brief outline answer is given at the end of the chapter.

Activity 1.5 demonstrates the profound effect that the physical symptoms of LTCs can have on the day-to-day life of the person. Many of these, such as pain and fatigue, can be mentally exhausting to live with and can have a negative psychological impact on the person's mental well-being. Depression is known to disproportionally affect those with LTCs with one in four who have an LTC experiencing it (NICE, 2015a).

The psychological impact of living with an LTC

People living with a condition such as type 2 diabetes, hypertension, CVA, COPD or end-stage renal disease are two to three times more likely to develop depression than people who are in good physical health (Haddad, 2010). It is known that living with LTCs can both cause and increase a person's depression (NICE, 2015a). This **comorbidity** adversely affects the course and outcome of both their underlying LTC and their overlying mental health condition. Indeed, as the population ages and the incidence of LTCs increases for some people they will be faced with **multimorbidity**. For example, a person living with rheumatoid arthritis and type 2 diabetes, who is experiencing pain and reduced ability to manage their medication, has an increased risk of developing depression, which may, in turn, increase their pain and distress, creating a cycle of symptoms (NICE, 2015a). There is also evidence to suggest that depression can increase the likelihood of a person developing conditions such as heart disease (Nicholson et al., 2006) or type 2 diabetes (Mezuk et al., 2008). This is thought to be multifactorial – for example, a sedentary lifestyle and poor diet (risk factors for heart disease) may be related to symptoms of depression, low energy levels, reduced motivation and lack of interest in day-to-day activities. Treatment side effects may increase the likelihood of a person developing depression – for example, corticosteroids; this could be due to the fact that corticosteriods reduce serotonin levels. Additionally, antidepressant medication is associated with an increase in a person's weight (Kivimäki et al., 2010), which if not managed could increase the person's chance of developing type 2 diabetes (Kivimäki et al., 2010). It is known that depression has a negative effect on a person's health outcome, their level of disability and how well they utilise available resources (Haddad, 2010). Given this complex interaction and the potential negative effect, diagnosing and managing depression is an important part of your care of those living with LTCs.

A formal diagnosis of depression is made using either the ICD-10 classification system or the DSM-IV system, with symptoms having been present for at least two weeks and evident on most days. When using these systems there are some key symptoms that need to be present for a diagnosis of depression to be made. These are: low mood, loss of interest and pleasure or loss of energy (NICE, 2015a). However, for people living with LTCs, identifying depression can be challenging as many of the physical symptoms of depression (e.g., fatigue, insomnia and reduced appetite) may also be related to the LTC and its treatment. Therefore, it is important that you are alert to the possibility of a person developing depression. Although you will not be involved in diagnosing depression, your knowledge and understanding of an individual may alert you to changes in their mood that could indicate depression. NICE (2015a) recommends the Two-Question Screen Tool for people with LTCs who may have depression.

- During the last month, have you often been bothered by feeling down, depressed or hopeless?
- During recent months, have you often been bothered by having little interest or pleasure in doing things?

As these questions link to the key symptoms required for a diagnosis of depression to be made, this screening tool has excellent sensitivity (Haddad, 2010). If a person answers 'yes' to one or both questions, a more detailed assessment for depression should be undertaken. In situations where communication is difficult – e.g., sensory impairment or learning disability – a visual analogue like the distress thermometer can be used (NICE, 2015a). Using a picture of a thermometer and a scale of 0–10, it uses a single question screen: *How distressed have you been during the past week on a scale of 0–10?* If any significant level of distress is identified, a score of 4 or more, this should be reported and investigated further. If necessary, a referral to specialist services – e.g., community learning disability services – should be made. Once a diagnosis of depression has been made, appropriate treatment and management are required. NICE (2015a) recommend the use of the stepped care framework, as outlined in Table 1.2.

Focus of the intervention	Nature of the intervention	Place of care
Step 4: Severe and complex depression, risk to life, severe self-neglect	Multiprofessional inpatient care, medication, high intensity psychological interventions	Specialist mental health in patient services
Step 3: Moderate to severe depression, persistent symptoms, poor response to treatment	Collaborative care, further assessment, combined treatments (medication/ psychological interventions)	Primary care, general hospital setting, access to specialist mental health services
Step 2: Mild to moderate depression, persistent symptoms	Low intensity psychosocial and psychological interventions, medication, further assessment and active monitoring	Primary care, general hospital setting, self-management
Step 1: All known or suspected presentations of depression	Assessment, monitoring, support, psycho-education and referral for further assessment	Primary care, self-care and self-management

Table 1.2   Stepped care for depression in LTCs

Source: NICE, 2009

Activity 1.6   Reflection

Reflecting on your recent clinical experience, can you identify a situation where it would have been appropriate to ask the questions in the Two-Question Screen Tool described above?

> If these questions had been asked, would the person's response to these have altered your care? If so, how?
>
> *As the answers will be based on your own observations, there is no outline answer at the end of this chapter.*

Many people find discussing mental health issues uncomfortable; this applies to the person with the LTC and the healthcare professionals involved in their care. Activity 1.6 will have highlighted that in some cases addressing mental health issues relies on you having the confidence to discuss mental health issues with those in your care. The information in Chapter 2 of this book can be used to support you to develop effective nurse–patient relationships, fostering a relationship that is open and non-judgemental. Developing trust in this way encourages those in your care to communicate their hopes and fears, and can assist you in recognising changes in a person's mental health.

Care across the lifespan: the transition from child to adult services

As mentioned at the start of this chapter, it is estimated that up to 10 per cent of children under the age of 10 are living with LTCs (DH, 2012). Many of these children are living into adulthood and require continuing support and care during their adult years to enable them to successfully manage their condition in order to live as healthy and as independent a life as possible. It is important, therefore, that you gain an understanding of the role of transition within the care and management of children living with LTCs. This will enable you to work with child health professionals and better support those in your care. Adolescence is a time of change for all young people, with many social and psychological changes taking place, peer pressure, pushing boundaries and increasing responsibilities. However, young people living with LTCs face particular challenges. Young people need age-appropriate services that are responsive to their changing needs as they grow into adulthood. NICE (2016b) describes transition as *The process to move from children's to adults' services*. It refers to the full process including initial planning, the actual transfer between services and support throughout.

The new clinical guideline sets out five quality standards.

1. Young people start planning their transition with health and social care practitioners by school year 9 (age 13 to 14 years), or immediately if they enter children's services after school year 9.
2. Young people have an annual meeting to review transition planning.

3. Young people have a named worker to coordinate care and support before, during and after transfer their transition.

4. Young people meet a practitioner from each adults' service they will move to before they transfer.

5. Young people who have moved from children's to adults' services but do not attend their first meeting or appointment are contacted by adults' services and given further opportunities to engage.

Transition should, at its heart, promote the **autonomy**, independence and aspirations of young people as they become young adults. This can be achieved if you place the young person at the centre of their transition being supported by collaborative care and management between health, social care and education. However, this is made difficult by the fact that some services stop at age 16, others at 18, and some will see young people past the age of 18 (CQC, 2014). It is known that organised transition programmes benefit young people and their families in many ways: improved follow-up, better disease control and improved documentation, resulting in improved communication and care. There is also evidence to suggest that poor transition and a lack of follow-up leads a young person to disengage from health services, and this can have a negative impact on their health (DH, 2008a). A report by New Philanthropy Capital (McGrath and Yeowart, 2009) noted that many of the needs of young people during transition were not being met by healthcare services, but were being met by charities instead. Within the UK the charity, Contact a Family (**www.contact.org.uk**) provides region-based information for families where a child has an LTC:

* *Preparing for adult life and transition: information for families, England and Wales;*
* *Preparing for adult life and transition – Northern Ireland;*
* *Preparing for adult life and transition – Scotland.*

The DH (2008a) recommends that transition from child to adult services should begin when a child is approximately 13 years old and support should continue until they are 25 years old. This is to tie in with an age when young people are already receiving advice regarding education and career choices. This approach allows the young person to plan their healthcare transition alongside planning for their future career and independence.

Health transition plans

Working with appropriate members of the healthcare team, health transition plans are developed by the young person and focus on what they can do to stay healthy, minimise their health need and maximise their independence. This collaborative approach allows the young person to identify their needs and work with healthcare professionals to write up an action plan to meet these needs. By engaging the young person in the early stages, there is the opportunity to increase their feelings of control and empowerment and to develop their self-management skills (DH, 2008a). A health transition plan should:

- assist the young person to become more knowledgeable and confident in making decisions that impact on their health and healthcare needs – e.g., action planning and self-management;
- support the young person in understanding their LTC and how to minimise the impact of their LTC on their future health and well-being – e.g., health education and health promotion;
- promote the sharing of information, where appropriate, between relevant health and social care services – e.g., health records being held by the young person;
- address transition in the context of the young person's life, taking into account all the person's needs – e.g., education.

In addition, the health transition plan should focus on the young person's strengths and include all areas of the person's life. There should be a clear focus on promoting health and well-being, and what is required to achieve this. The young person's physical, emotional (including sexual health) and social health should be assessed along with their ability for self-care, including any aids and adaptations required. The young person's ability to participate in the medical management of their LTC should also be assessed, including administration of medication. In the broader context of the young person's life, their education, training and leisure requirements should also be assessed, with the aim being to maximise the young person's independence (DH, 2008a).

Personal Folder or Health Passport

These are documents that are held by the young person and their family, and incorporate information about their LTC, medication and treatment, who is involved in their care and what is important to them. Its aim is to ensure that all relevant information about a young person's health and care requirements are kept in one place. It is designed to be a 'live' document and to be updated as the young person's circumstances change. This should be produced in the young person's preferred format. It is not a clinical record; however, it does ensure that relevant professionals have access to essential information about the young person, reducing the need for the young person and/or their family to repeat their health needs to different health teams (CQC, 2014). It may include:

- a one-page profile;
- information about their health condition, education and social care needs;
- their preferences about parent and carer involvement;
- emergency care plans;
- history of unplanned admissions;
- their strengths, achievements, hopes for the future and goals.

(NICE, 2016)

For the parents of a young person, the transition of care from child to adult health services can often cause anxiety. This is in part due to the increasing independence of the young person, who may now be making their own decisions, resulting in the parent feeling excluded (Allen et al., 2011). It is important, therefore, that transition planning incorporates not just the needs of the young person, but the needs of the whole family. If the young person and their family work effectively with child health services early in the transition process, this will enable the young person to develop the required knowledge and skills to successfully manage their LTC into their adult life and will support the family in their changing roles.

Activity 1.7   Reflection

Reflecting on your recent clinical experience and considering the information above, answer the following questions.

- What is your experience of how care has been provided and managed for young people?
- What were some of the challenges faced by both the young adult and their family?
- How might you have used a health transition plan/health passport to enhance their care?

As the answers will be based on your own observations, there is no outline answer at the end of this chapter.

Chapter summary

This chapter has provided you with an overview of the impact of LTCs across the lifespan. It has outlined the incidence of LTCs in both adults and children, and the impact this has on healthcare services and their design. In outlining the physical and psychological impact of living with LTCs, it has identified the importance of having a good understanding of the signs and symptoms of a variety of LTCs. It has emphasised the need for timely and focused transition planning to ensure that young people do not disengage from healthcare services at an important time in their health journey.

Having read this chapter and worked through the activities, you will have developed your knowledge and skills in relation to the impact of LTCs across the lifespan. How you use this new knowledge will depend on where you are working and your roles and responsibilities. By increasing your understanding of how the care and management of LTCs is delivered, you will be able to liaise with other members of the healthcare team to provide an appropriate level of care. You can better support people living with LTCs by developing your knowledge and understanding of the physical and psychological impact of living with a variety of LTCs. This will enable you to provide care that directly meets the needs of the person and will enable you to plan appropriate care for future needs. By working with your child health colleagues, you will be able to support young people during a crucial time in their healthcare journey, ensuring that they gain the necessary knowledge and skills to manage their LTC into adulthood.

Activities: brief outline answers

Activity 1.1 Critical thinking (page 7)

Some LTCs: asthma, arthritis (osteo and rheumatoid), diabetes (types 1 and 2), epilepsy, some cancers (prostate), chronic obstructive pulmonary disease (COPD), motor neurone disease (MND), cerebrovascular accident (CVA), dementia, depression, psoriasis, coronary heart disease (CHD), human immunodeficiency virus (HIV), Parkinson's disease, muscular dystrophy, hepatitis (B, C and D), chronic kidney disease, Crohn's disease, diverticulitis, cerebral palsy, cystic fibrosis, traumatic head injury, sensory impairment – e.g., deafness.

	Acute conditions	**Long Term Conditions**
Onset	Sudden and severe – e.g., appendicitis, meningitis, bone fracture	Generally, gradually over a period of time, though some conditions can progress rapidly
Duration	Short duration. Can result in long-term impairment – e.g., osteoporosis following bone fracture meningitis	Often life-long
Cause	Often single, identifiable cause – e.g., bacterial infection, traumatic injury	Factors include lifestyle, genetics, environment or unknown determinants
Diagnosis and prognosis	A diagnosis is usually made quickly and accurately	Diagnosis can take time, difficult to predict the outcome, can lead to uncertainty – e.g., a diagnosis of motor neurone disease usually takes between 12 and 18 months months from first symptom
Treatment	Usually effective in managing the condition – e.g., targeted use of antibiotics for bacterial infection	Often only able to manage symptoms, side effects present – e.g., triple therapy for HIV can cause fatigue and gastrointestinal upset
Outcome	Cure is possible	No cure is available

Activity 1.2 Critical thinking (page 9)

Over the course of his life, it is likely that Frazer and his family will have come into contact with the following health and social care professionals and services.

- Primary healthcare team (PHCT): GP and practice nurse for ongoing monitoring of his type 1 diabetes involving regular blood tests, weight and blood pressure monitoring, health promotion regarding smoking and alcohol consumption and wound care. Support from the specialist community diabetes team regarding self-management of type 1 diabetes and wound management. Access to community pharmacy for medication for regular medication prescriptions and for advice regarding taking over the counter medication. Input from the community podiatry/chiropody team regarding foot health, correct footwear and management of his ulcers.
- Secondary care services: regular review by outpatient services, both consultant and nurse specialist. Inpatient care for any severe foot ulcer infections and for negative pressure wound therapy and associated follow-up care.

This does not include access to services as a result of an emergency or for aspects of care not related to his type 1 diabetes.

Frazer's condition may affect his family in the following ways.

- Changing of roles and responsibilities within the family, both for Claire and Fiona, who may take on caring roles and responsibilities.
- Impact of Frazer's condition on Fiona, hospital and GP visits, not being able to play with her dad, not being as active.
- Making changes to the house to accommodate equipment that Frazer needs – e.g., wheelchair.
- Financial implications, cost of any adaptations, reduction in family income if Frazer is not able to work.
- Increase in stress for all family members, including the realisation that Frazer may become increasingly less able as a result of his disease.

Activity 1.3 Decision-making (page 12)

Linda – GP, Practice Nurse, Specialist Heart Failure Nurse, Community Pharmacist, Smoking cessation adviser. Working in different geographical locations, different preferred methods of referral, professional cultural differences, effective communication systems, not knowing who else is involved in care.

Peter – Flexible access to professionals – able to change appointments on a 'bad day', information about what the consultation will be about, how long to expect to be there, some questions he can prepare answers for in advance, opportunity to write down or record aspects of consultation, checking understanding. Advocate, carer or partner to support, specialist dementia nurse, Alzheimer's Society.

Temi – Use of patient-held records so that Temi always has information with her, good communication across teams – e.g., accident and emergency informing GP of admission, record of medication kept up to date, access to shared electronic records.

Activity 1.4 Critical thinking (page 14)

Physical noise

- There may be noise coming in from outside the room.
- Aroon may be crying/babbling.

Psychological noise

- They may be distracted by Aroon.
- They may have heard the words 'multiple sclerosis' and not listened to anything after that.
- They may be worried about each other.

Minimise physical noise

- Minimise disturbances, ensure phones are redirected, ask other staff to keep the area quiet.
- Offer to take Aroon out of the room while they are having their consultation.

Minimise psychological noise

- Spend some time ensuring that Aroon is happy and settled, offer to take Aroon out of the room for the remainder of the consultation.
- Observe their verbal and non-verbal communication for signs of confusion and distress. Note at what point in the consultation this was at – it may be necessary to go over information later. Listen to their questions/comments – they will provide you with useful information as to how much they have heard/understood and what may need to be recapped on.

Activity 1.5 Evidence-based practice and research (page 18)

Depression

Depression is a common mental health condition that is characterised by persistent low mood and lack of enjoyment in most activities. People may experience a range of physical, psychological and emotional symptoms, including fatigue, loss of energy, interrupted sleep pattern, thoughts of worthlessness, hopelessness, guilt, self-harm, suicidal thoughts, lack of appetite and concentration. People with LTCs are more at risk of experiencing episodes of depression. Some may experience a seasonal depression in the winter months, known as Seasonal Affective Disorder (NICE, 2015a).

Type 2 diabetes

Diabetes mellitus is a group of metabolic disorders charactersised by a persistent high level of blood sugar levels (hypergycaemia). Type 2 diabetes accounts for approximately 90 per cent of all cases and can occur at any age. Insulin is a hormone secreted by the pancreas as the level of glucose in the bloodstream increases, usually associated with digestion of food, and is responsible for moving glucose from the blood stream to the cells to be converted into energy (Simon et al., 2014). In type 2 diabetes, the body becomes resistant to the insulin or the pancreas does not produce enough, which results in a higher level of sugar circulating in the blood. Over time, even mildly elevated levels of glucose in the bloodstream can cause damage to the blood vessels, resulting in atheroma, visual disturbances due to damage to the small vessels of the retina and poor circulation, both peripheral and centrally. Symptoms of hyperglycaemia may include thirst, polyuria, blurred vision, tiredness and susceptibility to infections. Complications may result in cardiovascular disease, peripheral arterial disease, neuropathy and retinopathy. Type 2 diabetes can have an impact on quality of life, increase likelihood of anxiety and depression, and increased mortality (NICE, 2017).

Venous leg ulcers

Venous leg ulcers are defined as lower limb wounds that do not heal after two weeks; they become chronic if they fail to heal after four weeks. The cause of venous leg ulcers is sustained venous hypertension – high blood pressure within the veins. This is often due to an impaired calf pump function or continued venous insufficiency. Symptoms are a non-healing lower leg wound and prevalence of risk factors – obesity, immobility, venous insufficiency. Venous leg ulcers can have an impact on quality of life as they restrict a person's ability to do normal things, cause embarrassment, bad odour, pain, infection and difficulty sleeping.

People from lower socioeconomic backgrounds have longer healing times and recurrence rates. Treatment is long term with compression therapy, beyond wound closure (NICE, 2015b).

Further reading

Drennan, V and Goodman, C (2014) *Oxford Handbook of Primary Care and Community Nursing* (2nd edn). Oxford: Oxford University Press.

Contains a useful chapter on the care of people with LTCs, including signs and symptoms and management.

Useful websites

https://cks.nice.org.uk/#?char=A

A reliable source of practical evidence-based information on a range of common conditions managed in primary care.

www.contact.org.uk

This is a UK-wide charity providing information and support for families who are living with a disabled child.

www.bma.org.uk/qofguidance

This page on the British Medical Association website gives the most up-to-date information and guidance for the Quality Outcome Framework.

Chapter 2 The nurse–patient relationship in long term conditions

(Continued)

2.2 use clear language and appropriate written materials, making reasonable adjustments where appropriate, in order to optimise people's understanding of what caused their health condition and the implications of their care and treatment

Chapter aims

After reading this chapter, you will be able to:

- identify and describe the components of the nurse–patient relationship;
- explain the importance of engaging in a nurse–patient relationship with people living with LTCs and, if required, their carer and family;
- understand the role that emotional intelligence (EI) and resilience have in the care and management of those living with LTCs;
- recognise the importance of ensuring person-focused communication in the care and management of those living with LTCs.

Introduction

Cure sometimes: treat often: comfort always.

(Hippocrates 460–370 bc)

I will remember that there is art to medicine as well as science, and that warmth, sympathy, and understanding may outweigh the surgeon's knife or the chemist's drug.

(Hippocratic oath – modern version)

Engaging in, developing and maintaining caring and compassionate nurse–patient relationships is at the heart of effective nursing care. Doing this allows you to provide person-centred, individualised nursing care. The Nursing and Midwifery Council (NMC) places nurse–patient relationships and communication at the heart of nursing practice, and this is reflected in the *Code* (2015) and the NMC standards of proficiency (2018).

Those living with one or more LTCs can be in contact with healthcare professionals on many occasions and over a long period of time; this may take the form of a review with their practice nurse or when receiving inpatient care due to an exacerbation. At all stages of a person's journey, a key element of their care is your ability to foster holistic person-centred care, promoting **concordance** with treatment and management regimes, fostering autonomy in managing their own condition and increasing their satisfaction with their care. The development and maintenance of a person-centred relationship is central to this, which may involve not only forming a relationship with the individual, but also their family and carers. For those living with an LTC and those caring for them, it may not be the 'what' of the treatment (e.g., the intravenous anti-biotics for a chest infection) the person remembers but the 'how' of the treatment. 'How' the treatment was delivered: were they listened to, was the treatment explained to them, was a friendly face there, did they feel understood? To support you in your delivery of 'meaningful' care to those living with an LTC, this chapter will assist you in your development of the knowledge and skills required to successfully develop an effective nurse–patient relationship with those requiring your care. In order to do this, the chapter will help you to develop your knowledge, skills and attributes in relation to understanding what a nurse–patient relationship is, emotional intelligence and the relationship you have with carers. Some specific communication strategies that are useful when caring for those living with an LTC are also addressed.

Case study: Bill

Bill and his wife were struggling to manage his long-term conditions (angina and COPD); through working with Bill's community matron they have become more actively involved in the management of Bill's cardiac and lung problems. Both Bill and his wife have regained their confidence and are now able to live more independently. Bill told his story to Patient Voices, a programme founded to support the telling of individuals' stories of health and social care. Figure 2.1 is a word cloud of Bill's story, allowing you to see the words that appeared most frequently.

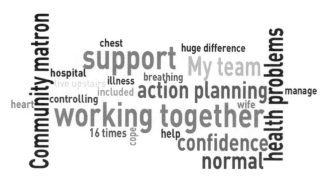

Figure 2.1 Bill's word cloud

Source: Patient Voices website, reproduced with permission

*To listen to Bill's story, follow the link: **www.patientvoices.org.uk/flv/0029pv384.htm***

An effective nurse–patient relationship enables us to *work together* as a *team* with individuals and their carers. This will improve their *confidence* in their ability to *manage* their condition. To *support* this, the qualities of care and compassion should be present in everything you do.

Care and compassion

The findings of the public enquiry into the events at Mid Staffordshire NHS Trust (2013) between 2005 and 2008 still inform healthcare delivery today. Recent publications (NHS, 2016) have focused on evidencing the impact of strategies such as *Compassion in Practice* (2012), which was borne out of the events at Mid Staffordshire. Findings indicate that the majority of staff across mental health (51.2 per cent), primary care (63.5 per cent) and acute care (59.3 per cent) were aware of the Compassion in Practice strategy and the role of the 6Cs. However, it is recognised that work still needs to be done – e.g., supporting leaders – to ensure that compassion is fully embedded as a key aspect of care into the NHS.

In addition, the use of temporary staff and 12-hour shift patterns can contribute to the 'pressures' felt by front-line staff. A study carried out by Ball et al. (2015) concluded that 12-hour shifts have some negative effect on either the quality of care delivered or the health of staff, with fatigue-related outcomes evident – e.g., needle-stick injuries. To address these issues, organisations, as identified in *Compassion in Practice: Evidencing the Impact* (NHS, 2016), should have strong leadership and governance that values the contribution that staff make, and the role of regulatory bodies should be more robust.

Care and compassion are human rights and should be enshrined throughout health and social care. People living with LTCs should be equal partners in their care, confident to say when care is not right. Staff should be engaged with the people they are caring for, putting them first and having the courage to speak up on behalf of patients. However, it is recognised that this will not be easy; compassionate care takes time and in a climate of pressures on the health system, 'time' is a precious commodity.

Compassion, a core value at the centre of healthcare practice (Department of Health and NHS Commissioning Board, 2012), is described as how, through the formation of a therapeutic relationship, care is delivered. This relationship is based on empathy, respect and dignity, and is central to how people perceive the care you provide.

Research summary: Compassion

In 2014, Bramley and Matiti set out to understand patients' experience of compassion. Their qualitative study used in-depth semi-structured interviews to gather data from ten patients. While the sample size is small, limiting transferability of the findings, the data gathered provides insight into how patients experience compassion. Data was analysed using thematic analysis, with the following main themes emerging: what is compassion, understanding the impact of compassion and being more compassionate. Participants described compassionate care as care when they were seen as a unique individual, where nurses took time to be with them and provide encouragement in adversity. To achieve this, participants stated that it was important for nurses to be emphathetic, for nurses to ask themselves: 'How would I feel in their shoes?' However, participants disagreed about whether compassion was integral to who a person is or whether it can be taught.

Arguably, if compassion can be taught, then education has a role in developing students' caring qualities. Research by Terry et al. (2017) used a book, a poem and a film to explore nurse educators' understanding of care and compassion. Forty-one nurse educators working across five universities in the UK participated in the study. They were asked to select one text that impacted on them most as a caring, compassionate practitioner and complete a questionnaire relating to their chosen text. Each text (n=39) and completed questionnaire was analysed through discourse analysis using a tool developed by the lead researchers. This was used to minimise bias that can occur in discourse analysis such as, under analysis, taking sides (Terry et al., 2017). Analysis of the texts and questionnaires identified ways in which care and compassion can be expressed in practice, including: compassionate care means seeing the other person and their suffering (n=25); compassionate people do not abandon suffering human beings (n=24); being able to connect with the other person is necessary to give good care (n=17), and caring can place a heavy burden on the carer (n=10).

While these two studies explore compassion from different perspectives, the findings from both can be used to inform your practice. Bramley and Matiti's work can help you understand how compassion is experienced by patients. By exploring how caregivers express compassion Terry and colleagues (2017) give you an insight into the emotional investment required.

Activity 2.1 Reflection

Having read the research summary above, consider how you can incorporate compassion into your day-to-day clinical practice. Write down your thoughts so that you can return to them when you have finished working through this chapter and see if you wish to change anything.

As this activity is based on your own observations, there is no outline answer at the end of the chapter.

Activity 2.1 may have highlighted the role that compassion has in your communication and the development of the positive relationships you make with those in your care. This type of nurse–patient relationship differs from 'social' relationships.

The nurse–patient relationship

The nurse–patient relationship is a professional, purposeful relationship, the aim of which is to meet the needs of the patient. Through development and maintenance of this relationship, a therapeutic focus is maintained that fosters autonomy and promotes patients' health and well-being. So why is the nurse–patient relationship so important to nursing? The Royal College of Nursing (RNC) defines nursing as:

> *The use of clinical judgement in the provision of care to enable people to improve, maintain or recover health, to cope with health problems, and to achieve the best possible quality of life, whatever their disease or disability, until death.*

> (RCN, 2014, p3)

Inherent within this definition is the notion of **enabling**. While the above quote emphasises clinical judgement, if you are to truly enable those in your care and provide person-centred care that meets and addresses their needs, then the development and maintenance of an effective nurse–patient relationship is essential. This relationship is dynamic, displaying positive characteristics of open communication, a feeling of connection and empowerment; negative characteristics include a disconnect between the nurse and the patient which result in disempowerment and vulnerability (Halldorsdottir, 2008). Developing the positive characteristics of this relationship will allow you to ensure that the focus of your nursing interventions is on the whole person and their response to the situation (RCN, 2014). Engaging in, through listening and questioning, and developing, through supporting, a positive nurse–patient relationship allows you to recognise the uniqueness of the person (Bach and Grant, 2018). Its success depends on your ability to make and maintain a professional relationship with those in your care. The characteristics that define a successful nurse–patient relationship (Chilton et al., 2004) include:

- maintaining appropriate boundaries;
- meeting the needs of the person;
- promoting the autonomy of the person;
- ensuring a positive experience for the person.

We will now look in more detail at each of these.

Maintaining appropriate boundaries

The maintenance of boundaries is crucial: boundaries define and manage expectation, and they ensure all parties are clear about what can reasonably be expected from each other. The Nursing and Midwifery Council (NMC, 2015) states that you will respect professional boundaries at all times; therefore, it is your responsibility to ensure that appropriate professional boundaries are maintained. For nurses involved in the care and management of those with LTCs, the nature of their relationship may vary: specialist nurses may be involved in delivering short-term interventions, while case managers may be involved in longer term care and care planning. These types of interactions will involve different levels of relationship building. Those involved in shorter interventions may focus on the intervention and its success, while those involved in longer term care may be more likely to emphasise the development of a connected relationship, where you view the individual as a person first and foremost (Hallsdordottir, 2008).

The development of a nurse–patient relationship is not without its challenges, and for the majority of nurses boundaries are maintained, allowing for the delivery of more person-focused and person-led care. However, given the ongoing nature of the nurse–patient relationship in the management of LTCs, there may be the potential for boundaries to 'blur'. The role that social media has in how we communicate with each other has the potential to 'blur' these boundaries further. It is important, therefore, that you do not put yourself in a position where this could happen – e.g., accepting a request to join a patient or a family member on a particular social media platform. It is about being personable rather than personal, possessing and using effective communication and interpersonal skills while maintaining professional boundaries. Table 2.1 outlines some useful questions (Chilton et al., 2004) to ask yourself to promote appropriate boundaries.

Question	Response
Is the focus of this relationship on the person and their needs?	If the answer is no, use the questions below to ensure that the focus remains on the person and their needs. • Have you undertaken a person-focused assessment? • Were you listening to the person and using this information to plan their care? • Have you let what you believe is right for the person influence their plan of care?
Is this person beginning to rely on me too much?	If the answer is yes, then it may be helpful to consider the following: ask the individual why they are relying on you, discuss this with them and let them know you may not always be available. Relying on one person can promote overdependence, a potential negative where a large focus of care and management in LTCs relates to self-management.
Am I becoming too emotionally involved in this person's care?	If the answer is yes, then you need to ask yourself if this is affecting the care you are delivering. (As part of forming nurse–patient relationships you invest part of your 'self' in that relationship. Discussing aspects of your personal life may be appropriate if they are used to either help build a relationship or to demonstrate to a person how a situation was managed. However, the focus of that discussion should be the individual and their needs, and not be used as an opportunity for you to discuss your needs.)

(Continued)

Table 2.1 (Continued)

Question	Response
Is the person and/ or their carer/family viewing me as a member of their family?	If the answer is yes, is this appropriate? (Individuals and/or carers may promote a friendship with you as this 'normalises' the relationship and allows them to forget the true nature of their relationship with you. This may be part of their coping mechanism and it may be appropriate for you to discuss this with them in order to find other ways in which they can be supported or accept their current situation. This may be especially true for those who are receiving ongoing care in their own homes.)

Table 2.1 Questions to ask yourself to ensure that appropriate boundaries are maintained

Meeting the needs of the person

In a nurse–patient relationship, the needs of the person are assessed at the outset to identify mutually acceptable goals and who is responsible in the achievement of those goals. The needs of the person are paramount and should be the focus of the relationship. Actively listening to the person, to find out their concerns, worries, etc., reminds us that the nurse–patient relationship is there to benefit the person, not the nurse. Asking a simple question such as 'What is the most important thing I can do for you today?' or 'Can you tell me why I have been asked to come to see you today?' demonstrates to the individual that your focus is on them and their needs, rather than your interpretation of what their needs might be. This is especially true when caring for those living with an LTC, where one of the main cornerstones of management is self-care: in order to promote self-care and management, you must devise a plan of care that clearly reflects the person's needs, as this will increase feelings of empowerment and autonomy.

Promoting the autonomy of the person

Autonomy is the freedom to determine one's own actions and behaviours. A relationship where you encourage active involvement of the individual promotes their autonomy and ensures that they are better able to understand their own situation and take active steps to participate in their care. For those living with an LTC, finding out their level of knowledge and understanding about their condition and how much they want to be involved in managing their own care will allow the level of personal autonomy that reflects their wishes. Many people living with an LTC are experts in their care and will possess a great deal of knowledge regarding their care and management. Indeed, it may be you that is asking the person questions about their care and management, rather than them asking you.

It must be recognised, though, that not all individuals will want to be actively involved in their care to the same degree. Some people may take the attitude that managing their condition is the responsibility of the healthcare team: 'That's what they get paid for', whereas others may actively seek to be more involved in their care: 'I would like to have access to a nebuliser at home and have a clear protocol written that enables me to manage my condition myself should I have an acute asthma attack'. Neither of these approaches is wrong or right, they are just different. By developing a nurse–patient relationship, you will begin to know what is right for that person and how to ensure a positive experience for that individual.

Ensuring a positive experience for the person

Meeting the needs of those living with an LTC in a caring and sensitive manner will promote a positive experience for the person. This person-centred approach will not only increase their ability to participate in self-care and management, but it will also assist them in maintaining a more positive outlook in relation to their condition and future.

In order to promote effective nurse–patient relationships with individuals living with an LTC, it is important to understand the concept of emotional intelligence. Put simply, emotional intelligence is about understanding your own emotions and those of others around you. Recognising and developing your own emotional intelligence will impact on the way you deliver care; recognising and developing the emotional intelligence of those living with an LTC has the potential to influence how they live with their condition.

The nurse–patient relationship and emotional intelligence

Case study: Linda

Linda is 78 years old and has been living with chronic heart failure since the age of 73. Linda started smoking at the age of 19 and has not managed to give up – she smokes ten cigarettes a day. Since her diagnosis she has made some positive changes in her diet, though she realises that she could do more to help improve her health – for example, take some exercise.

To ensure that Linda's care is delivered in a non-judgemental manner, you need to have an understanding about how your emotions might impact on the care delivered:

- you may feel that Linda is to blame for her current health issues due to her smoking and lack of exercise;
- you may feel that Linda is being selfish and lazy, and that she should stop smoking and take some exercise to prevent her condition deteriorating further.

(Continued)

(Continued)

Linda's own emotions may also be impacting on her attitude to her health:

- she may feel that as her health is already damaged, there is no point in stopping smoking;
- she may feel embarrassed and reluctant to ask for help in making a change in her lifestyle.

As you can see from the scenario above, there is the potential for our emotions and feelings to impact negatively on our interactions with those in our care. There is also the possibility that a person's emotions can have a negative impact on their condition and how they manage it.

To understand emotional intelligence as a concept, we need to go back to Howard Gardner's 'multiple intelligence' theory (Gardner, 1983) to see the first recognition of emotional intelligence, described by Gardener as intrapersonal intelligence. Intrapersonal intelligence is concerned with your capacity to understand yourself, to recognise and appreciate your emotions and to use this information to regulate your life (Gardner, 1999). Acknowledging Gardner's work on intrapersonal intelligence, Salovey and Mayer (1990) developed emotional intelligence as a concept. In their theory, intrapersonal intelligence is seen as being part of emotional intelligence. Salovey and Mayer define emotional intelligence as being:

*the ability to monitor one's own and **others**' feelings and emotions, to discriminate among them and to use this information to guide one's thinking and actions.*

(Salovey and Mayer, 1990, p189; emphasis added)

Emotional intelligence abilities	Application to practice
Self-awareness	Being aware of your strengths and weaknesses and looking to managing these.
	You may feel uncomfortable when being asked about a patient's prognosis, recognising that you do not know what to say. The important thing is to act on this and to put strategies in place to address this; one might be to discuss this with your mentor and ask her how she responds.
Self-regulation	Being aware of your 'self' and your emotions, and being able to regulate these and not become overwhelmed by them.
	When faced with a patient asking about their prognosis, your first response might be to change the subject; recognising this and refocusing on the question the patient has asked will increase your confidence in these situations. Working on your communication skills, such as asking reflective questions, will help you manage this.

Emotional intelligence abilities	Application to practice
Motivation	Your ability to use self-awareness and self-regulation of your emotions to inspire yourself and others.
	Recognising that you find discussing a patient's prognosis with them difficult and having a desire to improve your practice will motivate you to undertake activities that will increase your skills in this area.
Empathy	Your capacity to understand another's situation, to identify with their emotions and to use this to respond in an appropriate manner.
	By developing your communication skills and confidence, you will increase your ability to respond appropriately, support patients, develop a positive nurse–patient relationship and respond appropriately to individuals/relatives/carers who may be angry.
Social skills	Your capability to influence, maintain and improve interpersonal relationships through the use of effective and supportive communication skills.
	Through reflecting on your experience of talking to a patient about their prognosis and through the development of your communication skills, you have increased your ability to respond positively in these situations.

Table 2.2   Emotional intelligence abilities and their relation to nursing practice

The difference between intrapersonal intelligence and emotional intelligence is the ability to recognise and respond to *others'* emotions. In 1998, the Consortium for Research on Emotional Intelligence in Organisations (Cherniss, 1998) listed the abilities required for emotional intelligence as: self-awareness, self-regulation, motivation, empathy and social skills (see Table 2.2).

As you can see from Table 2.2, emotional intelligence influences many aspects of nursing care. The utilisation and development of emotional intelligence in relation to you and those in your care will have a positive impact on the nurse–patient relationship. In addition, reflecting on your practice using the emotional intelligence abilities will encourage problem solving and will develop your resilience. Resilience is the ability to persist, regroup and grow in a positive way, despite stressful experiences, which is an important factor when working with people who have complex needs. Developing resilience can help protect you against fatigue and burnout, and promote overall personal well-being, improve your work relationships and job satisfaction (Delgado et al., 2017).

Resilience and long-term conditions

Not only is it important, both personally and professionally, for you to develop your resilience, given the day-to-day challenges people living with one or more LTC face, it is important that they are supported to develop their own resilience. The role that resilience has in supporting those living with LTCs to adapt positively to their situation has been explored both in relation to specific LTCs, such as Parkinson's disease

(Shamaskin-Garroway et al., 2016), and across a range of LTCs (Robinson et al., 2017). The study by Shamaskin-Garroway et al. (2016) concluded that those reporting high levels of resilience demonstrated greater quality of life and better adjustment to their diagnosis. They also found evidence, however, to demonstrate that the degree of non-motor symptoms a person experienced contributed to their ability to adjust to their diagnosis. Focusing on a specific strategy to increase resilience, Robinson et al. (2017) reported on the impact of a six-week mental health resilience course. The course taught mindfulness techniques and cognitive behavioural therapy to older people living with a range of LTCs. Their findings demonstrated that at the end of the course and three months later participants reported significant improvement in their perceived resilience, evidenced by improved well-being, self-management and social interaction. However, it was recognised that due to the short nature of the course, maintaining this over a longer period of time might be challenging for participants. Therefore, finding approaches that can be used on a day-to-day basis is important. The following diagram (Figure 2.2) outlines one such approach and has been applied to a situation in which someone living with an LTC may encounter.

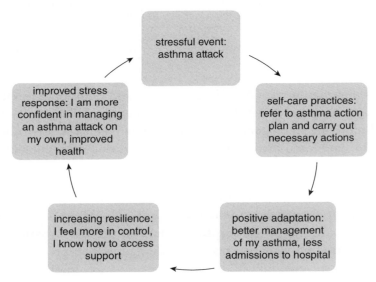

Figure 2.2   An approach to develop resilience based on work by Tebes et al. (2004)

Activity 2.2   Critical thinking/reflection

Using the approach to develop resilience outlined in Table 2.1, reflect on a situation from practice that you found stressful. Use the steps of the approach to structure your reflection and consider what strategies you could have used to improve how you responded in this situation.

As this activity is based on your own observations, there is no outline answer at the end of the chapter.

Completing Activity 2.2 will have provided you with the opportunity to develop your resilience when faced with a challenging situation. This is also important for people living with LTCs, where maintaining a positive attitude and displaying emotional responses can influence how effectively people engage in health-promotion activities and how well they cope with difficult situations – for example, a deterioration in their condition and how they manage the resulting stress (Telford et al., 2006).

The nurse–carer relationship

There are approximately 6.5 million carers in the UK involved in the direct care of family, friends and partners (Carers UK, 2015) and it is estimated that by 2037 this will increase to 9 million. One of the main aims in the care and management of LTCs is to promote self-management and to maintain people in their own homes for as long as possible, supported by primary care services. This increased emphasis on care in primary care and changes in service provision at local government level has resulted in many aspects of care now being delivered by informal carers. Therefore, carers play a pivotal role in the care and management of those living with an LTC. They are involved in many aspects of care from coordinating medical appointments and managing financial matters to providing personal care and administering medication (Carers UK, 2015).

This level of ongoing care, day after day, has an impact on many aspects of the carer's life – e.g., financially, socially and health-wise. All carers in the UK have the right to an individual assessment of their needs; this assessment must ensure that their work, lifelong learning and leisure activities are considered. Carer assessments are arranged through the local council, which should explain who will carry out the assessment; this may be done face to face, over the phone or via a self-assessment questionnaire. The assessment provides a baseline assessment of how the carer is coping and what they perceive their needs to be in relation to the following.

1.   Any aspect of caring: tasks involved in caring; how is your relationship with the person you are caring for and what practical help do you need?

2.   The health and well-being of the carer: how is your health? Do you have any other pressures – e.g., young children, and do you have any free time?

This assessment needs to be handled sensitively, with the carer being aware that the information supplied will be used to provide support for them and ultimately the person they are caring for. Therefore, it may be necessary for information to be shared with other members of the health and social care team. For example, if the carer is requesting specific support regarding a nursing intervention, then you, along with a community nurse, may provide the relevant support. Other practical support offered may be advising about benefits that may be available, providing information about local support groups and having access to **respite care** services.

Children who are carers also have the right to an assessment that will focus on the amount and level of care being delivered by the child, and the impact this has on their leisure and school life. It should be recognised that caring as a child can have a significant impact on both the physical and mental health of the child, and can impact on their choices and future life achievements. As part of the child assessment, it may also be relevant to find out from the parent they are caring for the impact their condition is having – e.g., how does your condition affect your children and how can we support you in your role as a parent?

Despite the fact that this has been the case since the early part of the twenty-first century, evidence shows there is still a lack of available support and information, with one in five carers saying they receive no practical support (Carers UK, 2014b). A systematic review undertaken by Washington et al. and published in 2011 concluded that carers still receive insufficient information to support them in their caring role. Their review identified specific areas relating to the type and timing of providing information:

- general information, that included treatment options, services available (including financial guidance);
- specific information, including disease progression that was tailored to the person's individual situation;
- changes in information requirements over time – e.g., after diagnosis the information required focused on prognosis and treatments; later, this changed to a need for information on social support;
- information to be provided proactively, knowing what to expect in the future, increasing symptoms, respite care and advance care planning.

In relation to how information is provided, the review evidenced that information was not always provided in a way that the carer could understand, emphasising the need for information to be presented clearly, avoiding technical language, and that any information provided should be discussed with the carer to ensure understanding. To be able to provide information to carers that reflects the person's individual situation, developing a positive relationship with the carer is key.

Coping and support

As a nurse, it is your responsibility to have an awareness of the role that stress and caring have in the provision of care for those living with an LTC. In your role, you can help carers manage stress by increasing your understanding about the situations that can increase carer stress and by providing carers with information about how to manage their stress. Some degree of stress can be productive; indeed, stress can increase our motivation to undertake activities – e.g., as a student nurse, a stress response to a forthcoming examination may be to plan and undertake a programme of revision. However, it should be noted that too much stress can have a negative impact on our ability to cope. Stress can affect a carer both psychologically and physically: psychologically, it can affect their ability to deliver care sensitively and responsively; physically, it can determine their ability to safely provide care, especially that requiring physical interventions, such as bathing. Carer stress is a possibility for any carer; however, those caring for individuals where there is significant physical burden or reduced cognitive ability may be particularly vulnerable. Research (Katbamna et al., 2017) exploring the burden of care on carers looking after people post-stroke, found that carer stress was increased due to the uncertain and unpredictable nature of stroke. For carers of a person with dementia, stress can be increased due to a range of reasons, in particular, changes in behaviour, carers needing to repeat information and situations where the person's behaviour does not conform with social norms (Feast et al., 2016). Being alert to the needs of carers and providing them with information and support to manage their stress will have a positive impact both on them and the person they are caring for. It can be seen, therefore, that stress can affect a carer both psychologically and physically. Psychologically, it can affect their ability to deliver care sensitively and responsively; physically, it can determine their ability to safely provide care, especially that requiring physical interventions, such as bathing.

Carers undertake many nursing-based activities when caring for people living with an LTC and want to be able to carry these out safely and effectively (Bee et al., 2008). Providing carers with adequate education and information regarding nursing activities relevant to them will enhance the care delivered. Some of the key areas identified by Bee et al. (2008) are as follows.

- Medication and pain management – education regarding awareness and understanding of the medication being taken, including side effects, how and when it should be taken, understanding of assessment and management of pain.
- Personal hygiene – education and advice regarding skin observation and assessment, and use of pressure-relieving aids, management of continence and bathing, and use of technical equipment such as hoists.
- Nutrition – information regarding a healthy diet and specific dietary requirements.
- Management of symptoms – information and advice regarding fatigue, weakness and awareness of a person's mental health status.
- Emergency situations – education and advice regarding recognising the signs of an emergency – e.g., myocardial infarction and who to contact.

Taking the time to provide practical support and training to carers will increase carer confidence, reduce stress and enhance their coping mechanisms.

Case study: Mary

Mary is 91 years old, takes medication to manage hypertension – she does not know what this is – and had a stroke 15 years ago, leaving her with a left-sided weakness.

(Continued)

(Continued)

She lives alone in a flat above a newsagent's shop that her daughter runs. It is a family business that Mary and her husband ran when he was alive. She has three daughters, two of whom live very locally and one who lives a few hours away and visits regularly. Mary has a carer three times a day to help with personal care and assist with meals. She spends lots of time in a chair or bed, but is able to transfer with her zimmer frame and a carer. Mary had a fall recently and was not wearing her pendant alarm, so was on the floor overnight. She sustained a skin tear to her forearm and developed a grade 2 pressure sore to her hip. Her daughters are anxious about her safety when there is no one in the flat, as this is not the first fall she has had. They have decided to put a rota in place so that one of them is there overnight with their mother. After assessment in A&E, she is sent home and referred to the district nurse team for wound care and review.

Activity 2.3   Decision-making

You are spending the day with the district nurse; one of her visits is to Mary (see the case study above). Considering Mary's needs and the key areas identified by Bee et al. (2008), what information would you provide?

A brief outline answer is given at the end of the chapter.

As you can see from this case study, while Mary has a carer who attends her three times a day, her daughters are also involved in her care. As Mary's daughters are new carers, it may be worthwhile for them to register as unpaid carers with their GP. Registering will allow them to access a range of support, including providing free annual health checks and flu vaccinations to involving them in Mary's care planning. As Mary's daughters are working, registering as unpaid carers would mean that appointments could be made at a time to suit them, minimising disruption.

It is estimated that there are over 3 million working carers in the UK (Carers UK, 2014b). Since June 2014, all UK employees, apart from those in Northern Ireland, who have worked for the same employer for at least 26 weeks, have the right to request flexible working. Employers must deal with the request in a 'reasonable manner', and assess the advantages and disadvantages of the request. However, employers do have the right to refuse if there is a clear business need that prevents flexible working.

Working carers and non-working carers often have concerns about financial security, which can be due to many factors. The extra cost of heating, transport, hospital parking charges and care services can mean that carers and their families cut back on essentials (Carers UK, 2014a). Financial support is available in the form of the Carer's Allowance and additional benefits; however, this is often a complex area to negotiate. Research by Carmichael and Hulme in 2008 identified the complexities of financial support for carers, especially in relation to the working/benefits paradox, where carers either felt they had to work as benefits were insufficient, or they did not work, as this would affect the benefits received. Allowing flexible working to support working carers has the potential to reduce the financial burden placed on carers. Flexible working has been shown to reduce sick leave and improve productivity, which are benefits for both the employee and employer.

While there are negative aspects to being a carer, for most carers, most of the time, their caring is a positive part of their life. Research by Pallant and Reid (2013) explored the positive and negative aspects of being a family carer, with their research concluding that carers perceive caring as worthwhile and value their role. Taking the time to positively recognise the role that carers play, and the positive and negative aspects, has the potential to increase the carer's feelings of self-worth, giving them the confidence to carry on as their role changes.

The very nature of LTCs makes it likely that a carer's role will change over time. Most people do not set out to become carers, but rather over a period of time find themselves in that role. It can happen slowly over the course of months or years, due to a gradual deterioration in health – e.g., as a result of heart disease or Parkinson's disease, or it can happen suddenly due to an acute deterioration in health – e.g., as a result of a cerebrovascular accident or other rapidly developing neurological condition. Often, the assumption is made that carers are happy to undertake this role, as they are there and already involved. Developing a positive nurse–carer relationship will enable you to address their changing needs, allowing them to continue in their role as a carer for as long as they wish to do so.

As discussed above, it is important that a person-focused nurse–patient relationship is in place if you are to provide effective support to a person living with an LTC and their carer. In order to allow this to happen, there has to be an open and honest exchange of information, ideas and wishes that informs clear person-centred care and management.

Communication strategies in LTCs

In your role as a nurse caring for people living with an LTC, you may be involved in their care at different stages in their journey. This may take the form of helping them to understand their diagnosis, providing them with information during an exacerbation of their condition or caring for them during the end stages of their illness. The questions asked by individuals and the nature of the information given at different stages on a person's journey changes. The aim of this section is to focus on specific aspects of communication that relate to caring for people living with an LTC. To support you in the development of more general knowledge and skills regarding your communication, there are many other books available – e.g., *Communication and Interpersonal Skills in Nursing* (Bach and Grant, 2018). When caring for people with an LTC, it is important to recognise what some of the barriers to communication may be (see the box below).

Barriers to communication

For some of those living with an LTC and for those caring for them, there are potential barriers to communication that impact on their ability to communicate and to form an effective therapeutic relationship. This can take the form of sensory impairment – e.g., reduction in hearing and/or vision. Some simple strategies to improve communication in this situation are: ensuring that hearing aids have batteries and glasses are clean, and accessing support and equipment through either Action on Hearing Loss or the Royal National Institute of Blind People (RNIB). For those living with a neurological disorder, such as Parkinson's disease or cerebrovascular accident, their ability to use non-verbal means of communication, facial expressions and gestures may be limited. Language difficulties – e.g., where English is not the person's or carer's first language, accessing an interpreter service rather than using a family member to interpret is preferable in this situation, especially where sensitive information may be discussed. As a nurse, you may also be your own barrier to communication: in challenging situations, we may choose to 'close the patient down', enabling us to retain some sense of control. Changing the topic or engaging in small talk diverts what could be a difficult conversation on to more familiar, easy ground. However, this approach does not allow the person the opportunity to discuss their concerns. Being aware of these barriers, utilising the nurse–patient relationship and developing your emotional intelligence will help you develop effective communication skills.

Due to the ongoing nature of their condition and the focus on promoting self-management, it is important that people living with an LTC are enabled to actively take part in the discussions regarding their treatment and management. To facilitate this, you can encourage them to use the steps outlined below in the acronym PART – for example, before they attend a consultation with a member of their health and/or social care team.

- **P**repare – identify your main concerns, prioritise them and write them down before the consultation. Try to be open in sharing thoughts and feelings, be prepared to concisely describe your main concern, why this is a concern and bring a list of any medication.
- **A**sk – ask questions about your condition, treatments, plan of care and any follow-up; ensure you get answers you understand.
- **R**epeat – repeat key points in the consultation, to verify your understanding and ensure that the consultation has been understood; this also allows the professional to check your understanding.

- **T**ake action – make sure that you understand what is going to happen next, ask for instructions to be written down. If the advice given is not going to be easy to follow, then let the professional know why to see if an alternative can be given.

Case study: Peter

Peter was diagnosed with Alzheimer's disease about 12 months ago. His main symptoms are difficulty in finding the right words and struggling with remembering directions and the sequencing of events. He has been started on Aricept and has noticed some improvement in his symptoms, though he is very frustrated and has expressed a wish for 'assisted suicide'. He is due to attend an outpatient appointment next week. He wants to manage this on his own, though his wife Sarah is keen to go with him.

Activity 2.4   Communication

Read through the case study above. How could you use the acronym PART to support Peter to attend his consultation independently?

A brief outline answer is given at the end of the chapter.

As you can see from Activity 2.4, it is important to listen to the person to understand their perspective and their needs: in understanding their perspective, you will be able to deliver person-centred care. However, in Peter's case it can be challenging for Sarah to allow Peter to attend his appointment on his own. Supporting Sarah to accept this and providing ways in which Peter can share what has been said with her will demonstrate your ability to develop therapeutic relationships with both of them. Actively listening to the individual is a key aspect of this: Epictetus (Greek philosopher, ad 55–c.135) said: *We have two ears and one mouth so that we listen twice as much as we speak.*

Your listening skills can be improved by paying attention to verbal and non-verbal communication, and by asking open-ended questions that encourage the person to give details and prompt you to follow them up. Use paraphrasing, which involves reflecting back to the person a summary of what they had been saying. Paraphrasing allows you to verify the accuracy of your listening and accurately demonstrates that you have been listening. Listen first and advise second: if an individual comes to you with a problem, you may be tempted to provide a solution; however, allowing the person to talk may allow them to find their own solution. This committed approach to listening enables you to focus on the person and their needs, demonstrating your commitment to them. An effective strategy that can be used in the care of those living with an LTC is digital story telling.

Digital story-telling: a communication strategy for LTCs

Story-telling can be viewed as a 'children's activity', yet it is through the use of stories that we understand, experience, communicate and create ourselves. Our stories, like our lives, are constantly changing; they consist of the process of telling the story as well as the end product – the story itself. This chapter started with Bill whose digital story, recorded by Patient Voices, allowed him to describe how the input of a community matron had improved his care. Digital story-telling, like Bill's, is a way of encouraging people to share their stories using digital tools. Their first-person narratives may include words, photographs, music and the person's own voice, and can be created using a range of digital platforms; they are usually between two and five minutes long. Patient Voices outlines a good digital story as one having the following characteristics.

- Brief: a good digital story is a short digital story.
- Simple: low-technology using a few carefully chosen images, voice-over and/or music and simple titling.
- Personal: reveal something personal about the storyteller.
- About the story: a way of developing associated skills.
- Respectful of others' feelings and experiences.
- Created in the spirit of collaboration and partnership.

This narrative approach focuses on the person and uses their narrative to understand the importance of the illness from their perspective. This person-centred approach promotes empowerment, placing the person at the heart of the issue, ensuring that the care provided reflects their needs (Matthews, 2014). Using technology in this way, by providing a people with different ways in which they can tell their story, allows you to ensure that you are using communication strategies best suited to the person and their needs – for example, someone with low levels of literacy, who has been asked to keep a food diary, may feel more comfortable narrating this, rather than trying to write it down.

Activity 2.5   Reflection

Access the Patient Voices site: **www.patientvoices.org.uk/find-htm** and using the find facility search for: morning express, and listen to this narrative

Using a model of reflection such as the Davis Model of Reflection (Davis, 2011), reflect on one aspect of this narrative (see the further reading section for the full reference).

As the answers will be based on your own observations, there is no outline answer at the end of the chapter.

As you can see from Activity 2.5, while patient or carer narratives can support us to improve our practice, they are not always easy for us to hear. Developing your emotional intelligence and resilience will support you to safeguard your own emotional health. However, the information provided by a narrative provides you with useful information that encourages empathy, and promotes understanding of the person and their needs. It may supply you with useful clues that can contribute to a holistic assessment of those in your care, allowing you to set a person-centred agenda.

Chapter summary

This chapter has provided you with an overview of the role of the nurse–patient relationship in relation to LTCs; it has also outlined the importance of emotional intelligence as a factor in this, both for you and for those in your care. In emphasising how the 6Cs can be applied to the care and management of people living with LTCs, a key message in recent healthcare delivering is recognised. It has focused on the importance of recognising the role of carers and working with them to support both carers and those living with an LTC. Some specific communication strategies that are useful in the care and management of LTCs have been discussed and related to clinical practice.

Having read this chapter and worked through the activities, you will have developed your knowledge and skills in relation to the nurse–patient relationship and long-term conditions. You can improve communication with those in your care and their family/carer in many ways. By increasing your level of emotional intelligence, you can be yourself, be open and honest, recognise and acknowledge your limitations and take personal responsibility. By engaging in a nurse–patient relationship with individuals and/or their carers, you can work as part of a team by listening and responding to their needs. By using communication strategies like narrative-based care, you can increase the well-being of the person/carer, improve physical and mental state, promote a better adjustment to illness and increase an individual's sense of control.

Activities: brief outline answers

Activity 2.3 Decision-making (page 44)

Medication and pain management – access information from the GP in relation to Mary's medication, it may be that a medicines review needs to take place with Mary to ensure that she understands her medication, what she is taking and why. Undertake a pain assessment using a recognised pain assessment tool to assess Mary's baseline level of pain (if any). Use this information to inform any further treatment/referrals.

Personal hygiene – discuss with Mary the importance of keeping her skin clean and dry. You may need to meet with Mary's carer to go over the care of Mary's skin tear and grade 2 pressure sore to ensure effective healing. Ensuring that Mary's skin is kept moist can reduce skin tears, so applying moisturiser would be appropriate.

Nutrition – provide Mary with information about the importance of a healthy, balanced diet; this information may also have to be provided to both her carer and daughters. Due to her age and possible reduced appetite, it may be more appropriate for Mary to have six small meals a day rather than three larger ones.

Management of symptoms – Mary had had a history of falls, therefore referral to occupational therapy and physiotherapy may be relevant.

Emergency situation – discuss with Mary the importance of wearing her pendant alarm and using it; it may also be relevant to discuss the signs of infection with Mary, her carer and daughters.

Activity 2.4 Communication (page 47)

To help Peter prepare for his consultation, you could assist him to identify his main concerns, to write these down and to identify any specific questions he has that he would like answered. These may relate to his medication and the likely progression of his Alzheimer's disease. You could encourage Peter to share how he is feeling, especially in relation to talking about 'assisted suicide'; it could be that Peter is depressed and would benefit from some treatment, either pharmacological, therapeutic or both. Help Peter to write down his questions and remind him to take some paper and a pen, or a dictaphone, with him so that he can write down the answers or record them for Sarah. Remind Peter that this is his consultation and that before he leaves he should review with his consultant what has been said.

Further reading

Grant, A and Goodman, B (2018) *Communication and Interpersonal Skills in Nursing* (4th edn). London: Sage/Learning Matters.

A useful introduction for nursing students to the complexities of communication skills.

Davis, N (2011) Reflection, in Davis, N, Clark, AC, O'Brien, M, Sumpton, K, Plaice, C and Waugh, S (eds) *Learning Skills for Nursing Students*. Exeter: Learning Matters, pp. 173–92.

Edward, K (2013) Chronic illness and wellbeing: using nursing practice to foster resilience as resistance. *British Journal of Nursing*, 22(13): 741–46.

An article exploring comorbid LTCs with mental illness and the role that nurses have in developing resilience to promote self-management.

Tremayne, P (2013) Using humour to enhance the nurse–patient relationship. *Nursing Standard*, 28(30): 37–40.

Using humour in daily interactions with patients can help develop the nurse–patient relationship and build resilience; recommendations for including humour in patient care are included.

Useful websites

www.carersuk.org

Provides a gateway to all carer UK sites – e.g., Scotland, Northern Ireland and Wales; offers advice and information for carers.

www.patientvoices.org.uk

Using digital story-telling, Patient Voices provide insight into the experiences of patients, carers and staff to promote change both individual and organisational.

Chapter 3 Health promotion in long term conditions

Chapter aims

After reading this chapter, you will be able to:

- explain the importance of health promotion for people living with a LTC;
- understand the influence of health determinants in the care and management of people living with an LTC;
- identify, describe and apply approaches to health promotion in the care and management of LTCs;
- understand and describe the process of motivational interviewing and its role in the care and management of LTCs.

Introduction

Health promotion enables people to increase control over their own health. It covers a wide range of social and environmental interventions that are designed to benefit and protect individual people's health and quality of life by addressing and preventing the root causes of ill health, not just focusing on treatment and cure.

(World Health Organization, 2016)

Health promotion is a key strategy for use in the care and management of people living with an LTC. Simple approaches, such as reducing the amount of salt in your diet, stopping smoking or taking some exercise, can help reduce the burden of LTCs globally. The World Health Organization (WHO) identify in their definition of health promotion above, that a person's ability to positively affect their health can improve their quality of life by addressing not just physical but mental and social well-being (WHO, 2016). In order to successfully engage a person with a LTC in health-promoting behaviour, it is important that you know and understand them and their lives. Using the nurse–patient relationship (see Chapter 2) as your means of providing person-centred communication and care will contribute to your ability to include health promotion as part of your care and management of people living with an LTC. It should also be recognised that for many carers, the act of caring for a person with an LTC can impact negatively on their own health; therefore, engaging them in health promotion, as required, will support them in the role as a carer. See Chapter 2 for information on supporting carers and improving their health and well-being.

Activity 3.1 reminds you about the health promotion interventions you may have been involved in with people in your care who are living with an LTC. This may include, for example, advising someone with a respiratory LTC such as asthma or COPD to have an annual flu vaccination or to give up smoking. These interventions encourage people to learn about their condition, understand the importance of self-care, and then to actively participate and be involved in their care. This approach empowers the person, increasing

Activity 3.1   Reflection

Thinking about your clinical practice and your role as a health promoter, answer the following questions.

- Have you been in a situation when the opportunity to promote good health and well-being to a patient has arisen?
- Have you been involved in any heath promotion activities that related to a person living with an LTC?
- How did you carry out your health promotion?
- How did you evaluate the effectiveness of your health promotion?

If you have not been involved in any health promotion intervention, reflect on the health promotion you have seen your mentor involved in or on potential opportuntities you may have to promote health.

As this activity is based on your own observations, there is no outline answer at the end of the chapter.

their sense of control over their situation. If we look at the example above, it also minimises the risk of seasonal respiratory infections which may exacerbate their condition and reduces the risk of hospital admission. In order for your intervention to be a success, it is important that you understand about empowerment, health promotion approaches and their use, and how to evaluate your intervention. Health promotion is not just about an individual's health and well-being. A global approach, promoting health and well-being for all, is essential, and interventions should target whole populations and communities. The United Nations (UN) have identified 17 goals – the Sustainable Development Goals (SDGs) – which are a blueprint to achieve a better and more sustainable future for all. In 2015, all 193 member states of the UN committed to the ambitious agenda for a safer, fairer and healthier world by 2030 through the SDGs.

You can read about the 17 SDGs following this link: **www.un.org/sustainabledevelop ment/sustainable-development-goals/**

Activity 3.2   Reflection

Consider the 17 Sustainable Development Goals and consider three ways in which nurses can contribute to them within your daily clinical practice.

As this activity is based on your own observations, there is no outline answer at the end of the chapter.

The WHO recognise that good health is a foundation to achieving these goals and individuals require support to achieve this as a universal right and essential resource for everyday living (WHO, 2017).

Health promotion should play a key part of your day-to-day activity as a nurse and this is endorsed by our professional bodies as well as in UK policy. Public Health England (PHE) is an executive agency of the Department of Health, created in 2013. They have responsibility in England to protect and improve the nation's health and well-being, as well as to reduce inequalities in health. There are similar agencies in Scotland, Wales and Northern Ireland with the same role. Web links to each country's strategy for reducing health inequalities can be found at the end of this chapter. PHE recognise that every nurse has a contribution to make in public health, which includes engaging in health promotion. Public health is a proactive approach, with its services aimed at early diagnosis, preventative treatment and the development of social policy to ensure that all people have a standard of living that supports the maintenance of their health. In all countries in the UK, public health is a high priority on the health agenda, with each national government's public health strategy focused on reducing health inequalities. Having an understanding of the determinants of health and the role that public health has in minimising health equalities will enable you to provide effective health promotion for people living with a LTC.

To support you in your ability to promote health in people living with an LTC, this chapter aims to develop your knowledge and understanding of health promotion in relation to the care and management of LTCs. To do this, the chapter will focus on developing your knowledge, skills and attributes in relation to health promotion approaches and how to use these to empower people with an LTC to manage their own health condition. First, though, to enable you to better support people living with an LTC, this chapter will discuss the factors that contribute to a person's overall health and well-being (Naidoo and Wills, 2016) and how public health strategies can minimise these.

The influence of health when living with an LTC

As discussed in Chapter 1, the majority of care and management you will be involved in when supporting people living with an LTC takes place in primary care. It may be that, during an acute episode or deterioration in their condition, a person is admitted to secondary care where you are involved in delivering specific care and management. However, on a day-to-day basis, people living with an LTC manage their condition either independently or with support from their primary healthcare team. Their care and management takes place in their own home; they live their life in their local community and contribute to the local area. It is important, therefore, that you have an understanding of how their 'life' (behavioural, social, economic, emotional and spiritual) can influence and affect their LTC and their overall sense of health.

Determinants of health

There are many factors that affect the health of a person and their community. These factors are called 'determinants of health' and can determine how healthy a person is at the present and may be in the future. The health of a person depends on many factors that influence and impact on their life – e.g., genetics, education, environment (WHO, 2010). Figure 3.1 identifies the determinants of health (Dahlgren and Whitehead, 1991).

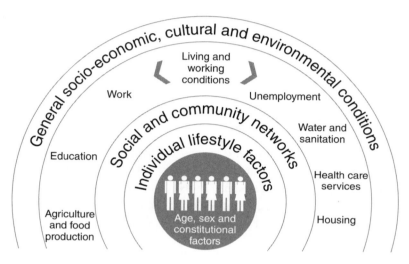

Figure 3.1   The main determinants of health

Source: Dahlgren, G and Whitehead, M (1991) *Policies and Strategies to Promote Social Equity in Health.* Sotckholm, Sweden: Institute for Future Studies.

Case study: Mary

Mary, who is 91 years old, has had several more falls at home over the next few months and, during a recent admission to hospital, it was decided that she would be safer and better cared for in a care home. She is assessed on the ward as having nursing needs, as her mobility has decreased to needing hoisting to transfer, she is having some continence issues and recent weight loss means that she is at very high risk of developing pressure sores. She continues to have left-sided weakness following the stroke she had many years ago.

Mary's daughters are given the details of some local nursing homes and have picked one nearby for Mary to live in. They are initially worried about how this will be paid for, but Mary has some savings from the family business and currently lives in a property that she owns.

(Continued)

(Continued)

Mary is a little anxious about having lots of different people take care of her. She is particular about her appearance, always choosing a smart blouse to wear, enjoying having her hair done and still applying a little make-up each day. She also has a small appetite and needs encouragement to eat and drink. Mary is a horse-racing fan – in fact, she enjoys all sports on television and also enjoys the company of others. She is well known in the small town where she lives, having run the local newsagent with her husband for years. Mary is a Roman Catholic; her faith is important to her, but she has not been able to attend church in some years.

Activity 3.3   Critical thinking

Read Mary's case study above and consider how her current situation might influence, either negatively or positively, the determinants of health, as depicted in Figure 3.1; age, sex and constitutional factors; individual lifestyle factors; social and community networks; living conditions; and general socioeconomic, cultural and environmental conditions.

A brief outline answer is given at the end of the chapter.

As Activity 3.3 demonstrates, determinants of health are personal to individuals and their situation, and can have both a negative and positive effect on a person's health. As a result, there can be large variations in the health of different groups within the population. This can lead to stark inequalities in health. For example, in 2010–12, male life expectancy at birth was highest in East Dorset at 82.9 years and lowest in Glasgow City at 72.6 years (Office of National Statistics (ONS), 2014). If there are no changes to mortality rates from those in 2010–12, then 91 per cent of boys in East Dorset will reach their 65th birthday, whereas in Glasgow City this percentage is only 75 per cent (ONS, 2014). It is these inequalities in the health of the population and how to minimise the impact of them, that is the remit of public health.

Health promotion and LTCs

As a nurse caring for people living with a LTC, the health promotion you deliver will focus on improving that person's health whatever the stage of their disease progression. Health promotion will be a part of your care and management from diagnosis through to the palliative stages of their illness. In the early stages of a diagnosis, your health promotion may focus on supporting the person to increase their knowledge and understanding about their LTC and how to manage their symptoms, so that they can minimise the risk of long term complications – for example, educating a person with diabetes how best to maintain optimum blood glucose control (HbA1C) and how this will, in turn, help to reduce the likelihood of them developing diabetic peripheral neuropathy. As a person's LTC progresses, the health promotion activities you support the person to engage in may be aimed at restoring their highest level of physical, social and emotional function following an exacerbation. For example, for a person living with COPD, this may focus on pulmonary rehabilitation and supporting them to engage in some level of physical activity that maintains their lung function. Finally, in the palliative stages of their illness, the health promotion implemented could focus on improving their quality of life in relation to symptom management through effective use of both pharmacological and non-pharmacological means – e.g., massage, acupuncture. While health promotion may be part of your care and management at different times in a person's health journey, and have a very different focus as a result, the underlying principles remain the same. The process of working together with a person living with an LTC relies on that person being able to understand and to act on the information you provide, and to use this to maintain and maximise their health. This level of engagement will allow the person to actively participate in the health promotion process, empowering them to take control of their health and well-being. The ability of a person to do this is dependent on their level of health literacy – that is, their capability to access, understand and use information to maintain their health (Sykes et al., 2013). Berkman et al. (2010, p9) describes health literacy as:

the degree to which individuals can obtain, process, understand, and communicate about health-related information needed to make informed health decisions

By improving health literacy, there is the potential to motivate people and to empower them to take a more active role in managing their health. Low health literacy can have a negative effect on a person's ability to engage in health promotion and ultimately on their health. Programmes to support healthcare professionals to tackle the issue of poor health literacy are available across the UK – for example, Health Education England (HEE) (2017) have launched a free educational toolkit to raise awareness and upskill the health workforce (the website to access this is included at the end of the chapter). HEE (2017) estimate that 43 per cent of working-age adults in the UK do not have the health literacy skills to understand health information, and this increases to 61 per cent when the information involves numbers. It is important, therefore, that you present health promotion information in a format and manner that is relevant to the person, their level of health literacy and their situation. A person's level of health literacy will also influence what approach you use to deliver the health promotion intervention.

Approaches to health promotion

As your reflections from Activity 3.3 may suggest, how you use health promotion activities varies; you may use different approaches at different times, depending on what the aim of the health promotion is. For example, you may use an educational model when teaching a person how to administer their medication correctly or you may use a behaviour change model when supporting a person to make a change in their behaviour by reducing the amount of alcohol they drink. Being able to use a variety of approaches is particularly relevant when you are working with people living with an LTC who may require health promotion to be delivered using more than one approach and over a long period of time. In order to provide health promotion in a way that is meaningful, it is important to have an understanding of these different approaches and their relevance in the care and management of people living with an LTC (see Table 3.1). For further reading on health promotion, see the reading list at the end of the chapter.

Approach to health promotion	Description
Medical approach	Treatment and prevention of ill health: patients are encouraged to comply with preventative and early detection measures such as vaccination and screening.
	Living with an LTC is complex and the medical model does not necessarily address the role that society and the environment play in promoting a person's health.
Behaviour change approach	Encourages patients by persuasive education to make what are perceived by the health promoter to be healthy lifestyle choices.
	For people living with an LTC, behaviour change approaches can be used successfully once particular needs have been identified and the intervention is targeted to meet those specific needs.
Educational approach	Respects a patient's right to make an informed choice by information provision. Encourages exploration of a person's own values and beliefs, and supports them in decision-making.
	Providing people living with an LTC and their carers with relevant information regarding their condition and how to manage it can increase their sense of control and empowerment.
Empowerment approach	Patient-centred approach: patients identify their own learning needs and gain the knowledge to make their own decisions about health needs.
	An example of this might be the use of life story work and reminiscence therapy for people living with dementia. The aim of the intervention is to increase the person's sense of who they are and to enable those involved in their care to see more of the person, allowing for planning and delivery of more person-centred care. Evaluation of these types of approaches can be difficult as results are hard to measure.
Social change approach	This does not focus on the individual but on society as a whole. It concerns the creation of an environment, through political and social action, that acknowledges the rights of each individual.
	An example of this may be the dementia-friendly communities initiative by the Alzheimer's Society, supported by everyday settings to be dementia aware.

Table 3.1   Health promotion approaches

Source: Naidoo and Wills, 2016.

Research summary: Life story work

Life story work (LSW) is a person-centred intervention that can aid communication and well-being for older people living with dementia. It involves constructing a biography of an individual using their help and that of those close to them. The process usually results in a product, which may take the form of a book, film or photo album, and can include items and memorabilia (McKinney, 2017). It can aid communication and understanding for carers by enabling them to learn about the individual behind the dementia (Kellett et al., 2010). LSW helps carers to develop a therapeutic relationship with the people by enabling them to understand their biography, thus appreciating the individual's value as a person (McKeown et al., 2010). Chan et al. (2013) explored engagement with life story work for older people in China, living in the community. The participants all experienced mild to moderate symptoms of depression. The intervention group engaged with an eight-week programme of collating their life stories with a facilitator and the control group did not. This study identified a measurable reduction in symptoms of depression for those participating. A multiple case study design piece of research looking at individuals' engagement with LSW demonstrated benefits for the person living with dementia, their family members and the staff involved in their care (McKeown et al., 2010). The researchers, using a constructivist design, found that LSW enabled the voice of the person with dementia to be heard, evoked a sense of pride for all engaged in the work and supported family members to 'uphold' their relative's personhood, when they may have found themselves losing sight of it due to the disease. A fascinating intergenerational project that paired older people with adolescents for a 12-week project to compile a life story review book for the older person found positive effects for both groups (Knight et al., 2017). Themes to emerge from the study included stereotypes being challenged from both groups, enhanced well-being and a positive impact on depressive symptoms.

To enable you to apply the above health promotion approaches to your clinical practice, take the time to read the following case study and undertake Activity 3.3. This will allow you to critically apply the above approaches to a person living with an LTC.

Case study: Sian

Sian Jones is a 20-year-old student who has been living with asthma since the age of 11. After taking a year out after finishing school to work in a local sports centre, Sian has just started a Sports Science degree at university and has moved away from home

(Continued)

(Continued)

for the first time. Sian enjoys playing hockey and netball, and plays for the university teams in both these sports. She is enjoying her studies and is taking full advantage of 'student life'; she lives in a shared house with four other students who are on the same course as her.

This morning during hockey practice Sian became breathless and began wheezing. Sian became concerned as her breathlessness did not resolve as quickly as usual and decided to make an appointment at her GP surgery. You are working with the practice nurse when Sian comes in to see her. During this consultation Sian admits that she has not been taking her Beclazone inhaler regularly, which she keeps forgetting to do; she has noticed that she has been taking her ventolin more regularly.

Activity 3.4   Critical thinking

Plan a health promotion intervention to support Sian to manage an aspect of her asthma more effectively. Using the sample layout below, complete a chart that includes your approach and intervention, and the rationale for your choice.

Approach	Intervention	Rationale

A brief outline answer is given at the end of the chapter.

In participating in Activity 3.4 it may have been evident that your intervention incorporated more than one health promotion approach. Taking the time to consider your rationale will have supported you to think more critically about your choice, promoting evidence-based practice. In addition, it will support the development of your problem-solving skills, allowing you to apply these principles to other clinical situations.

Motivation and health promotion

Dixon (2008) recognises that the success, or not, of a health promotion intervention can relate to how motivated a person is to participate and, in turn, how committed they are to making the change. It can be seen, therefore, that a person's motivation to participate in health promotion can influence how successful they are going to be in maintaining their health change. Motivation can either be intrinsic or extrinsic. Intrinsic motivation comes from within: I have a desire to change my behaviour; I am self-motivated and I know the change will improve my health. Extrinsic motivation comes from external influences: I have a desire to change my behaviour because if I stop smoking I will save money. To maximise a person's participation in their health promotion it is important to understand what factors influence their motivation to change – are they extrinsic and/or intrinsic (Dixon, 2008). One of the more popular models that addresses motivation in relation to health promotion is the transtheoretical approach (DiClemente, 2007), which identifies stages that a person progresses, and relapses, through while making changes in their health behaviour. People can join at any stage and it is often represented in a cyclical way. Table 3.3 describes the stages of the transtheoretical model and outlines some of the strategies and their aims that may be implemented. To assist you in relating this to your care and management of people living with an LTC, the transtheoretical model has been related to Frazer, one of the case studies you are following in this book. See the box for further information.

Case study: Frazer

Frazer is 47 and living with type 1 diabetes. In the past, he has not always managed his diabetes as effectively as he should; this has resulted in diabetic peripheral neuropathy. Frazer has an ulcer on his foot that is not healing; and has had extensive treatment for this to prevent amputation. Five years ago Frazer managed to stop smoking; however, he still drinks alcohol on a daily basis. Attempts by his practice nurse to encourage Frazer to reduce his alcohol intake and have three non-drinking days a week have failed; he drinks two pints of beer a day.

What stage is Frazer at?	Your aim is . . .	Your strategy is . . .
Pre-contemplation – here Frazer is not intending to make a change in his health behaviour. He may be unmotivated or resistant to making a change, though he may also be concerned about his health behaviour.	To raise awareness with Frazer of the impact his alcohol intake is having on his diabetes.	To provide Frazer with relevant information in an appropriate format; this may be written, audio or visual. You would then revisit this information with Frazer at follow-up visits.
Contemplation – at this stage Frazer may be stating to you his desire to change his health behaviour by reducing his alcohol intake. Frazer may be weighing up the pros and cons of this.	To allow Frazer to see the benefits of reducing his alcohol intake – both in relation to his diabetes and his general health.	To explore the advantages of reducing his alcohol intake with Frazer. However, you will need to acknowledge with him some of the disadvantages, the loss of something he enjoys, challenges and increased stress he may face.

(Continued)

(Continued)

What stage is Frazer at?	Your aim is . . .	Your strategy is . . .
Preparation – here Frazer is stating his intention to change his health behaviour by reducing his alcohol intake. Frazer now has to commit to a plan that will enable him to change his health behaviour.	To assist Frazer to manage and overcome any challenges to reducing his alcohol intake.	To form a plan of action with Frazer that will enable him to change his behaviour. This may involve providing him with information in relation to alternatives to drinking alcohol – e.g., low alcohol lager, swapping an alcoholic drink for a non-alcoholic drink and how to manage any withdrawal symptoms. Establishing links with a support group would also be beneficial for Frazer.
Action – at this stage Frazer has made a recent change (within six months) to his health behaviour by reducing his alcohol intake. At this stage Frazer's new behaviour is established.	To use an effective therapeutic relationship to support Frazer to adapt and maintain his health behaviour change.	To review Frazer's plan of action with him, to provide positive reinforcement of his success to date. To encourage Frazer to maintain contact with support group for ongoing support to enable him to keep his consumption of alcohol down or even to stop.
Maintenance – here Frazer has maintained his health behaviour change and has reduced his alcohol consumption and has three days a week where he does not drink. He has integrated the change into his lifestyle.	To provide ongoing support to Frazer.	To minimise the risk of Frazer relapsing by evaluating his success so far and to plan coping strategies that would limit the risk of a relapse – e.g., relaxation techniques, creating rewards for the new behaviour.

Table 3.2 The transtheoretical model and its relevance to your practice

Source: DiClemente, 2007.

It should be recognised that the successful behaviour change is not always maintained and that relapses may occur. To minimise this, it is important that you ensure that each stage is addressed comprehensively and that the aim identified is supported with appropriate strategies. This will give the person the best opportunity to succeed; however, should they relapse they will have to revisit the stages, paying particular attention to any that were not fully addressed (DiClemente, 2007). The transtheoretical model provides a useful framework for targeting health promotion interventions depending on how ready, or otherwise, Frazer is to change his behaviour. However, it does not provide you with a specific strategy that you could use in your health promotion intervention to enable Frazer to make changes. One such strategy is motivational interviewing.

Motivational interviewing: a behaviour change strategy to promote health in people living with an LTC

Motivational interviewing (MI) is an evidence-based approach for helping people to change behaviour. It is person-centred, compassionate, directive and is accepting of an individual's status. The professional listens for opportunities to encourage and strengthen the desire to change (Miller and Rollnick, 2012). By enabling a person to explore their feelings in relation to their behaviour change, and giving them the time to work through these, it is likely that their intrinsic motivation to change is going to increase. This is due to the fact that they have reached the decision to change their behaviour themselves and have therefore increased their motivation and **self-efficacy**. Your role in motivational interviewing is to understand why a person might resist change, to actively listen to them and understand their motivations (what are the pros and cons of changing) and in doing so empower them to make their change. The skills you would use and their application to your practice (Carrier, 2015) are outlined in Table 3.3.

MI skill	How you would use it in your practice
Using open questions	Using open questions encourages a person to explore how they feel about a particular behaviour. For example, rather than ask the question 'Do you smoke after each meal?', you could ask, 'How do you feel about having a cigarette after each meal?' This not only allows the person to explore their feelings, but also helps you to understand the person, their motivation and their feelings better.
Active and reflective listening	By actively listening to a person and reflecting back what they have said, you can demonstrate that you have understood what the person has said. For example, hearing the statement 'I would like to take more exercise – I have put on some weight over the past few months', and by reflecting back to the person like this, 'You are able to see the connection between your lack of exercise and your weight', you will encourage the person to explore their feelings further.
Rolling with resistance	There will be times during discussions about behaviour change where a person is resistant to what you are saying. In MI it is important that you 'roll with the resistance' and respond in an understanding way. Resistance can be reduced by reassuring a person that they are under no obligation to change: 'I am here to support you to lose weight, I am not going to force you to change'. Resistance can also be reduced by recognising when a person may not be ready to discuss a situation: 'From what you are saying, you don't sound ready to talk about this today. Shall we discuss this at another meeting?'

Table 3.3   MI skills and their application to your clinical practice

Using these skills will enable you to find out if a person is ready to make a change in their behaviour. If they are ready to make a change, then it is useful to find out what changes they feel able to make as this places control with the person. You can help by breaking a major change down into smaller more achievable steps to maintain the person's self-efficacy (Carrier, 2015). The use of MI places the person at the centre of the decisions in relation to changing their behaviour. Through the use of open questions you can encourage them to set the agenda. In sharing information with them, by finding out what they know and then providing relevant information, you can encourage them to think about how the information applies to them. This approach encourages person-centred health promotion that acknowledges the role that the person has to play in maintaining a successful behaviour change.

Making Every Contact Count

Making Every Contact Count (MECC) is an approach to behaviour change that encourages staff to use opportunities arising during routine interactions with patients to have brief conversations on how they might make positive improvements to their health and well-being.

> *The delivery of very brief or brief interventions and signposting by frontline professionals has been shown by NICE to be both effective and cost-effective in supporting people to reduce their tobacco and alcohol use, and in improving their physical activity levels and diet.*

(Making Every Contact Count (MECC) Consensus statement, 2016)

MECC is a straightforward health-promoting strategy that you can engage in during your next patient interaction and within the majority of your interactions. It is about systematically promoting the benefits of healthy living to all. You may be asking individuals about their lifestyle and any changes they may wish to make, responding appropriately to the lifestyle issues raised and then taking the appropriate action to either give information, signpost or refer service users to the support they need. For example, during the admission of a patient you may routinely ask 'Do you smoke?'. If the patient responds 'yes', then using a MECC approach you could ask, 'Have you ever considered stopping smoking?'. Then, dependent on the answer (a) 'Oh no, dear', or (b) 'Yes, I have tried but I always go back to it' or even (c) 'No! Leave me alone!', you can signpost as appropriate with (a) 'Well, if you do think about giving up, let us know or your GP, and we can refer you to a smoking cessation service' or (b) 'Well done for trying; did you know you are more likely to be successful with help? Would you like some more information?' or (c) 'Just let us know if you would like to discuss it in the future' – and that is MECC in a nutshell.

The benefits to this approach include patients potentially having better treatment outcomes – for example, if they lose weight prior to surgery or give up smoking. They may end up feeling better, quicker, gaining in confidence and motivation and feeling supported. It is a person-centered approach to care and it will contribute to the reduction of health inequalities, as it enhances the opportunity for patients to gain access to additional health services and support.

Activity 3.5   Critical thinking

Can you think of any potential barriers to staff using the MECC approach in practice?

A brief outline answer is given at the end of the chapter.

Health promotion for people with learning disabilities (LD)

We know that people with LD experience inequalities in health in relation with people having reduced access to health screening and health promotion services (Cooper et al., 2018; Mafuba and Gates, 2015). People with LD have more health needs than the general population, and the risk of exacerbations of LTCs are increased due to the potential impact of their cognitive impairment, affecting their ability to identify health risk and recognising deterioration in their condition (Codling, 2015). The approaches and strategies discussed in this chapter are relevant to the promotion of health in this group of people, but be aware of the potential for poor engagement due difficulty in understanding, organisational barriers and limited social support for this vulnerable group (Cooper et al., 2018). Understanding the barriers that might prevent people with LD access health promotion will help you to plan and deliver appropriate interventions.

- Learning and communication difficulties – a person with LD may not understand or appreciate the significance of a healthy lifestyle or understand the importance of health screening. This can result in the person not participating in the health-promotion activity or not mentioning when they feel unwell, as they may not realise the significance of the symptoms. By providing information in an appropriate format – e.g., a picture book – it gives people with LD the opportunity to learn about their health. An example of this is a health-promotion educational strategy aimed at enabling people with LD to learn about managing long term conditions (Codling, 2015). Topics include communicating with healthcare professionals, pain and symptom control, and recognising red flags for their condition.
- Poor carer and professional awareness – carers may not be aware of the importance of a healthy lifestyle, and healthcare professionals may misinterpret changes as being due to the LD rather than another health need. By working with carers to improve their knowledge and understanding, you will enhance both the health of the carer and person with LD.
- Discrimination – there is discrimination and difficulty accessing health services for people with LD. Developing an understanding of your attitudes and beliefs, and that of society's, will influence the care you deliver.

Most areas of the UK have access to community learning disability teams; these teams are available for you to access and will be able to provide you with specialist information, resources and support. A key role of these teams is to advise and support primary care trusts in delivering annual health checks for people with LD.

Case study: Daniel

Daniel is 30 years old and is living with Down's syndrome. He lives in supported accommodation with three other people who are also living with learning disabilities. Daniel relies on convenience foods the majority of the time, though his support worker is trying to improve his diet. He does not work and takes limited exercise; as a result, he has been putting on weight. Daniel is attending his GP surgery for his annual health check. At this visit it is noted that his weight has increased and his BMI is 28 (it was 24 last year). This is concerning to Daniel's GP, as his weight gain will increase his chances of developing type 2 diabetes and heart disease. The GP has asked the practice nurse to work with Daniel to reduce his weight.

Activity 3.6   Critical thinking

Go to **www.rcn.org.uk/professional-development/publications/pub-005769** where you can find the RCN learning disability guidance for pre-registration nurses. You will find this a helpful resource.

- How could you work with Daniel to improve his health?
- How might you best communicate with him effectively?
- What approaches might you use to help him change his diet? What approaches might you use to encourage him to increase the amount of exercise he takes?

A brief outline answer is given at the end of the chapter.

By supporting Daniel to improve his health you will be able to increase his sense of autonomy and minimise his health complications in the future.

Chapter summary

This chapter has provided you with an overview of the role of health promotion in the care and management of people living with an LTC. The importance of determinants of health and public health in relation to LTCs has been outlined and the necessary role that health promotion has in the care and management of people living with an LTC. It has focused on health promotion approaches and how to effect change in a person's health behaviour to enhance their health and well-being. Some specific behaviour change strategies that can be used in promoting health for people living with an LTC have been discussed and related to your clinical practice.

Having read through this chapter and worked through the activities, you will have succeeded in increasing your knowledge and skills of health promotion in relation to the care and management of people living with an LTC. How you will use your knowledge and skills will depend on where you are working, and your roles and responsibilities. Nevertheless, you can increase the appropriateness of your health promotion by using the knowledge and skills developed in this chapter. By increasing your knowledge of health determinants and health-promotion approaches, you will be able to provide health-promotion interventions that address the holistic nature of health. By understanding motivation in relation to health promotion and how to relate this to a person's readiness to change, you will provide health-promotion information appropriate for that person. In using a strategy like MI, you will place the person at the centre of your interactions with them, ensuring that they are driving the health promotion.

Activities: brief outline answers

Activity 3.3 Critical thinking (page 56)

- Age, sex and constitutional factors – Mary has a history of cardiovascular disease living with hypertension and previously having a stroke. While statistically speaking, as a woman, Mary is likely to live longer than her male counterparts, her frailty is negatively influencing her current health and is a contributing factor to her mortality. She can be formally described as frail due to her decreased mobility, continence difficulties and increased risk of falling. As her condition progresses, her symptoms are likely to worsen, resulting in poorer health and increased need for nursing care.
- Individual lifestyle factors – Mary has reduced mobility, requiring carers to help her move. The result of this includes increased dependency, increased risk of pressure sores and a deterioration of mental well-being. The transition from living at home to going into a long term care facility can also have a negative impact on well-being. This can be offset by ensuring that social and emotional needs are met adequately and important family connections are maintained. Person care planning from the nursing team with the home and engagement in advance care planning can help Mary maintain a sense of control over her life.
- Social and community networks – Admission to a nursing home can be a barrier to maintaining important social links, which can have a negative impact on an individual's well-being. Loneliness in older people can result in deterioration in health and well-being, and contribute to a shorter life span. For someone who has been effectively house-bound by their physical state, admission to a care home may result in an increase in social contact, the formation of new networks and friends, and supported access to activities that had been previously unattainable. In this instance, there could be a positive impact on well-being.
- Living and working conditions – Mary will be moving to a home that can cater for all her physical and social needs, and may be able to access facilities such as a bath, social

activities and outings. There will be a loss of independence and privacy in shared living and 24 staffing. There will be a significant impact on her financial status, as she has savings over a threshold level that require her to pay for nursing care. UK nursing homes can cost upwards of £1,000 weekly, which will quickly decrease a lifetime of savings. There is also the possibility that her family home would have to be sold if the savings run out. The implications of this expenditure will affect the whole family.

• General socioeconomic, cultural and environmental conditions – Due to global financial difficulties, Mary may find that her pension and any savings she has have decreased as interest rates remain low.

Activity 3.4 Critical thinking (page 60)

Examples are given here of how all health promotion approaches may be used with Sian.

Approach	Intervention	Rationale
Medical	To discuss with Sian's GP if she should have a regular flu vaccine.	It is recommended that people with asthma, who take regular steroid preventer inhalers like beclazone, have a yearly flu vaccine administered between early September to early November.
Educational	To provide Sian with comprehensive information regarding her medication – when to take, how to take and why she needs to take it.	Explaining to Sian how her medication works in controlling her asthma and the need to take this regularly to ensure that the medication is effective, will increase her knowledge about her asthma.
Behavioural	Work with Sian to develop a routine so that she remembers to take her medication regularly.	Working with Sian, by asking her to outline her daily routine and encouraging her to identify when the best time to take her beclazone would be, and how she can remember to do this, means that Sian is more likely to adopt a new approach as she has found the solution that fits in with her life.
Empowerment	Provide Sian with education regarding her medication and behavioural change strategies.	Using both the educational and behavioural approach has the potential to empower Sian to self-manage her condition more effectively. Placing Sian at the centre of the plan supports her to take more control over her situation.

It is important that the impact of these strategies are evaluated, therefore it would be important to follow these up in a review meeting with Sian.

Activity 3.5 Critical thinking (page 65)

Lack of staff knowledge about MECC or services available, lack of confidence, poor communication skills, time (is MECC another addition to workload?), worry about offending people, perception that it is not your role, concern about your own position as a role model.

These are well-documented barriers to implementing MECC, but they can all be overcome. On your next placement, ask your mentor about MECC. Do they use it? Do they know about it? Talk about some of the barriers mentioned above.

Activity 3.6 Critical thinking (page 66)

Both you and the practice nurse will need to consider how you deliver information to Daniel in a format that he will understand. The British Institute of Learning Disabilities provides a range of books focusing on good health, which includes titles on healthy eating and exercise. If providing written material, try to ensure that you address Daniel directly – e.g., playing football will help you lose weight and this is good for your heart. Using diagrams and pictures to illustrate the words will help reinforce the message. When discussing either healthy eating or exercise with Daniel, speak clearly and allow him time to answer. Provide your information in a positive way – e.g., don't say, 'Don't eat crisps every day', say 'Have crisps on a Monday'. Always make sure that Daniel has understood the conversation and check at the end. Good collaboration with Daniel's support worker and the local Community Learning Disability Team will ensure that Daniel is well supported.

Further reading

Bennett, C, Parry, J and Lawrence, Z (2009) Promoting health in primary care. *Nursing Standard,* 23 (47): 48–56.

An overview of the role of health promotion in primary care.

Dixon, A (2008) *Motivation and Confidence: What Does It Take to Change Behaviour?* London: King's Fund.

A paper that discusses the role that personal motivation and confidence have in relation to behaviour change.

Darch, J, Baillie, L, Gillison, F (2017) Nurses as role models in health promotion: a concept analysis. *British Journal of Nursing,* 26(17): 982–88.

An interesting exploration of what it means to be a good role model when promoting health.

Jenkins, C and Mckay, A (2013) A collaborative approach to health promotion in early stage dementia Nursing standard 27(36): 49–57.

A series that explores how health promotion interventions are adapted across the span of an LTC.

Useful websites

www.gov.uk/government/organisations/public-health-england

This link takes you to an index page where relevant information relating to health inequalities in England is listed; this includes how to reduce health inequalities and makes reference to local initiatives.

www.health-ni.gov.uk/topics/public-health-policy-and-advice

This link takes you to the main page where the Northern Ireland government's information in relation to public health and health inequalities is.

www.healthscotland.scot

This link takes you to the main page for NHS Health Scotland's information about health inequalities and how the NHS in Scotland is planning to reduce these.

www.publichealthwalesobservatory.wales.nhs.uk/home

The home page for inequalities and equalities, this contains information from Public Health Wales Observatory and additional resources relating to health inequalities.

http://www.makingeverycontactcount.co.uk

This link takes you to the main site for MECC; here you will find resources about MECC, training and elearning activities to support you to deliver MECC as part of your day-to-day inter-actions with people.

www.hee.nhs.uk/our-work/health-literacy

This link enables access to free educational resources in relation to health literacy awareness for healthcare professionals.

Chapter 4 Self-management in long term conditions

NMC Future nurse: Standards of proficiency for registered nurses

This chapter will address the following standards:

Platform 1: Being an accountable professional

At the point of registration, the registered nurse will be able to:

1.9   understand the need to base all decisions regarding care and interventions on people's needs and preferences, recognising and addressing any personal and external factors that may unduly influence their decisions

1.11 communicate effectively using a range of skills and strategies with colleagues and people at all stages of life and with a range of mental, physical, cognitive and behavioural health challenges

Platform 2: Promoting health and preventing ill health

At the point of registration, the registered nurse will be able to:

2.1   understand and apply the aims and principles of health promotion, protection and improvement and the prevention of ill health when engaging with people

2.4   identify and use all appropriate opportunities, making reasonable adjustments when required, to discuss the impact of smoking, substance and alcohol use, sexual behaviours, diet and exercise on mental, physical and behavioural health and wellbeing, in the context of people's individual circumstances

2.8   explain and demonstrate the use of up to date approaches to behaviour change to enable people to use their strengths and expertise and make informed choices when managing their own health and making lifestyle adjustments

2.9   use appropriate communication skills and strength-based approaches to support and enable people to make informed choices about their care to manage health

(Continued)

(Continued)

challenges in order to have satisfying and fulfilling lives within the limitations cause by reduced capability, ill health and disability

Platform 3: Assessing needs and planning care

At the point of registration, the registered nurse will be able to:

3.16 demonstrate knowledge of when and how to refer people safely to other professionals or services for clinical intervention and support

Platform 7: Coordinating care

At the point of registration, the registered nurse will be able to:

7.5 understand and recognise the need to respond to the challenges of providing safe, effective and person-centred nursing care for people who have co-morbidities and complex care needs

NMC Annexe A:

Communication and relationship management skills

At the point of registration, the registered nurse will be able to safely demonstrate the following skills:

2 **Evidence-based, best practice approaches to communication for supporting people of all ages, their families and carers in preventing ill health and in managing their care**

2.2 use clear language and appropriate, written materials, making reasonable adjustments where appropriate in order to optimise people's understanding of what has caused their health condition and the implications of their care and treatment

2.6 use repetition and positive reinforcement strategies

3 **Evidence-based, best practice communication skills and approaches for providing therapeutic interventions**

3.1 motivational interviewing techniques

Chapter aims

After reading this chapter, you will be able to:

- explain the difference between self-care and self-management ;
- understand the importance of self-efficacy and patient activation in promoting self-managemet for people living with LTCs;

- identify the key components of self-management;
- recognise the role that self-management can play in the care of people living with dementia.

Introduction

Self-management is the cornerstone of effective LTC care and management; options for self-management should be made available at the time of diagnoses right the way through to palliative and end-of-life care. Self-management is important both for the person living with an LTC and for the NHS. It is known that people who are not supported to self-manage are disempowered, feel abandoned and may experience increased exacerbations and health crises (McDonald, 2014). It is thought that around 20 per cent of emergency admissions to hospital are potentially preventable, with many of these involving people living with an LTC (Blunt, 2013). The aim of self-management in the care and management of LTCs is to promote self-care in people living with an LTC, thereby enabling them to self-manage their condition in a way that allows them to maintain as much control over their life and future as they would like to have.

The terms 'self-care' and 'self-management' can be used interchangeably, although there are some differences in these terms. Self-care refers to the resources used by patients to promote their health and manage their health conditions; these can include knowledge of their condition, determination, managing minor ailments and maintaining health following acute illness (Department of Health, 2006). Self-caring people display the following positive behaviours: healthy lifestyle, concordance with treatment regimens, effective use of services, and being able to understand and respond to symptoms and problems (Forbes and While, 2009). Self-management requires the person living with an LTC to make changes in their behaviour to improve their health and well-being. Therefore, it is likely that you will use some of the health promotion approaches and some of the behaviour change strategies discussed in Chapter 3 to support people living with an LTC to self-manage. This is certainly what happened to 18-year-old Amy, who has type 1 diabetes; this is how she describes her experience of living with the condition.

It's not easy having a long-term condition. When I was younger, I didn't want people to see me as being 'different'; all I wanted was to fit in, to be the same. However, having type 1 diabetes made me feel different. I was always having to check my blood glucose levels, watch what I ate, when I ate. My parents tried to keep me on track, but it wasn't easy. I'd 'forget' to check my blood glucose levels, eat (and drink) things I wasn't supposed to, basically winging it a bit, but that was OK, right? Wrong. It all came to a head after I'd finished college. I'd been out with friends, yes, I'd been drinking, and hadn't checked my blood glucose levels all night. By the time I got home, I was feeling unwell. I was dizzy, sweating and feeling a bit 'out of it'. I tried to check my blood glucose levels but couldn't because I was shaking so much. My friends panicked and took me to hospital. It was a wake-up call, to be honest. I realised that I had to take control. I had to manage my diabetes so it didn't manage me! Now I'm much more organized. I have an app on my phone where I record my blood glucose levels, carbs, exercise, and I have a 'night out' plan which I adhere to. Most importantly, I showed my friends how to measure my blood glucose and what to do. It's made me realise I'm not so different after all.

In the quote above, it is evident that Amy made a conscious decision to take control of her type 1 diabetes rather than allowing it to control her and her life. However, it should be recognised that not all people living with an LTC will feel able to, or want to, participate in their own self-management. Oskar is 37, is obese and has hypertension. He has been told by his GP that in order to help control his blood pressure, he needs to lose weight.

Why should I lose weight? So, my blood pressure is a bit high. I take the tablets my GP gives me – they'll keep it OK. Anyway, I'm still young; it's at least another 10 years until I need to think about that. I work full time, I keep up with the kids, what's the problem?

It is clear from this quote that Oskar does not consider that he needs to change his lifestyle to help self-manage his hypertension. People with LTCs, like Oskar, may wish to manage their condition but are unable to do so. This could be for a variety of reasons – e.g., feeling that they are not being listened to, a lack of knowledge and understanding about their condition, or their social situation. Engaging people like Oskar in the self-management of their LTC requires you to address the underlying reasons for their reluctance to actively participate in their own self-management. Using the knowledge and skills discussed in Chapters 2 and 3, such as engaging in a therapeutic relationship and using effective communication skills, will support you in being able to address these underlying reasons for their reluctance.

To support you in effectively enabling people living with an LTC to self-manage, this chapter will develop your knowledge and skills in relation to the fundamental role that self-management has for people living with an LTC. To do this, the chapter will define self-care and self-management, and discuss the relationship between the two. Self-efficacy and patient activation will be discussed in relation to self-management and how you can, through therapeutic actions, support people to self-manage their LTC. There will be a focus on the skills required to become an effective self-manager. Finally, the importance of promoting self-management in dementia will be discussed, with some strategies for care being outlined.

Self-care and self-management in LTCs

There is no way you can avoid managing a chronic condition. If you do nothing but suffer, this is a management style. If you only take medication, this is another management style. If you choose to be a positive self-manager and undergo all the best treatments that healthcare professionals have to offer along with being proactive in your day to day management, this will lead you to live a healthy life.

(Lorig et al., 2006, p1)

Self-care and self-management can often be used to mean the same thing. When considering these terms in relation to supporting people to live well with one or more LTC, it is important to be clear about what they both mean.

Activity 4.1   Reflection

Consider what the terms 'self-care' and 'self-management' mean to you and write down a definition of each.

As this activity is based on your observations, there is no outline at the end of the chapter.

When completing Activity 4.1, you might have found it quite difficult to differentiate between self-care and self-management. This illustrates that if you are to support people living with LTC to become active partners in their care, you need to understand what self-care and self-management are and how they can be promoted. Self-care can be defined as the actions that healthy people take in order to develop, protect, maintain and improve their health and well-being (Self Care Forum, 2018). On some level, we all participate in self-care, whether brushing our teeth, taking regular exercise or managing minor illnesses. These activities demonstrate positive self-care behaviours: lifestyle, managing therapy regimens, accessing services appropriately, understanding symptoms and responding to them. The Self Care Forum depicts self-care as a continuum (see Figure 4.1).

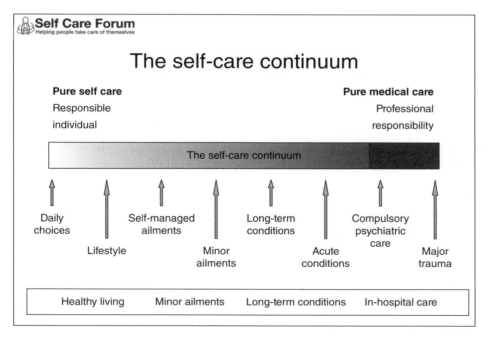

Figure 4.1   The Self Care Continuum (The Self Care Forum, 2018)

While self-care behaviours can be attributed to both healthy people and those living with an LTC, self-management is the day-to-day management that people with LTCs engage in to manage their illness. There has been much debate about what self-management is and what it encompasses. Corbin and Strauss (1985) identified three tasks: the medical management of the condition, behaviour management and emotional management. While the tasks identified by Corbin and Strauss outlined the areas for self-management, they did not include how these could be achieved. To address these, the following core processes were outlined (Lorig and Holman, 2003):

- problem solving;
- decision-making;
- resource utilisation;
- partnership with healthcare providers;
- taking action.

More recently, descriptions of self-management have integrated the work by Corbin and Strauss, and Lorig and Holman, putting forward three main areas: focusing on illness needs, activating resources and living with chronic illness (Schulman-Green et al., 2012). What is evident in all these definitions is that, if patients are to be effective self-managers, they need to be engaged in their care and informed about their care and management. However, as can be seen from the examples earlier in this chapter, people may not want, or feel able, to take a more active role in managing their own health and working in partnership with health and social care professionals. If you intend to work with people to support them to address the areas identified by Schulman-Green (2012), then building their 'self-efficacy' is key.

The role of self-efficacy in self-management

Self-efficacy can be defined as the extent to which a person believes they can exercise control of their health habits successfully (Bandura, 2004), influencing their goals and aspirations. A systematic review carried out by the Health Foundation (De Silva, 2011) concluded that as a person's self-efficacy increased, this had a positive effect on their attitude, behaviour, use of healthcare resources and quality of life. Bandura (2004) identifies four modes of influence in which a person's belief in their self-efficacy can be developed:

1. Mastery experiences: successfully self-managing an aspect of their LTC strengthens a person's sense of self-efficacy. However, those who experience easy successes may not develop the resilience required to self-manage more complex aspects of their LTC. Prompting patients to recall previous successes and the strategies they used will enable you to promote problem- solving skills, in turn increasing resilience.

2. Social modelling: seeing people with similar LTCs, who are facing similar challenges, succeeding in self-managing their condition, increases others' beliefs in their own ability to self-manage. This is the rationale behind peer support programmes, such as those provided by Self Management UK

(www.selfmanagementuk.org). It should be recognised that social modelling may not take place face-to-face, because with the increase in digital resources, people can access information across a range of platforms.

3. Social persuasion: if people are encouraged to believe in themselves, they will try harder, increasing their chance of success. This includes providing supportive feedback about a patient's progress and achievements, highlighting their achievements – for example: 'It's great to see that you have managed to self-administer your insulin this week. I know that you have found this difficult in the past.'

4. Psychological responses: how a person interprets their emotional and physical response to an LTC will also influence their self-efficacy. For instance, a person with COPD may not want to undertake physical activity that maintains lung function because they are anxious about becoming breathless. You can help to increase self-efficacy by acknowledging this fear, explaining the benefits of exercise and the body's response to this, and providing guidance on how to manage any anxiety.

Activity 4.2   Critical thinking

Revisit Linda's case study in Chapters 1 and 2 (pages 12 and 37). We pick up her story below.

Linda continues to smoke. However, she was able to make some changes to her lifestyle and until recently had been walking twice a week with a cardiac rehab group who meet at her local community centre. She enjoyed the company and had begun to lose some weight. However, over the past two weeks Linda has lost confidence in her ability to manage episodes of chest pain, triggered by a recent episode when she was out shopping. She did not have her GTN spray with her and was admitted, via ambulance, to the Emergency Department. This has increased her anxiety about leaving her house, increasing her social isolation; she has not met with her walking group since the incident. Over the past ten days she has requested a home visit three times for a range of physical symtoms. Using Bandura's four modes of influence, identify ways in which you could increase Linda's self-efficacy.

Once you have completed this activity, turn to the outline answer at the end of the chapter and identify any areas requiring further work.

As you can see from Activity 4.2, developing Linda's self-efficacy is one of the first steps in supporting her to take a more active role in self-managing her LTCs. However, improving Linda's self-efficacy, in isolation of any other factors that may contribute to her ability to become a more active self-manager, may not be sufficient. Understanding how 'active' Linda is, or would like to be, in managing her own health will ensure the sustainability of her self-management.

Patient activation to support self-management in LTCs

Patient activation is a behavioural concept and is defined as the knowledge, skills and confidence a person has in managing their health and healthcare (Hibbard et al., 2005). Hibbard et al. (2007) used the Patient Activation Measure (PAM) to explore if increased patient activation improved self-management. Their research concluded that increased patient activation was accompanied by positive changes in self-management behaviours. Importantly, they also evidenced that positive patient activation was sustained over time, resulting in better health outcomes.

The Patient Activation Measure (Hibbard et al., 2005) is the most commonly used measure of patient activation. It is a self-reporting measure that contains a series of 13 statements designed to assess the scope of a person's activation. The measure is subdivided into four stages of activation – low to high (Hibbard and Gilburt, 2014). Individuals are asked to state how much they agree or disagree with a range of statements relating to their health, these statements relating to the different stages of activation.

- Stage 1: individuals are passive, lacking confidence or knowledge; adherence to medication may be poor. Statements on PAM exploring this include: *taking an active role in my own healthcare is the most important thing that affects my health.*
- Stage 2: individuals have some knowledge, but may not be able to connect this information together, resulting in gaps, though they are able to set simple goals. PAM statements addressing this include: *I know what each of my prescribed medications does.*
- Stage 3: individuals have the key facts and are developing self-management skills; they are goal orientated and view themselves as part of their healthcare team. Statements on PAM acknowledging this include: *I know how to prevent further problems with my health condition.*
- Stage 4: individuals are self-managing, though they may struggle in times of change or stress. PAM statements addressing this include: *I am confident that I can tell whether I need to go to the doctor or whether I can take care of a health problem myself.*

Exploring patient activation addresses the left-hand wall of the House of Care (Coulter et al., 2013; see Chapter 1 for further information), where the aim is for those living with LTCs to be informed and engaged in their care. This is further supported by research carried out by McDonald in 2014, in which 77 per cent of the participants in the study indicated that they should be able to manage more of their healthcare independently at home, but that a lack of support and information prevented this.

As you can see from Activity 4.3, getting people to the point of being able to self-manage their LTC more effectively may take some time. As a healthcare professional, you have an active role to play in supporting people living with LTCs to develop the skills they require to self-management their health.

Activity 4.3 Critical thinking

Reflecting on the quote by Oskar, included at the start of this chapter, and using the information in this chapter, consider the following questions.

- What stage of activation is Oskar at?
- How might you be able to increase this?

Once you have completed this activity, turn to the outline answer at the end of the chapter and identify any areas requiring further work

The components of self-management in LTCs

As self-management is multifactorial, it is important to ensure that the approaches used address all aspects of self-management – for instance, self-efficacy. Figure 4.2 demonstrates this; here different strategies focus on supporting people to develop a range of self-management skills. What is important to recognise is that placing these strategies on a continuum recognises that self-efficacy and activation are gained over time and as part of a continual process.

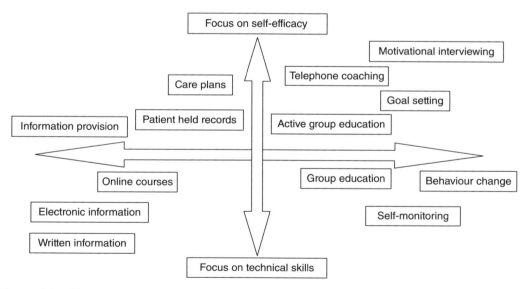

Figure 4.2 The continuum of strategies to support self-management

Source: de Silva, 2011, reproduced with permission

Being aware of the strategies available ensures that you are able to tailor your approach to meet the needs of the person and what area of self-management it is they want to address. Given the breadth of the strategies that may be needed to support self-management, referral to other members of the health and social care team may be required. For instance, specialist nurse services may be required to provide people with more detailed knowledge about their disease trajectory and management. Health psychologists may be involved in behaviour change approaches, such as motivational interviewing. At the start of this chapter, the following key areas of self-management were mentioned: focusing on illness needs, activating resources and living with chronic illness (Schulman-Green et al., 2012). We will now explore them in more detail.

Focusing on illness needs

This aspect of self-management addresses the tasks and skills necessary for people living with LTCs to care for illness-specific concerns – for instance, using a GTN spray for an episode of angina. This includes learning about their LTC and the treatment regimes in order to manage their LTC on a day-to-day basis. Additionally, performing health-promotion activities and maintaining behaviour change to minimise the impact of their LTC forms part of focusing on illness need. This aspect of self-management may be addressed by the person independently or with input from family/carers and/or healthcare professionals. The time and attention this aspect requires will depend on the person's illness trajectory and their life context.

Case study: Frazer

See Chapter 1, p. 8, for further information about Frazer.

Eight months ago, negative pressure wound therapy was used as a rescue therapy for Frazer's non-healing ulcer; this was carried out to prevent amputation. Initially, there was some improvement in Frazer's foot, but he is experiencing severe pain in his leg and has had further infections, which are now healed. Despite the ongoing issues with his ulcer, Frazer is not always concordant with carrying out his foot health checks, which are an important part of his self-management.

Activity 4.4   Critical thinking

You are spending the day at the diabetic foot clinic where Frazer has an appointment. Based on what you know about Frazer and his previous history, consider which self-management strategies (see Figure 4.2) could be used and why to support Frazer to engage more actively in his care.

Once you have completed this activity, turn to the outline answer at the end of the chapter and identify any areas requiring further work.

As identified in Activity 4.4, understanding a person's illness journey and their previous responses to self-management will ensure that the approaches you use are tailored to the individual needs of the person.

Activating resources

This refers to the people, community and services that are available to support people to self-manage. This includes individuals, such as family, friends, health and social care professionals. In addition, resources also include community resources and services – e.g., spiritual resources and community groups. Social prescribing is not a new idea – occupational therapy has long been supporting people to participate in meaningful activities as part of their care. Social prescribing allows GPs and other frontline healthcare professionals to refer people to 'services' in their community alongside their medical treatment. Services available include art classes, cooking groups and gardening. Further information on the impact of social prescribing can be found in the further reading list at the end of the chapter.

Activity 4.5   Reflection

Where you live, consider what services are available in the local community that could support social prescribing for people living with LTCs. Remember to consider those living with both physical and mental health conditions.

As this activity is based on your own reflections, no sample answer is provided at the end of the chapter.

In reflecting on Activity 4.5, you may have realised that many of the services you identified were run by third-sector organisations such as charities. This demonstrates the interrelationship between health, social care and tertiary services to ensure that those living with LTCs have access to a range of services to address their individual needs.

Living with chronic illness

This area of self-management concentrates on the tasks and skills related to coping with the LTC, both psychological and physical, as well as integrating the LTC into the context of the person's life. As discussed in Chapter 1, living with an LTC impacts on a person both physically and psychologically. Therefore, addressing a person's emotions is an important part of supporting them to adjust to live their new 'normal'. In addition, adjusting to 'living with chronic illness' involves modifying lifestyle, balancing maintaining 'normalcy' and taking appropriate action to manage illness needs.

If we consider Frazer (see Activity 4.4), it can be seen that in addition to addressing illness needs, goal setting will also support Frazer to self-manage to ensure that he acts to manage his LTC. One approach that could be used to support effective goal setting is action planning. For instance, the goal that you set with Frazer could be to 'minimise the risk of further deterioration in foot health'. The purpose of action planning is to break down the goal into smaller tasks (how is Frazer going to achieve this; what does he have to do?). Therefore, while the overall goal might be quite large, the action plan breaks it down into manageable pieces, enabling the person to see that they are working towards their overall goal. Lorig et al. (2014) state that it should:

- be reasonable – is this something that the person can expect to achieve in a reasonable time, such as in a week or two?;
- be behaviour-specific – giving the person an identified behaviour to address, something they can actually see changing (e.g., rather than saying 'losing weight', say 'no eating after your evening meal');
- answer the following questions: What is the person going to do? How often are they going to do this? When are they going to do this?
- inspire confidence – how confident is the person that they are going to achieve this? They could rate this on a scale of one to ten, one being no confidence and ten being most confident. If a person rates their confidence below seven, they should ask themselves why their confidence is low and review their action plan in a way that will increase their likelihood of success.

When completing an action plan, a person may experience problems that affect their ability to achieve what they had set out to do. This could be for a variety of reasons: the overall goal was unrealistic, the action plan was too ambitious or their condition deteriorated. What is important here is that the person does not give up but finds ways to solve the problem that is preventing them from reaching their goal. This could take the form of reviewing their goal or giving themselves longer to complete their action plan. Supporting people living with an LTC to find solutions to their problems will increase their knowledge and understanding of their LTC, increase the skills required to manage their LTC, and increase their self-efficacy in managing their LTC.

Action plan
Goal: to minimise the risk of further deterioration of foot health
Aim: to monitor my feet for signs of change – every morning this week I will: • *examine my feet assessing colour, swelling, breaks in the skin and pain or numbness;* • *wash and dry my feet carefully;* • *apply moisturiser to my feet.* This week I will avoid: • *walking around barefoot;* • *hot-water bottles, hot baths, etc.*

This week I will remember to: • *ensure that my socks and shoes are well fitting;* • *use my wheelchair when out and about to reduce pressure on my feet.*		

This week I will be aware of the danger of:

• *skin removal – corns;*
• *knocking or banging my feet against objects.*

What to do if anything changes:

• *If I notice any changes in my feet, I am to notify healthcare professionals immediately to ensure appropriate treatment and management.*

How confident am I that I will achieve this? 8 out of 10		
Day of the week	*Achieved*	*Any comments*
Monday	*Yes*	*Inspected my feet today, used a mirror to help me check the soles of my feet, remembered to dry and apply moisturiser after my shower.*
Tuesday	*Yes*	*As Monday*
Wednesday	*Yes*	*As Monday, did notice that some of my socks were a bit worn out; will buy new ones tomorrow.*
Thursday	*Yes*	*Slept in this morning; no shower today but did inspect them; will wash, dry and moisturise them tonight.*
Friday	*Yes*	*As Monday*
Saturday	*No*	*Took Fiona swimming today; had to take my outdoor shoes off in the changing rooms; forgot to dry my feet before I put my shoes on.*
Sunday	*Yes*	*Noticed that there was an area of redness and swelling on my right foot. Contacted the out-of-hours service and was advised to attend GP; antibiotics prescribed; appointment with practice nurse to be arranged.*

Table 4.1   Action plan for Frazer

As you can see, Frazer's action plan focuses on practical advice that he can incorporate into his day-to-day activities, encouraging him to adhere to his plan. In addition, there are clear instructions for him to follow should there be any deterioration in his foot health.

Activity 4.6   Critical thinking

Reflecting on Activity 4.2 and your input with Linda, using the format of the action plan detailed on page 82 and taking into consideration Linda's concerns, work with Linda to support her to compile an action plan to

(Continued)

> (Continued)
>
> enable her to return to her walking group. It may not be possible for the goal
> on the first action plan you compile with Linda to state that she will rejoin
> her walking group; you may have to break this down in to a smaller goal first.
> This approach will ensure that the goal set is achievable, increasing Linda's
> chance of success in this.
>
> *Once you have completed this activity, turn to the outline answer at the end of the*
> *chapter and identify any areas requiring further work.*

As you can see from Activity 4.6, successful self-management relies on the person who is living with the LTC being able to identify specific goals they would like to achieve, and planning and implementing a course of action to enable them to succeed. However, it should be recognised that, for some people, there may be times where some goals are unachievable. In this situation it is important to support the person to compile another action plan that will enable them to return to their first goal. Alternatively, it may be appropriate to find other goals that are more achievable for the individual at that time. This flexible, positive approach will focus on what the person can do rather than on what they cannot do.

Given the components of self-management discussed above, it can be seen that self-management is a complex process. It is not about the person living with the LTC managing their care in isolation. It is about working in partnership with the health and social care team, accessing relevant information and education, and then using what they have learned to manage their condition in the way that best suits their lifestyle (Lorig et al., 2014). This can be particularly challenging for people living with dementia who may have to consider modifying their lifestyle early in their disease trajectory. The next section of this chapter will focus on specific self-management approaches that can be used to support people living with dementia and their family/carers.

'Living well' for people living with dementia

Although almost ten years old, the *Living Well with Dementia: A National Dementia Strategy* (DH, 2009) is still relevant today. Its underlying principles of good quality early diagnosis and easy access to care and support for carers are echoed in the *Prime Minister's Challenge on Dementia 2020* (DH, 2015). Both these publications emphasise the need for people living with dementia to be enabled to 'live well'. There are many factors influencing the ability of a person living with dementia to live well and be able to participate in their care decisions. Supporting the person living with dementia to maintain communication channels with healthcare professionals, their family and carers is a key aspect of living well; additionally, the use of assistive technology that maintains and promotes independent living is key. As mentioned in Chapter 2, carers play a significant role in the care and management of LTCs; caring for a person with dementia has its own challenges, so supporting carers to maintain their role impacts positively on the well-being of the person with dementia.

Communication

People living with dementia should have their hearing and vision checked regularly, and professionals should ensure that, when communicating, they take into consideration the individual's ability to communicate. Verbal communication should be person-centred, match the person's level of cognitive ability and focus on the communication ability the person has, rather than focusing on their communication deficit. Listening and adapting your rate of speech, tone and words used to find what gets the best response ensures that communication continues to be a two-way process.

Memory books containing images and simple statements can be used to aid communication and memory recall. A memory book may include a family photograph with the names of the people in the photograph next to them. They can also be used when the same question is asked repeatedly, by providing a simple answer to the question through words and pictures. Another useful resource is Talking Mats; this is a relatively low-cost communication tool developed by speech and language therapists. It uses specifically designed communication symbols that can be used by all ages.

Research summary: Talking Mats

Research by Murphy and Oliver (2013) and Reitz and Dalemans (2016) explored how Talking Mats could be used to support shared decision making for people living with dementia. Both studies focused on how Talking Mats could be used to support discussion around daily living, with both studies recruiting small numbers of participants – 18 couples in the research by Murphy and Oliver (2013) and 6 couples in the research by Reitz and Dalemans (2016). Both research studies divided their participants into an intervention (using Talking Mats) and control (not using Talking Mats) group.

Results from these studies demonstrated that using Talking Mats meant that the person living with dementia was better able to participate in decisions about their care. Both research studies concluded that people living with dementia found that using Talking Mats helped them to remember what they were talking about and remind them of the things they could still do. For carers, Talking Mats helped them to understand what the person with dementia was trying to say by keeping the conversation focused. Additionally, using them reduced confrontation, as the person with dementia could look back at the Talking Mat and see what had been discussed (Murphy and Oliver, 2013).

(Continued)

(Continued)

In addition to being used to support decision making for people living with dementia, Talking Mats have also been used to support frail older people with communication difficulties to express their views (Murphy et al., 2004). While some of the participants in this study had dementia, others had different communication difficulties, such as deafness. In this study, the Talking Mats were used to explore four areas of the person's life: activities, people, environment and self. All ten participants were resident in care homes (within six months). The nature of the areas explored addressed both internal – health and appearance – and external factors – the care home environment. When considering activities, analysis of the data evidenced that the most popular activity was listening to music, though it should be acknowledged that a range of activities were enjoyed. When considering the environment and people, there were more positive than negative comments. The study concluded that Talking Mats is an enjoyable method of allowing frail older people to express views they might otherwise not be able to do.

As can be seen from the research summary, Talking Mats have been shown to improve communication between the carer and the person living with dementia. To further improve communication between the person living with dementia and the health and social care team, carers could be provided with a diary that includes the following information: changes in memory ability, drastic mood changes, unusual behaviour, health-related changes to sleep, appetite, etc., and any health complaints of the person. Identifying changes early that may signify an acute illness, such as an infection, or deterioration in the person's dementia can ensure that prompt action is taken. This may include undertaking a health assessment of the person, addressing acute episodes and reviewing ongoing care plans to support person-centred care. Not only does this approach support the person living with dementia to 'live well', it also supports the carer to 'care well'.

Supporting carers

It is known that people who care for a person living with dementia provide more day-to-day assistance, report increased stress and have less time for family and friends. In addition, those caring for a person with early onset dementia experience increased work-related challenges (Brodaty and Donkin, 2009). Providing support for carers to allow them to continue in their role is an important part of ensuring that a person living with dementia 'lives well'. Providing carers with training and education about activities of daily living (ADLs) will enable the carer to provide appropriate physical care for the person living with dementia. Offering carers the opportunity to practise activities such as manual handling and washing and dressing under supervision of experienced healthcare professionals ensures that these activities are carried out correctly (DiZazzo-Miller et al., 2014). This has the potential to reduce the likelihood of injury to the carer in the case of manual handling, and maximise functional independence for the person living with dementia in the case of washing and dressing. Top tips can include the following (DiZazzo-Miller et al., 2014).

- Nutrition – remember that people with cognitive deterioration do not always recognise when they are hungry or thirsty, therefore always offer food and drink. However, keep choices limited so that it is easier for the person to make a decision.
- Manual handling – do not rush, but make sure that the person is listening to what is being said and understands what is going to happen. Reduce clutter, make sure that the environment is safe, e.g., no extension cables lying on the floor, and use the equipment that is available.
- Personal hygiene – develop a routine for both morning and evening (this provides familiarity and reduces stress), use the aids available, e.g., perching stool, and if these are not available consider requesting an occupational therapy assessment. If the person does not want a wash, do not argue, leave them, wait a while and then try again later.

Supporting effective communication and providing practical support for carers has the potential to support them to carry out their caring role. Assistive technology can also be used to support people living with dementia to maintain their independence and self-manage their condition.

Assistive technology

Assistive technology refers to equipment that may increase the range of activities and the independence and well-being of people living with a disability, either physical or cognitive; this includes adaptive aids and environmental modifications (Royal Commission on Long Term Care, 1999). Assistive technology can be used to support a range of LTCs, equipping people with the resources and information they need to self-manage. For a person living with dementia, it is important to keep the technology simple and appropriate to a person's level of need. For a person with dementia, this might focus on technologies to assist them to move around their own environment. For example, a picture of a bed on the bedroom door, a wardrobe with clear doors or a notice saying 'tea and coffee' on a kitchen cupboard can assist a person with dementia to be more independent in their activities of daily living. Using memory aids such as calendars, diaries and a schedule of their daily routine can all contribute to improving a person's independence. Large-faced clocks or clocks that say 'It's Friday afternoon' rather than the time allow the person to intuitively understand where they are (Gibson et al., 2014). Medication dispensers can be connected to a telecare system that alarms and unlocks automatically when medication is to be taken; they can also alert carers or the telehealth operator when a dose is missed. This technology does rely on the person being able to recognise what the alarm means and take their medication. Therefore, ongoing and regular review of the person's ability to use this technology should be carried out.

Telecare is the delivery of care to people living in their own home via computers and telecommunications systems (Gibson et al., 2014). It involves a range of services including household safety, such as carbon monoxide detectors, fire or smoke detectors and flood detectors. Telecare also includes services to ensure personal safety such as fall detectors and bed or chair occupancy sensors. Fall detectors can sense a serious fall and will raise the alarm at the monitoring centre; the monitoring centre will then contact the registered emergency contact number, ensuring that the incident is responded to. Bed or chair occupancy sensors can be used at night; they can be programmed to switch on lights, minimising the risk of falls, an important aspect to consider if the person is known to experience nocturnal wandering. Many of the devices do not require the person with dementia to remember where they are or how to use them. It should be remembered, though, that devices, such as the fall detector, rely on the person putting them on every day; this may not be suitable for people living on their own. It is clear that assistive technology has a role to play in promoting the independence of people living with dementia; however, it should be used alongside other forms of care, such as a day hospital and support groups, and not as a substitute for these.

Mobile technologies, such as MP3 players, can also be used as assistive technology. It is known that music has a positive effect on the general function of people living with dementia and, perhaps most importantly for carers of people with dementia, it has been shown to reduce agitation, wandering and irritability (Janata, 2012). Research carried out by Lewis et al. (2015) investigating the impact on carers of MP3 player use by people living with dementia found that the MP3 players were used throughout the day and night, with the average length of time that the MP3 player was listened to being one hour. During this time carers reported that they were able to catch up on household chores or spend some time relaxing. Participants overwhelmingly commented on the positive effect that listening to music had on the person living with dementia, with this having a knock-on effect on their own personal health and well-being.

Using the above strategies relating to communication, assistive technology and supporting carers has the potential to allow the person living with dementia to stay in their own home for as long as possible and live as independently and as 'well' as possible.

Activity 4.5   Reflection

Using a model of reflection, such as the one by Driscoll (1994), consider the following questions.

- What? – reflect back on a situation when you have cared for a person with dementia and identify aspects of self-management and 'living well'.
- So what? – reflect on your feelings at the time and how you feel about the situation now; consider the positives and negatives of the

situation and whether any of the strategies discussed in this chapter were used; consider how your experiences compared to those of your colleagues.

- Now what? – take the time to think about what you might do differently/ the same if faced with the same situation; would you use any of the strategies discussed in this chapter? If so, why and how, and where could you access further information in the future?

Using a model of reflection will assist you to structure your reflection, ensuring that you stay focused on a specific topic. Using the questions listed will further increase your level of analysis of the situation, developing your ability to critically analyse your practice and the practice of colleagues.

As the answers will be based on your own observations and discussions, there is no outline answer at the end of the chapter.

Chapter summary

This chapter has provided you with an overview of the role of self-management in the care and management of people living with an LTC, a key element of recent health policy. It has outlined the difference between self-care and self-management, and has discussed the key components of self-management. There has been a clear focus on the person with the LTC and supporting them to develop their skills in relation to self-management. Specific ways in which to do this have been discussed and applied to your clinical practice. The importance of self-management in dementia has also been discussed, with some specific areas of good practice being identified.

Having read through this chapter and undertaken the activities, you will have developed your knowledge and skills about the role of self-management in LTCs and how you can support individuals to take a more active role in managing their LTC. As a nurse, you can improve a person's self-management by developing the skills required to become an effective self-manager. You can utilise goal setting, action planning and problem-solving to enable a person with an LTC to regain control of their condition and their life. By having an increased awareness of some of the strategies available to support self-management, you will provide holistic care for those living with an LTC. Self-management is not about the person living with the LTC managing their care in isolation. It is about the person living with the LTC working with members of the healthcare team, accessing relevant information and education, and then using that information to manage their condition in the way that best suits their life.

Activities: brief outline answers

Activity 4.2 Critical thinking (page 77)

Mastery experiences: you could discuss with Linda the successful changes she made in relation to taking exercise, asking reflective questions such as 'What was it that prompted you to join the cardiac walking group?', 'What made you successful in doing this?' and 'How did it make you feel?'. This approach will encourage Linda to reflect on her successes, support her to develop problem-solving skills and consider ways in which she can return to her previous activity.

Social modelling: given Linda's anxiety, it might not be appropriate to signpost her to another peer support group; encouraging her instead to rejoin her walking group where she knows the other participants may be more suitable. If she is not ready to do this, then you could arrange for peer support at home either face-to-face or via the telephone. In addition, depending on Linda's IT skills, it may be possible to introduce social support via a digital resource.

Social persuasion: this aspect of self-efficacy links in with mastery experience; providing Linda with positive feedback on her previous achievements, particularly in relation to increasing her level of activity, may encourage her to continue with self-managing her condition.

Psychological responses: acknowledging Linda's anxiety about leaving the house and how it manifests itself physically and psychologically, will encourage you to provide guidance on how this can be managed – for example, relaxation techniques, ensuring that she has her GTN spray with her and having a clear plan of what to do if she experiences chest pain. Emphasising the benefits of exercise both physically and psychologically may also improve Linda's self-efficacy.

Activity 4.3 Critical thinking (page 79)

Oskar is at stage 1 of the Patient Activation Measure; he does not feel that he has to make any changes to his behaviour to manage his hypertension. At the moment, he views his condition as being treated by his medication and is not something to worry about until he is older. When meeting with Oskar, you could use some of the PAM statements as reflective questions to encourage him to think about how he manages his health. It may be that you are not able to increase Oskar's activation in a single meeting, but that you have to use a framework such as Making Every Contact Count (see Chapter 3 for further information) and discuss Oskar's health with him over a period of time.

Activity 4.4 Critical thinking (page 80)

Given Frazer's previous lack of involvement in his care, you may choose to focus on developing his level of self-efficacy. Developing a plan of care with Frazer that he would then 'own' could support him to realise that he is able to make positive changes. As one of your aims is to affect behaviour change, which has not always been successful in the past, you may decide that motivational interviewing (see Chapter 3) and goal setting would be appropriate strategies to use. Goals should be set in partnership with Frazer and should be SMART: specific, measureable, achieveable, realistic and timely. For further information on goal setting, see the article by Furze (2015) in the further reading section at the end of the chapter.

Activity 4.6 Critical thinking (page 83)

Action plan
Goal: to go outside in to the garden every day
Aim: to be able to feel confident about going outside.   Each day I will do the following.   • *Remember to keep my GTN spray with me at all times.*

- *Go outside into the garden every day.*
- *Carry out the relaxed breathing before I go outside.*

Every day I will keep a diary and will include the following.

- *How comfortable I felt before carrying out the relaxed breathing and going outside, scored out of 10. How I felt when I was outside and how comfortable I felt after being outside, scored out of 10. How intense the craving for a cigarette was, what I was doing, how I was feeling, whether I had a cigarette and, if so, how I felt after I had smoked; if not, how I felt after the craving had passed.*

Befire going outside I will carry out the following relaxed breathing for 3–5 minutes.

- *Sit in a comfortable chair in a relaxed position with my head and arms supported.*
- *Breathe in deeply, filling my lungs from the bottom as if I am filling a bottle.*
- *Breathe in through my nose and out through my mouth.*
- *Breathe out slowly, counting from 1 to 5.*
- *Keep doing this until I feel calm, breathing without holding my breath or stopping.*

What to do if anything changes: *N/A*

How confident am I that I will achieve this? *7 out of 10.*

Day of the week	Achieved	Any comments
Monday		
Tuesday		
Wednesday		
Thursday		
Friday		
Saturday		
Sunday		

Further reading

Chesterman, D and Bray, M (2018) Report on some action research in the implementation of social prescribing in Crawley. Paths to greater well-being: 'sometimes you have to be in it to get it'. *Action Learning: Research and Practice*, 15(2): 168–81.

This article explores the benefits of social prescribing to promote health and well-being.

Furze, G (2015) Goal setting: a key skill for person-centred care. *Practice Nursing*, 26(5): 241–4.

This article provides practical advice about goal setting, which you can use when supporting people living with LTCs with action planning.

Hibbard, JH (2017) Patient activation and the use of information to support informed health decisions. *Patient Education and Counseling*, 100(1): 5–7.

This article outlines how PAM can be used to provide tailored support to people living with LTCs.

Toms, GR, Quinn, C, Anderson, DE and Clare, L (2015) Help yourself: perspectives on self-management from people with dementia and their caregivers. *Qualitative Health Research,* 25(1): 87–98.

This article discusses the findings of a study exploring the views of people living with dementia, and their family, on self-management.

Useful websites

www.selfmanagementuk.org

The home page for the EPP and other resources relating to self-management.

www.nhs.uk/IPG/Pages/AboutThisService.aspx

Information prescription service: this is the home page, with external links, that allows you to create information prescriptions about a range of LTCs that include local support and services.

www.nhs.uk/Planners/Yourhealth/Pages/Yourhealth.aspx

The home page for Your Health, Your Way, providing lots of relevant information in relation to courses and support, healthy living, etc., in relation to LTCs.

www.scie.org.uk/publications/dementia/about.asp

This website focuses on information to support people living with dementia to maintain their independence.

Chapter 5 Quality of life and symptom management in long term conditions

(Continued)

Annexe B:

Nursing procedures

Use evidence based, best practice approaches to take a history, observe, recognise and accurately assess people of all ages:

10 Use evidence based, best practice approaches for meeting needs for care and support at the end of life, accurately assessing the person's capacity for independence and self-care and initiating appropriate interventions

   10.1 observe, and assess the need for intervention for people, families and carers, identify, assess and respond appropriately to uncontrolled symptoms and signs of distress including pain, nausea, thirst, constipation, restlessness, agitation, anxiety and depression

   10.2 manage and monitor effectiveness of symptom relief medication, infusion pumps and other devices

   10.3 assess and review preferences and care priorities of the dying person and their family and carers

   10.5 understand and apply DNACPR (do not attempt cardiopulmonary resuscitation) decisions and verification of expected death

11 Procedural competencies required for best practice, evidence based medicines administration and optimisation

   11.1 carry out initial and continued assessments of people receiving care and their ability to self-administer their own medications

   11.2 recognise the various procedural routes under which medicines can be prescribed, supplied, dispensed and administered; and the laws, policies, regulations and guidance that underpin them

   11.3 use the principles of safe remote prescribing and directions to administer medicines

Chapter aims

After reading this chapter, you will be able to:

* explain what quality of life (QoL) is and its importance in the care and management of LTCs;
* recognise the importance of medicines management in supporting people living with LTCs to manage symptoms effectively;
* recognise the role that care planning has in effective symptom management.

Introduction

Chronic illnesses come with symptoms. These symptoms are signals from the body that something unusual is happening. They cannot be seen by others, are often difficult to describe to others, and are usually unpredictable.

(Lorig et al., 2006, p39)

Many symptoms of LTCs can be managed and minimised by person-centred health promotion and health education and by effective self-management. However, for some people living with an LTC their disease progression is marked out by changing, and often worsening, signs and symptoms. A sign is something that is noticed by other people and is generally objective and can be seen, heard, felt or measured. This could be pyrexia, high blood pressure or an increased BMI, or, for example, a daughter may notice her mother having increased lower leg swelling as a sign of worsening heart failure. A symptom is experienced by the person with the LTC, is generally subjective and cannot always be measured, seen, heard or felt. This may be pain, nausea or hunger. An example could be a person living with eczema experiencing a severe itch, though on observation there may be no noticeable cause of the itch. A feature of an LTC may be both a sign and a symptom – e.g., increased pain in a venous leg ulcer is a symptom for the person with the leg ulcer, but is a sign to the nurse that infection is present. The ability of a person living with an LTC to recognise relevant signs and symptoms, and to effectively manage these improves their health outcome and quality of life, and is one of the key aspects in the promotion of self-management in LTCs.

Activity 5.1   Evidence-based practice and research

Research the following LTCs: cardiovascular disease (CVD), depression and type 2 diabetes, and write down your answers to the following questions.

- What are the main signs and symptoms of these LTCs?
- Why do these signs and symptoms occur?
- Briefly describe how these signs and symptoms can be managed.

Some useful resources:

- your preferred applied anatomy and physiology text books;
- Clinical Knowledge Summaries from NICE – available at: **https://cks. nice.org.uk/#?char=A** – a useful website for healthcare professionals providing evidence-based information on managing common conditions seen in primary care.

A brief outline answer is given at the end of the chapter.

As you can see from Activity 5.1, there are many signs and symptoms that require effective management when caring for people living with an LTC. Many people will experience more than one symptom, and will be taking medication and using other therapeutic interventions to manage these. Previous chapters in this book have recognised the importance of engaging in a therapeutic relationship, the role of effective health promotion, and the importance of self-management in the care and management of LTCs. If someone with COPD smokes, health promotion will play a part in supporting them to change their health behaviour. Working with someone living with type 2 diabetes and helping them to formulate an action plan to change their diet will enable them to self-manage their condition. Through supporting the development of your knowledge, skills and attributes in relation to quality of life and symptom management, this chapter will help you to improve the quality of life of people living with an LTC. Using the nursing process and the principles of care planning, pain management and anxiety will be discussed; having an understanding of these principles will enable you to use this process to address other symptoms.

Quality of life in LTCs

Quality of Life (QoL) is a term that is used often in healthcare, where the aim of care is to 'improve', 'promote' or 'maintain' a person's QoL. However, it is a term that can be difficult to quantify, as it can mean different things to different people and can be assessed against many things – for example, QoL in relation to health and QoL in relation to employment opportunities. These factors are broad-ranging and can be related back to the determinants of health (Chapter 3). The World Health Organization provides a holistic definition of QoL which focuses on how a person sees their place in life in relation to the culture and value system they live in, and their goals, expectations, standards and concerns (WHO, 1997). Many factors can influence and affect your QoL, such as health – both physical and psychological – relationships and opportunities. Over your lifetime, it is likely that some of the factors influencing and affecting your QoL will change. It is this subjective aspect of QoL that makes it challenging to measure and quantify. However, it is also likely that there are some key factors that are important to your QoL, whatever your age and/or stage of life.

To assist you in your care of people living with an LTC, it is helpful to understand how QoL can be measured. Many QoL assessment scales are available: some focus on specific LTCs (e.g., post-myocardial infarction and mental health), while others are generic and can be used across a range of LTCs. Generic scales are useful as they allow you to undertake an initial assessment of a person's QoL, which may or may not result in referrals being made to other members of the healthcare team. Understanding the impact of an LTC on a person's QoL will enable you to work with them to put in place a plan of care that will maintain QoL as their condition progresses.

Activity 5.2   Critical thinking

Select one of the LTC's from Activity 5.1, or a condition that a patient you have cared for is living with, and do a library search to see if there are any Quality of Life measurement scales specific to those conditions.

- What areas of an individual's life do they attempt to measure?
- What questions within the scales are particularly important to that specific LTC?
- How can you use these scales within your assessment and care of people with that LTC?

Discuss your findings with a colleague or your mentor to see how it may enhance your own assessment and care of someone with an LTC.

As this activity is based on your own choice of LTC, there is no outline answer at the end of the chapter.

Symptom management in LTCs

Activity 5.1 has shown you that people living with an LTC will experience many symptoms depending on the LTC they are living with. Effective symptom management requires an appropriate person-centred plan of care to be in place that addresses these symptoms. There are many ways that you can put together a plan of care for a person – e.g., an action plan. Traditional care plans may be either pre-printed or handwritten, core or individualised and may include care pathways. Working in collaboration with the person allows a personalised care plan to be drawn up. This has the benefit of ensuring that the care and management planned clearly meets their individual needs. Rather than achieving a 'best fit' for the person and their needs you achieve a 'perfect fit'. As they are time-consuming to write, however, a compromise may be to use core care plans that are personalised to the individual person and their needs (Barrett et al., 2009).

Personalised care planning and symptom management in LTCs

People who are living with an LTC play an important role in the management of their own heath. This management involves a complex set of skills that require confidence and knowledge. It can involve managing medication, monitoring of own health, making lifestyle changes and developing coping strategies. Personalised care planning is an approach in which healthcare professionals work with the person to provide support to identify their own needs and set their own goals (Coulter et al., 2015). A Cochrane

Systematic review found that this approach could lead to some improvements in disease management, and support individuals to develop the skills and confidence required to manage their LTC. The review also demonstrated lower levels of depression for those involved in their own care in this way (Coulter et al., 2015).

As a nurse involved in the care and management of people living with an LTC, using a scheme of care planning that incorporates the nursing process will enable you to work with the person, their family and carers to successfully manage their symptoms. The nursing process is the means by which you implement your model. Over the years, this process has been adapted and refined: Barrett et al. (2009) developed the nursing process to aid problem solving:

- assess;
- systematic nursing diagnosis;
- plan;
- implement;
- recheck;
- evaluate.

This six-step process can be remembered by the acronym ASPIRE. When using the nursing process, it is important to remember that all steps are interrelated. A plan cannot be made unless an assessment has taken place and a systematic nursing diagnosis has been made; care cannot be evaluated unless a plan has been implemented and rechecked. For the nursing process to be used effectively, you must possess effective communication skills, have developed a positive therapeutic relationship, have a sound knowledge of the LTC the person is living with, and how the symptoms of this can be managed. Used efficiently and in partnership with the person living with an LTC, good care planning can ensure holistic symptom management.

Medicines management

Symptoms of LTCs require comprehensive assessment and treatment to enable people to manage them. A holistic approach that encompasses biopsychosocial interventions can enhance quality of life and well-being. The most common intervention for patients to manage medical conditions is medicines (Royal Pharmaceutical Society, 2016). People living with LTCs are taking an increasing number of medicines, with **polypharmacy** becoming the norm for those with multi-morbidities. As mentioned in Chapter 1, many people living with LTCs live with one or more – e.g., diabetes and coronary heart disease. Polypharmacy is when an individual is prescribed multiple medicines to be taken at the same time, which can create additional risk for patients (NICE, 2018). Polypharmacy can be both appropriate and problematic; appropriate polypharmacy is when the patient's experience is understood and that medicine use is as safe as possible, taking into consideration best evidence (Kaufman, 2014). However, problematic polypharmacy is when medications are prescribed inappropriately, increasing the risks of medicines interacting with each other and causing harm, or an unacceptable 'pill burden' for the person, resulting in poor adherence or increased prescribing to counteract side-effects of existing medicines (NICE, 2018).

Medicines optimisation is a person-centered approach to safe and effective use of medicines to help people get the best from their prescriptions (NICE, 2015c). This approach supports shared decision-making with the person. As a nurse, it is important to understand what the person understands about their medicines: Do they know what they are taking? What it is for? How to take it? How long to take it for? It is about ensuring that medication decisions are based on the best evidence base and are also a cost-effective solution. It is known that between 30 and 50 per cent of people living with an LTC do not take their medication as prescribed (NICE, 2009b). When patients do not take their medicine correctly, the consequences can include ill health, poorer life expectancy, longer recovery times and poor quality of life. There is also an economic impact of wasted medicines and increased hospital admissions. To support medicines optimisation, it is important that you understand how people living with LTCs view their medication and what might result in non-adherence to their medication regime. For young people living with an LTC, it might be that they are in denial about their diagnosis or that they feel stigmatised. People who have been on a medication for a long time and who are now asymptomatic may decide that their medication is now unnecessary and stop taking it. Older people, or those with an LTC that affects manual dexterity, may find that they are not able to open the packaging. People with cognitive decline may forget to take their medication.

The acronym AIDES (Bergman-Evans, 2006) can help you to work with patients to support the correct and safe use of their medicines. The following table lists the questions to be considered in helping older adults to manage their medicines.

	Questions to consider
A: Assessment	Does the person have cognitive ability to manage medicines?
	Review all medicines, including any over-the-counter or alternative remedies.
	Can the person self-administer their medicines?
I: Individualised	Does the medicine regime fit with the person's lifestyle?
	Does the person understand which medicines are for which symptom?
D: Documentation	Ensure accurate records of a full medication list are completed in patients' notes.
	Ensure the patient has an up-to-date list, in a format they understand. Consider using IT to support hand-held information.
E: Education	What does the patient already know about their medicines?
	What else do they need to know?
	Do they know how the medicine will treat their symptoms?
	How will you give them the information?

(Continued)

Table 5.1 (Continued)

	Questions to consider
S: Supervision	When will the medicines next be reviewed?
	Does the patient need a follow-up appointment with their GP?
	Do they attend annual medicines reviews?
	Does their pharmacy offer a review service?
	Do they know what to do next?

Table 5.1 Questions used in the AIDES model to improve medication adherence in older adults (Berman-Evans, 2006)

The NMC *Future Nurse: Standards for Proficiency for Registered Nurses* (2018) details the breadth of skills and competence that you require at point of registration with regard to medicines management (see the start of the chapter). These responsibilities go beyond safe administration, and incorporate the assessment and diagnosis of symptoms, the ability to effectively monitor the efficacy of medicines given and assess the ability of those in your care to manage their own medicines. You also need to demonstrate an understanding of the professional, legal and ethical frameworks that guide the supply, dispensing, prescribing and administration of medicines. Some useful websites are listed at the end of this chapter to help your journey to proficiency.

Activity 5.3 Decision-making

The community matron is undertaking an annual medicines review in Sunnydale care home for all the residents. Since her last visit there is a new resident, Mary, who is 91 years old. Mary takes a lot of daily medication and tells you that she does not know what they are all for, since her last few hospital admissions, she is on much more. Her current list of medication is in the table below.

Medication	What it is for?	Instructions	Possible side effects
Co-codamol 30/500mg	*Pain*	*4 x daily, ensure 4–6 hours between doses*	*Constipation, confusion, drowsiness, dizziness*
Furosemide 40mg			
Clopidogrel 75mg			
Alendronic Acid 10mg			
Mirtazapine 30mg			
Senna 15mg			
Atorvastatin 20mg			
Aspirin 75mg			

- Using the latest BNF and relevant NICE guidelines, complete the table to support the care home staff to help Mary with her medication.
- Consider what information may help Mary understand her medications and support their proper use.
- What are the polypharmacy issues relating to Mary's medication?

A brief outline answer is given at the end of the chapter.

As you will see from Activity 5.3, older people are susceptible to the risks of polypharmacy. Medication has an important role to play in the management of symptoms for LTCs, but how you communicate about the type of medication, how it should be taken and how to recognise potential side effects will have a significant impact on how the person living with an LTC will be able to use it effectively.

The management of pain in LTCs

Activity 5.4   Critical thinking

According to the International Association for the Study of Pain (1986), pain is *an unpleasant sensory and emotional experience associated with actual or potential tissue damage.* The perception of pain evolved in humans to warn us of danger so that we can take action to avoid damage. For example, we withdraw our hand from a flame to avoid getting burnt. However, for people with an LTC, it is not possible to withdraw from the pain, as the pain may be caused by the condition. To help you to provide effective pain management to people with LTCs, it is important to have an understanding of the mechanisms of how we feel pain and the different types of pain. To support you to do this, answer the following questions.

- How do we feel pain?
- What is the difference between nociceptive and neuropathic pain?
- What are the body's natural analgesics?

A brief outline answer is given at the end of the chapter.

As you can see from Activity 5.4, there are differences in the way that pain is experienced, whether it is acute and chronic, and in how the pain is transmitted via the nervous system. It is therefore important to know if the person is experiencing acute or

chronic pain, and whether it is nociceptive or neuropathic, as this will influence how
you manage their pain. However, it should be noted that pain is not purely a series of
physiological processes.

Pain is what the patient says it is. (Thomas, 2003, p124)

Pain is experienced by people and families – not nerve endings. (Dame Cicely Saunders)

Pain is a common symptom for people living with an LTC; for many people, it is their
major concern and for many their pain will be chronic. The Chronic Pain Policy
Coalition aims to develop an improved strategy to prevent, treat and manage chronic
pain. They recognise chronic pain as an LTC and that the care and management of
chronic pain could be improved. A report published in 2011 identified that:

- clear standards should be agreed for the identification, assessment and initial
  management of chronic pain;
- a campaign should be organised to increase understanding in health and social care
  professionals about the impact of chronic pain and how to prevent and treat it;
- nationally agreed commissioning guidance should be developed that describes best
  care;
- an epidemiology of chronic pain working group should be set up to gather data
  and monitor chronic pain.

Pain has many causes and means different things to different people: it changes during the course of an LTC, and its treatment and management vary from person to
person (Endacott et al., 2009). This highlights the individual nature of pain. In the
1960s, as a result of her research with terminally ill people, Dame Cicely Saunders
developed the concept of 'total pain'. Total pain incorporates the physical, social,
spiritual and psychological aspects of a person; these aspects then interact to produce
a person's individual pain experience (Clark, 2002). Table 5.2 outlines some of the
factors that can influence a person's total pain as applied to the case study Mary (see
Activity 5.3).

Aspects	Influencing factors	Application to practice
Physical	The condition The person's functional capacity Side effects of treatment Disfigurement	Mary's pressure sore on her hip cause her pain and discomfort; pain has reduced her ability to mobilise – she uses both a zimmer frame and a wheelchair.
Social	Family issues Loss of role at work Loss of role at home Finances Change in appearance due to condition Sense of helplessness	Mary has had to move into a nursing home for care, which has reduced her ability to see family and friends. She is now reliant on people visiting her. The nursing home fees will have a significant impact on her savings, which she was hoping would provide ongoing security for her daughters.

Aspects	Influencing factors	Application to practice
Spiritual	Purpose Religion Meaning Uncertainty about future Hope Fear of pain/death	Mary is facing a different future now that she is living in a nursing home and being dependent on others to meet her needs. She is a member of the local Roman Catholic church and hopes to be able to stay in contact with others in the community. Mary is particular about her appearance and clothes, and enjoys wearing a little make-up. She hopes that this will continue in the care home.
Psychological	Anger Delays in diagnosis Coping ability Control and sense of usefulness Failure of treatment	The transition to dependence on others may cause Mary some anxiety. She has been on an antidepressant medication for a long time, but does not describe herself as feeling depressed. She will be taking on a different role within her family.

Table 5.2   Total pain: aspects, influencing factors and application to practice

This personal construct of pain means that pain is subjective, making an unbiased objective assessment of it complex and challenging. You must remain objective at all times, and recognise how your perceptions and the individuality of the person can impact on pain perception. If you use the nursing process to structure your care and management of a person's pain, then undertaking a comprehensive assessment of a person and their pain is the first step to successful management.

Assessing pain in long term conditions

Case study: Anisa

Anisa was diagnosed with relapsing remitting multiple sclerosis 11 years ago. She is married to Kaldeep and has a young son, Aroon. Over the past 11 years Anisa has experienced several relapses of her MS, with two affecting her right leg. Anisa's last relapse eight weeks ago has left her with residual spasms in her leg, causing musculoskeletal pain and discomfort. Anisa now works part-time as a teaching assistant; Kaldeep works full-time as a software engineer; recent promotion has meant that he is away from home more than previously.

Since her last remission eight weeks ago, Anisa is still off work. You are spending time with the MS clinical nurse specialist (CNS) who is visiting her. During this consultation, Anisa mentions her residual spasms and musculoskeletal pain. Her pain is due to muscle spasm, caused by increased muscle tone due to nerve damage. This causes the stretch muscles in her lower leg to become hyperactive. Her spasms and associated musculoskeletal pain are worse at night.

Activity 5.5   Evidence-based practice and research

Reflecting on the concept of 'total pain', answer the following questions.

- What could be contributing to Anisa's pain in the case study above?
- What methods could you and the CNS use to assess Anisa's total pain?

A brief outline answer is given at the end of the chapter.

Activity 5.5 has demonstrated that there are many ways in which a person's pain can be assessed. It may be that you may have to try more than one method of assessment until you find one that is suitable. Consistency of pain assessment is important to enable a clear picture of a person's pain to be obtained. Therefore, it is important that the same method of pain assessment is used each time that a person's pain is assessed. In Anisa's case, you could ask her to keep a pain diary. Including Anisa's own assessment of her pain alongside your assessment will enhance the overall picture you obtain. For some people – e.g., those with cognitive impairment or a learning disability – ensuring effective pain assessment can be challenging and may result in pain being undiagnosed or undertreated.

Pain assessment in cognitive impairment

Undiagnosed or undertreated pain in people with cognitive impairment may be due to a variety of reasons. In Alzheimer's disease, for example, many of the areas of the brain that are affected – the hippocampus and the prefrontal cortex – are also involved in processing pain (Porth and Matfin, 2014). People with cognitive impairment may under-report their pain; they may not understand the questions being asked; in addition, due to lack or loss of communication skills, their ability to verbalise that they are in pain may be reduced (Achterberg et al., 2013). However, people with cognitive impairment can experience the same physical health conditions as those without cognitive impairment (e.g., diabetes, COPD, musculoskeletal problems), and therefore it is likely that they experience similar amounts of pain as people without cognitive impairment.

Many pain-assessment tools require the person to verbalise their pain, which people with a cognitive impairment find difficult. Therefore, as well as using picture scale tools, using specific pain-assessment tools for people with cognitive impairment is important.

- Abbey pain scale – this is an assessment tool for use with people who have dementia and are not able to verbalise. Assessment is undertaken by observing the person and reporting on a variety of indicators. These include behaviour changes – e.g., increasing confusion; facial expressions – e.g., looking frightened; and physical changes – e.g., contractures.

- Pain assessment in advanced dementia (PAINAD) – an observational tool that looks at the person's breathing, vocalising, facial expression, body language and how consolable they are.
- The disability distress assessment tool – this is used to help identify distress cues in people with cognitive impairment or limited communication. It describes the person's normal behaviour – for example, what vocal sounds they make when they are content and what sounds they make when they are distressed. A note is then made of what situations are known to cause the person distress. Once completed, this assessment tool can be used to identify times when a person is distressed. While this tool identifies distress, it can be a useful indicator of pain.

Working with the person's carer, especially to find out what the person's normal behaviour is, will enhance any pain assessment carried out. This section reiterates that it is the process of assessment and the knowledge and skills you use, and not just the assessment tool being used, that is important (Endacott et al., 2009).

Having used a holistic approach to assessing Anisa's pain, alongside an appropriate pain-assessment tool, you are now able to work with Anisa to plan and implement an effective plan of care.

Planning and implementing pain management in LTCs

Recognising the concept of 'total pain' and the factors that influence a person's pain, it is important to realise that there are many methods that can be implemented to manage pain in LTCs. These range from medication, both prescribed and over-the-counter, the use of physiotherapy and psychological care. The methods used will differ depending on the person and the type of pain being experienced. In the case of musculoskeletal pain, the management may focus on physiotherapy, relaxation and medication. The management of neuropathic pain may consist of physiotherapy, advice regarding posture and positioning, the use of antidepressant and anticonvulsant medication, and relaxation (Taverner, 2014). It may not be possible to achieve complete pain relief for everyone; if this is the case, the aim will be to reduce the pain to a level that is tolerable for the person.

Case study: Anisa

Anisa's pain assessment revealed that she was experiencing musculoskeletal pain, radiating down her right calf and into her foot, on six nights out of seven and occasionally during the day on four out of seven days. Anisa scored her pain as being

(Continued)

(Continued)

seven out of ten and described it as 'aching'; she was aware that this was disturbing her usual sleep pattern and was concerned that it would increase her fatigue. The aim of the plan of care agreed between Anisa and her MS CNS was to reduce both the frequency (to three out of seven nights and two out of seven days) and intensity (to four) of Anisa's pain, as well as to improve the quality of her sleep. Following consultation, they agreed a plan of care, as follows.

Physiotherapy

The MS CNS will refer Anisa to the community physiotherapist for an assessment and a planned programme of stretching exercises to help lengthen Anisa's calf muscles to reduce spasm and spasticity. Physiotherapy has been shown to improve mobility in people with MS; focusing on quality of life and not just pain is known to have a positive effect (Lalkhen et al., 2012). These exercises will need to be carried out on a daily basis and Anisa has agreed to write up an action plan (see Chapter 4) to ensure that she is able to do this. The MS CNS has also asked that the physiotherapist considers using transcutaneous electrical nerve stimulation (TENS) as a non-pharmacological means of managing Anisa's pain. The evidence surrounding TENS is varied; however, it is used in the management of pain in a variety of situations. TENS stimulates the nervous system through the use of transcutaneous electrodes; this stimulation is thought to reduce the transmission of pain signals to the brain, altering the person's perception of their pain.

Relaxation

The CNS has suggested that Anisa should try relaxation as part of her ongoing pain management. Anisa might find this particularly useful at night to improve the quality of her sleep. A simple technique that Anisa could use would be relaxed breathing; focusing on her breathing has the potential to break the cycle of pain and anxiety by providing the mind with something else to focus on.

Prescribed medication

As a qualified nurse/independent prescriber, Anisa's MS CNS is able to prescribe any licensed medication, within the sphere of her clinical competence (RCN, 2014). Based on her assessment of Anisa and her pain, she has prescribed an initial dose of Baclofen: 5mg, three times a day. This can be gradually increased, depending on the degree of relief that Anisa is experiencing. By reducing the transmission of electrical impulses along the nerves in Anisa's central nervous system, Baclofen will cause her muscles to relax, reducing the amount of spasm and pain. As well as outlining to Anisa how Baclofen works, the MS CNS has provided her with information regarding some of the common side effects:

- gastrointestinal upset: Anisa has been advised to take her Baclofen after eating food and in case of nausea to eat little and often;
- dry mouth: chewing sugar-free gum or sweets can help reduce Anisa's dry mouth;
- drowsiness: before driving, Anisa should make sure that her reaction time is normal; alcohol should be avoided as it may increase her drowsiness;
- dizziness: getting up from either lying or sitting slowly; if the feeling continues, Anisa could lie down for a few minutes until the dizziness passes.

The MS CNS also advised Anisa that if she is concerned regarding any aspect of this medication, she should contact her and not stop taking it suddenly, as sudden withdrawal can cause severe side effects. The MS CNS will visit Anisa weekly over the next six weeks to review the benefits of the treatment.

Over-the-counter medication

As well as taking her prescribed medication, Anisa may also be taking over-the-counter medication to help manage her pain – e.g., paracetamol or ibuprofen. If this is the case, it is important that the MS CNS identifies this, as it is known that ibuprofen reduces the rate at which Baclofen is excreted from the body, resulting in an increased risk of toxicity. Therefore, Anisa should be advised to use paracetamol in preference to ibuprofen.

Both Anisa and the MS CNS agreed that Angela should continue to assess her musculoskeletal pain on a regular basis and devise her own action plan (Chapter 4) to identify when and how this will be done. The effectiveness of the above plan of care will be rechecked against Anisa's initial pain assessment and her ongoing assessment of her musculoskeletal pain. This recheck will allow specific information, such as Anisa's assessment of her pain, to be linked to the plan of care that was implemented. In the initial stages, this recheck will be done on a weekly basis for the next four weeks, providing ongoing support for Anisa. A formal evaluation will take place at the end of four weeks.

It was decided not to refer Anisa to an occupational therapist for splinting at this stage, but to evaluate the above plan of care and refer if there is no improvement in Anisa's spasm and pain.

As you can see, Anisa and her MS CNS worked collaboratively to compile the above plan of care. Empowerment was maintained by incorporating action planning, enabling Anisa to fit her physiotherapy and pain assessment into her daily routine. Recognising the potential benefits of relaxation as a strategy Anisa could use in a variety of situations will positively reflect on her QoL. The role of the MS CNS was to provide specialist knowledge regarding the pharmacological management of Anisa's spasms and associated musculoskeletal pain, and to refer to other members of the multidisciplinary team to maximise Anisa's pain relief.

Evaluating pain management in LTCs

Evaluating the care implemented is the final stage of well-organised nursing care: the process of evaluation allows you to understand whether the care implemented has been successful in meeting the person's identified needs. Evaluating the care implemented requires a collaborative approach and should be based on how well the aims of the care have been met. Evaluating care requires you to be able to analyse all stages of the planning and implementation processes – e.g., was the pain assessment tool used appropriate, was the stated aim achievable and were the planned interventions suitable for the person and their needs (Barrett et al., 2009). By breaking the process down into its component parts, you are able to evaluate which parts were successful and which parts were not. Evaluating your care and management in this way allows you to reflect on your practice, prompting both personal and professional development.

Case study: Anisa

Four weeks after your initial visit to Anisa with her MS CNS, both you and the MS CNS are visiting her to evaluate the plan of care that was implemented. Anisa has continued to assess her pain as outlined in her action plan; she is now experiencing pain on four nights out of seven and on two days out of seven, with her pain intensity having reduced to between three and four. She also reports that while she is still experiencing pain on four nights out of seven, the quality of her sleep has improved.

Physiotherapy

Anisa has found the physiotherapy to be very beneficial and has worked hard to ensure that she carries out her exercises every day. As well as exercising her right leg, she has been doing the same exercises with her left leg and has noticed a reduction in the severity of the muscle spasms. Anisa feels this has contributed the most in reducing her musculoskeletal pain. She has not had any TENS yet, though the physiotherapist has recommended this.

Relaxation

Anisa finds this beneficial, especially in managing her levels of stress and improving the quality of her sleep. Despite being awake due to her pain, she is able to remain calm and relaxed, increasing the chances of her being able to get back to sleep.

Prescribed medication

Anisa continues to take 5mg of Baclofen three times a day; she experienced some side effects when she initially started taking the Baclofen – mainly nausea and some dizziness. However, she is able to manage these. Despite still experiencing pain on four out of seven nights, she is not keen to increase her dose of Baclofen yet.

Over-the-counter medication

Anisa has not been taking any regular over-the-counter analgesics.

Following the evaluation of the care implemented against the original aims of the care, both Anisa and her MS CNS note that while the severity of Anisa's pain has reduced and the quality of her sleep has improved, she is still experiencing pain on four nights out of seven. As Anisa is not keen to increase the dose of Baclofen, her MS CNS suggests that she asks her physiotherapist about using TENS at night. Anisa agrees to this suggestion and will discuss it with her physiotherapist at her next appointment. A further recheck meeting is planned for one week's time.

In this case study, the aims of the initial plan of care were not fully met, demonstrating the cyclical nature of effective care planning and implementation. During the process of evaluation, not only do you evaluate the care that has been delivered to date, you also undertake an assessment of the person's new baseline. This then leads into the planning, implementation and evaluation of further interventions.

Activity 5.6   Decision-making

Revisit previous chapters, pages 12 and 37, and re-read Linda's case study.

Linda is becoming more anxious; she does not go out on her own at all now and is relying on her son more frequently. She is frustrated by her situation and would like to feel more confident about herself and her health. Linda has come in to see the practice nurse at her GP surgery to talk about her situation. You are spending the day with the practice nurse and sit in on her consultation with Linda.

What plan of care could you implement to address Linda's anxiety and what members of the multidisciplinary team could you involve?

A brief outline answer is given at the end of the chapter.

As you will have seen from the scenarios above and Activity 5.6, the symptoms experienced by people living with an LTC can be multifactorial and can affect many aspects of their day-to-day life. Having an understanding of the common signs and symptoms of specific LTCs and how they are managed will assist you in your delivery of appropriate and effective symptom management.

Chapter summary

This chapter has provided you with an overview of QoL in people living with an LTC and the role that effective symptom management has in promoting and enhancing QoL. This chapter has explored the role of medication in managing symptoms and how the role of the nurse can enhance the benefits with effective communication and application of knowledge. By relating effective planning of care to symptom management, it has emphasised the importance of person-centred care in the effective management of symptoms in people living with an LTC.

Having read through this chapter and worked through the activities, you will have developed your knowledge and skills in relation to symptom management in the care and management of people living with an LTC. How you use this new knowledge and skills will depend on where you are working and your roles and responsibilities. However, as a nurse, you can improve the care you provide to people living with an LTC, and their carers, by recognising the importance of maintaining QoL and the factors that influence QoL. Using an effective framework for planning care, to work collaboratively with those living with an LTC, will ensure that the care and management you provide is based on a good assessment of the person's needs and is clearly focused on addressing those needs. It will also encourage you to reflect on your practice, further developing your knowledge and skills in relation to many aspects of person-centred care.

Activities: brief outline answers

Activity 5.1 Evidence-based practice and research (page 95)

Cardiovascular disease (CVD)

CVD is an umbrella term that covers any disease that involves the heart, blood vessels or both, and is caused by atherosclerosis. Atherosclerosis develops when atheroma form plaques on the lining of arteries; atheroma are a complex mixture of white blood cells, lipids and calcium. Over time, these plaques increase in size causing narrowing of the arteries resulting in reduced blood flow and hypertension (CKS, 2014). Due to the nature of CVD, people may experience many different symptoms, including those of angina, chest pain that may radiate to the left arm, jaw and neck, and stroke, which could include limb weakness, difficulty in speaking and facial weakness.

There are a number of known risk factors for CVD, which include smoking, lack of physical activity, increased alcohol consumption and being overweight. Advice should be given about smoking cessation, reducing the amount of saturated fat and increasing the amount of fish and fruit and vegetables in their diet to help reduce cholesterol, as well as taking regular exercise. It is important to ensure that any prescribed medication (e.g., statins, beta blockers) are taken as prescribed (CKS, 2014).

Depression

Depression is a mental health condition characterised by persistent low mood and a loss of pleasure in most activities. It is associated with a range of physical, emotional and behavioural symptoms (CKS, 2015). Symptoms may include fatigue and loss of energy, poor concentration, feelings of worthlessness, thoughts of death and suicidal thoughts, disturbed sleep – too much or too little – and changes to appetite causing weight loss or gain. People with depression may experience some or all of these symptoms at different times.

There is not a known pathophysiological reason for depression, and there are no biological diagnostic measures to determine the illness (McCarron et al., 2016). There are known factors that increase the risk of an individual experiencing depression: these include a personal or family history, alcohol dependence and living with one or more LTCs. Assessment tools can aid clinicians in measuring the severity of the depression from mild to severe and to assess the depressed person's risk of self-harm, including suicide (McCarron et al., 2016). This information and joint care planning with the person can aid treatment decisions.

There are two main treatments for depression – antidepressant medication and psychotherapy – and patients can be treated with one or both at the same time. Social prescribing of exercise and social opportunities such as befriending or gardening are also a tool that may help in primary care (King's Fund, 2017) to enhance the person's general well-being and quality of life. It is also important to help the person identify other sources of support such as friends and family, and other professionals such as a health visitor or bereavement counsellor (CKS, 2015). A comprehensive, biopsychosocial assessment and developing a therapeutic relationship will help you to identify some of the many causal factors behind the person's depression.

Type 2 diabetes

Type 2 diabetes is caused by insulin resistance and the reduced ability of beta cells in the pancreas to produce insulin. The resulting high blood glucose levels lead to further damage of the beta cells, resulting in a further reduction in the production of insulin (Muralitharan and Peate, 2013). Type 2 diabetes can remain undiagnosed for some time due to the fact that the degree of hyperglycaemia is not severe enough to produce symptoms. Some common symptoms include: increased thirst, blurred vision, weight loss and lethargy (CKS, 2017c).

Modifiable risk factors for type 2 diabetes include lack of exercise, obesity and smoking; therefore, health education/promotion around lifestyle changes should form part of the ongoing care and management. This should include dietary advice regarding carbohydrate intake. Once a person has been diagnosed and commenced on medication to control their blood glucose level, then ongoing monitoring of their HbA1c should take place to ensure this is within agreed levels. Information regarding complications should be provided, especially in relation to foot and eye care, with annual reviews taking place (CKS, 2017c).

Activity 5.3 Decision-making (page 100)

Medication	What it is for?	Instructions	Possible side effects
Co-codamol 30/500mg	*Pain*	*4 x daily* *Ensure 4–6 hours between doses*	*Constipation, confusion, drowsiness, dizziness*
Furosemide 40mg	*Diuretic – 'water tablet'*	*One tablet daily* *Take in the morning as it may cause frequent urination*	*Can cause urinary retention*
Clopidogrel 75mg	*Anti platelet – to thin the blood*	*One tablet daily* *Take with food at the same time each day*	*Abdominal pain, diarrhoea, bleeding disorders*
Alendronic Acid 10mg	*Bisphosphonate – for bone health*	*Take once daily* *Sit up and take on empty stomach 30 minutes before food*	*Constipation, diahorroea, dizziness*

(Continued)

(Continued)

Medication	What it is for?	Instructions	Possible side effects
Mirtazapine 30mg	*Antidepressant*	*Take at bedtime*	*Abnormal dreams, anxiety, confusion, dizziness, drowsiness*
Senna 15mg	*Laxative*	*Take at bedtime*	*Abdominal spasm, discoloured urine, pruritis*
Atorvastatin 20mg	*Statin – to lower cholesterol*	*Take once daily*	*Muscle tenderness/pain, back pain, epistaxis*
Aspirin 75mg	*Protect from stroke*	*Take once daily, dispersed in water*	*GI bleeding or irritation*

It is important that people understand what they are taking and why. Nurses need to use language that can be easily understood and check understanding – for example, it is for pain rather than an analgesic, or that is for your heart rather than for cardiac function. Writing information down means the patient does not have to remember it all. You should have the knowledge to be able to explain potential side effects and tell patients what to do if they suspect they are experiencing them, so that they do not stop important medication without medical advice. The risks of polypharmacy for older people are well documented and can result in them experiencing lots of side effects, poor medication adherence, increased confusion and risk of falls. For further learning, look up a medication management tool for older people such as STOPP/START toolkit and see if you can apply it to Mary and her current medication. Discuss your ideas with your mentor.

Activity 5.4 Critical thinking (page 101)

How do we feel pain?

There are pain receptors (nociceptors) within our skin, periosteum, arterial walls, joint surfaces and the lining of our cranium. Damage to these tissues stimulates local pain receptors, allowing pain to be easily localised and identified – for example, a person with osteoarthritis who has pain in their knees. Pain receptors in other parts of the body, mainly the organs, are supplied by a larger, more diffuse arrangement of pain receptors. This may make locating pain more difficult, as the pain can be experienced over a larger area. There are some organs in the body where there are almost no pain receptors – e.g., the liver parenchyma and the alveoli in the lungs. However, the liver capsule, the bronchi and parietal pleura are very sensitive to pain. Pain receptors are free nerve endings that are activated by stimuli such as pressure (mechanoreceptors), extremes of temperature (thermoreceptors) and chemical substances (chemoreceptors) (Porth and Matfin, 2014). Chronic pain is felt due to the fact that pain receptors do not adapt to sustained stimulation but keep on being activated and producing signals. This is because the body's natural analgesics need to be stimulated to remind the person to protect that area of their body to help manage the pain. Acute and chronic pain sensations are transmitted via sensory nerves to the thalamus and hypothalamus. Acute pain sensations are transmitted via larger A-delta fibres that are able to carry a larger number of impulses while chronic pain sensations are transmitted via smaller C fibres carrying a lower number of impulses (Porth and Matfin, 2014).

What is the difference between nociceptive and neuropathic pain?

Nociceptive pain is felt as a result of the activation of pain receptors (nociceptors). This type of pain is usually due to tissue damage – e.g., trauma, surgery or disease progression. It is often described as sharp, aching, crushing or throbbing. Neuropathic pain is felt when the nerve itself is damaged by compression or infiltration; the damaged nerve then sends signals to the rest of the nervous system. Due to damage to the sensory nerves, the pain may be experienced in an area where there is numbness. Neuropathic pain is often described as burning, stabbing or like pins and needles (Porth and Matfin, 2014). An example of this is shingles (herpes zoster infection), which can cause peripheral neuropathic pain. This pain is often described as hot, burning, stabbing, shooting or tingling.

What are the body's natural analgesics?

The body's natural analgesics are opioid peptides (dynophorins and endorphins) produced in the hypothalamus and pituitary gland. They are found in the nervous system in the areas of the brain associated with pain reception. They are also found in areas of the spinal cord. Their distribution corresponds to the areas of the brain where electrical stimulation can control pain, such as the thalamus. When a person experiences pain, these opioid peptides are released at the point where the pain signal enters the spinal cord and at the synapses in the thalamus, hypothalamus and cerebral cortex (Porth and Matfin, 2014).

Activity 5.5 Evidence-based practice and research (page 104)

Aspects	Influencing factors	Application to practice
Physical	The condition The person's functional capacity Side effects of treatment Disfigurement	Anisa may realise that this symptom could be permanent and that she may experience further deteriorations in her functional capacity. Her disturbed sleep may be a contributing factor.
Social	Family issues Loss of role at work Loss of role at home Finances Change in appearance due to condition Sense of helplessness	Anisa is currently off work; depending on her illness benefits, this may have a financial impact on her and her family. In addition, she may feel she is not able to fulfil her role as a mother.
Spiritual	Purpose Religion Meaning Uncertainty about future Hope Fear of pain/death	This relapse may be a reminder to Anisa of the ongoing nature of her RRMS and that it will become progressively worse.
Psychological	Anger Delays in diagnosis Coping ability Control and sense of usefulness Failure of treatment	Anisa may question her ability to cope with her condition; she may be concerned that as her condition worsens, she may become a 'burden'.

Some methods of pain assessment are as follows.

- Taking a pain history – assessing the site, nature and duration of the pain, as well as factors that relieve and exacerbate it.
- Physical examination – may help confirm the cause of the pain; will also allow examination of other aspects, such as nutrition.
- Body charts – pictures of the human body where the person can indicate and record the location of any pain; these can be updated.

- Numerical and visual analogue scales – includes 0–3 and 0–10 numerical scale and the no pain to worse pain, or no pain relief to complete pain relief visual analogue scale.
- Picture scales – use of faces with expressions ranging from happiness to distress.
- Pain questionnaires and inventories – these question the person on a range of factors relating to their pain – e.g., pain intensity, mood, pain relief.

Using communication skills, such as active listening, touch and observation, and engaging in a therapeutic relationship with Anisa, will enhance the assessment process, enabling you and Anisa to work together to manage her pain.

Activity 5.6 Decision-making (page 109)

The aim of your plan would be to increase Linda's coping strategies to reduce her anxiety and increase her confidence. To do this, you would need to undertake a holistic assessment of Linda and try to identify the trigger for her anxiety; this could be related to the sudden and unexpected nature of her husband's death. You would want to recheck Linda's progress and the suitability of your plan weekly, with a formal evaluation being arranged in approximately four weeks' time.

Using an action plan would be an appropriate way to ensure that Linda is in control of her care; however, due to her lack of confidence, you may need to work with her to compile this. The goal of Linda's action plan could be that she goes outside to the garden by herself; you would need to ensure that Linda's confidence level in achieving this is above seven to make it a realistic goal for her to achieve. You could incorporate relaxation into Linda's action plan – e.g., focused breathing and relaxation could reduce her anxiety, but in addition it could help manage her breathlessness. Initially, you may not involve other members of the multidisciplinary team in Linda's care; however, you may discuss her anxiety with her GP, heart failure CNS or community-based occupational therapist. Depending on whether there is an improvement in Linda's anxiety or not, you may need to refer on to more specialist support, such as cognitive behavioural therapy.

Further reading

Carmona-Torres, JM, Cobo-Cuenca, AI, Recio-Andrade, B, Laredo-Aguilera, JA, Martins, MM, Rodríguez-Borrego, MA (2018) Prevalence and factors associated with polypharmacy in older people. *Journal of Clinical Nursing,* 27(15 –16): 2942–52.

This European study explores how many older people are affected by polypharmacy and what the contributing risk factors are.

Fry, M, Arendts, G, Chenoweth, L (2017) Emergency nurses' evaluation of observational pain assessment tools for older people with cognitive impairment. *Journal of Clinical Nursing.* 26(910): 1281–90.

This study compares the efficacy of different pain assessment tools for people with a cognitive impairment in an emergency setting.

Osborne, LA, Bindemann, N, Noble, JG and Reed, P (2012) Changes in the key areas of quality of life associated with age and time since diagnosis of long term conditions. *Chronic Illness,* 8(2): 112–20.

This research article investigated the relationship between QoL, age and time since diagnosis. Results showed that the areas people feel important change over time; this has implications for how QoL might be assessed.

Shah, C, Lehman, H and Richardson, S (2014) Medicines optimisation: an agenda for community nursing. *Journal of Community Nursing.* 28(3): 82–5.

Useful websites

http://cks.nice.org.uk/#?char=A

The home page of Clinical Knowledge Summaries: a useful, evidence-based resource providing information about the care and management of a range of LTCs.

www.e-lfh.org.uk

E-Learning for Health offers free education and training for healthcare professionals. Modules include Pharmacology and Prescribing, Supporting self-care and end-of-life care that includes symptom management.

www.medicines.org.uk/emc/

The Electronic Medicines Compendium provides up-to-date information provided by the manufacturers of drugs and patient information leaflets.

www.prescqipp.info

PresQUIPP are an NHS-funded organisation that supports quality, optimised prescribing for patients by providing evidence-based resources for primary care professionals.

Chapter 6 Managing complex care in long term conditions

Platform 7: Coordinating care

7.4   identify the implications of current health policy and future policy changes for nursing and other professions and understand the impact of policy changes on the delivery and coordination of care

Chapter aims

After reading this chapter, you will be able to:

* understand the role case management has in the management of people with LTCs who have complex care needs;
* explain the roles and responsibilities of the case manager in the care of people living with an LTC;
* use care pathways to support person-centred care for those living with an LTC who have complex needs;
* recognise the importance of effective discharge planning for people living with an LTC and their carers.

Introduction

People are living longer and with multiple long-term conditions. We need to move away from an exclusive focus on body parts, biomarkers and pathology, and towards a more whole-person approach that responds meaningfully to what people value for their lives.

(National Voices, 2018, p10)

The ageing population of the UK means that between 2015 and 2035 the number of older people with four or more LTCs will double. Over 50 per cent of people aged 65 and older already have at least two LTCs (multimorbidity) (Kingston et al., 2018). While it is recognised that people living with one or more LTCs are intensive users of health and social care services, it is also known that increasing a person's sense of self-worth promotes their desire to manage their own health (DH, 2008b). The majority of people living with LTCs will have their condition managed effectively through appropriate health promotion and health education, self-management and timely symptom management. However, people living with multiple LTCs will have more complex health and social care needs, and are likely to experience a reduced QoL, polypharmacy and increased mortality (Kingston et al., 2018). They require a range of integrated services, and the delivery of proactive care and management which is coordinated by a suitably qualified person.

Case study: Andrew

Andrew is a 76-year-old widower who is living with chronic obstructive pulmonary disease (COPD). He lives alone in a one-bedroomed flat in a sheltered housing complex.

Over the last 12 months Andrew has been experiencing worsening health and has had two admissions to hospital for chest infections in the last three months. This is despite his district nurse working with Andrew to increase his level of exercise and improve his nutritional intake. After some initial success, Andrew was not able to maintain his level of exercise and, due to his increasing dyspnoea, he has been relying on meals on wheels to provide him with a hot meal. His recent chest infections have left him with worsening dyspnoea and associated reduction in his mobility. Care workers visit twice a day to assist him with washing and dressing, and a neighbour pops in to dust, vacuum and help with his laundry. At the weekly practice meeting, following his last admission, Andrew's GP transferred his care to the community matron for case management.

David will be Andrew's case manager. David is a community matron and a non-medical prescriber and, working as part of the practice team, will be responsible for coordinating Andrew's care and management. David will use a case management approach to ensure that Andrew's ongoing physical, social and psychological needs are met. By leading and taking responsibility for Andrew's care, David will coordinate input from other agencies, ensuring that Andrew's care needs are met. Through working with Andrew and as his single point of contact, David will support him to make informed choices about the care he receives. David will further work with Andrew to encourage him to be aware of changes in his condition that signal an exacerbation and to take action to address these.

Andrew's story demonstrates that the aim of case management is to streamline the care and management of complex needs that result from living with multiple LTCs. You may not be directly involved in the case management of people living with LTCs, though it may be that, when working with a community matron or specialist respiratory nurse, you observe the management of complex care needs for this group of people. Integrating the knowledge from previous chapters in relation to health promotion and health education, self-management and symptom management will enable you to assist in the delivery of effective case management and complex care. To further support you in your role, this chapter will develop your knowledge and understanding of case management and complex care. In order to do this, the chapter will discuss the roles and responsibilities of case managers and how the care of those requiring complex care is managed. The chapter also discusses the way in which care pathways can be used and examines the importance of discharge planning for those living with LTCs who have been admitted to secondary care.

Case management in LTCs

Case management originated in the USA where, in the 1950s, it was used as a means of providing care to people with severe mental health needs. From this, it was then rolled out and used with older people who had complex health and social care needs. The aim of case management is to provide coordinated care that is person-centred and responsive to the changing needs of people living with LTCs, that leads to higher quality and cost-effective outcomes, including reducing the need for long-term care (Park and Park, 2018). In the UK, case management has been used in mental health nursing since the 1980s; this was as a response to the shift from institutionalised to community care. Since then, it has formed part of the care and management of people living with LTCs. As well as streamlining the care provided, the aim of case management is to enable people living with LTCs who require complex care to avoid hospital admissions and to have more choice about their care.

Activity 6.1   Reflection

Case management is a key part of the care and management of people living with an LTC. On your own or with a group of colleagues, reflect on the areas where you have undertaken clinical practice and consider the following questions.

- What members of the health and social care team undertake the role of case manager?
- What are their roles and responsibilities in relation to managing the care of people with LTCs?
- How do they fit in with the wider multidisciplinary team?
- What advanced clinical skills do you think would benefit a nurse working as case manager?

As the answers will be based on your own observations, there is no outline answer at the end of the chapter.

Undertaking Activity 6.1 will have shown you that case management can be undertaken by a range of health and social care professionals. These may include district nurses, nurse specialists and community matrons, physiotherapists and social workers.

Roles and responsibilities of the case manager in LTCs

In completing Activity 6.1, you will have begun to identify some of the roles and responsibilities that case managers have, which are both strategic and patient-focused.

In the literature, the terms 'case manager' and 'community matron' are used interchangeably, and there is some overlapping of roles. Generally speaking, case managers are responsible for coordinating the care and management of people living with LTCs who have a complex single LTC or social need. They will be responsible for planning, monitoring and anticipating the needs of those living with one or more LTC. In this situation, the case manager is likely to be a qualified nurse, social worker or other healthcare professional. Community matrons are responsible for supporting high-intensity patients who require the input of advanced clinical skills (such as advanced health assessment) and clinical management as in, for example, management of hydration (Bentley, 2014).

Whereas the level of clinical nursing care may vary between case managers and community matrons, the roles and responsibilities of the case manager or community matron should be underpinned by the following core elements (Bentley, 2014):

- case finding or screening to identify suitable patients;
- person-centred assessment and diagnosis;
- holistic care planning and implementation of care;
- referral of patient to appropriate services and coordination of these;
- monitoring and evaluation of services and patient outcomes – e.g., independence maintained.

It is the responsibility of the case manager/community matron to ensure that the core elements listed above form the basis of their roles and responsibilities in relation to people living with an LTC. Using Andrew's case scenario, Table 6.1 provides you with some points to consider and applies these core elements to clinical practice.

Core elements	Points to consider	Application to practice
Case finding or screening	Identifying people through the use of referral criteria, who may benefit from a case management approach. Be aware of hidden populations – e.g., the homeless, asylum seekers and travellers. Some examples of referral criteria include: • must be over 18 years of age; • people who frequently use health/social care services; • people who have had two or more accident and emergency and/or hospital admissions in the past 12 months; • people who have one or more LTC; • people who are taking four or more medications.	Andrew has had two unplanned hospital admissions in the last three months. When at home, he has a care package for assistance with his personal hygiene and a neighbour cooks meals and helps with housework. His current health status means that he is eligible for a case management approach to his care and management.

Core elements	Points to consider	Application to practice
Assessment	Assessing a person's health and social care needs using recognised assessments. Using information gathered from the person, their carer and family and other services involved in the person's care. Be aware of obtaining consent to share information and confidentiality. This may include undertaking a physical health assessment, making a diagnosis and non-medical prescribing.	Working with Andrew, David will assess his current health and social care needs, including his concordance and compliance with his medication regime. Given Andrew's current health status, this is likely to include a physical health assessment. David will review the current level of support to ensure that it is meeting Andrew's health and social care needs. Areas highlighted in David's assessment may include improving his nutritional intake and educating Andrew about the signs that indicate that his condition is deteriorating.
Care planning	Formulating a personalised care plan to meet the needs identified in the assessment. This care plan may also address anticipated needs. If required, the care plan is agreed with the person's GP and consultant. Coordinates input from other members of the health and social care team who may also have some clinical input.	This will depend on the result of Andrew's assessment; it will be David's responsibility to coordinate the input of other agencies. David may refer Andrew on for further nutritional support; David may be required to prescribe nutritional supplements. David is also likely to provide Andrew with information regarding his condition.
Implementation of care plan	Maintaining contact with the person and monitoring input from other health and social care professionals. Provides clinical care if required.	David will become Andrew's single point of contact; he will remain visible to Andrew, ensuring that the care plan is well coordinated. David may also undertake ongoing monitoring of Andrew's physical health status.
Monitoring and reviewing	Monitoring the effectiveness of the care plan and reviewing the level of care if required. Using care pathways and protocols to streamline care.	David will review Andrew's care plan on a regular basis, depending on his current health status. David may use care pathways to support Andrew's care – e.g., acute exacerbation of COPD care pathway.

Table 6.1 Application of the core elements of case management (as described by Offredy et al., 2009) to your clinical practice

As you can see from Table 6.1, the core elements of case management allow David, as Andrew's community matron, to coordinate and guide his care. Ensuring a single point of contact will improve communication between all health and social care professionals involved in Andrew's care, and with Andrew himself.

Research summary

A meta-synthesis carried out by Askerud and Conder (2017) explored the experience of patients living with LTCs who were supported by nursing case managers. The researchers synthesised the results of 15 studies that aimed to gain an understanding of patients' perceptions of nursing case management. The studies represented over 1,000 patients across the qualitative studies included. Askerud and Conder (2017) appraised each identified study for quality and inclusion, and then used the combined results to answer the question. The research found that a nursing case management approach fostered therapeutic relationships based on trust and with participants having a high level of confidence in their nursing case managers. This encouraged patients to self-manage their LTCs. The ability to develop a long-term relationship with one healthcare professional was highly valued by the patients as it provided continuity of care (Askerud and Conder, 2017). These findings were reiterated in an earlier literature review by Sutherland and Hayter (2009) who found that case management was effective in improving a person's level of self-care and increasing their level of psychosocial support. In addition, through effective assessment and monitoring, the progression of their LTC was managed more effectively. They concluded that case management has the potential to improve health outcomes for people living with LTCs (Sutherland and Hayter, 2009).

According to Askerud and Conder (2017), it is the nursing case manager's ability to navigate the health and social care systems and communicate effectively across them that enhances both the quality and efficacy of care of people with complex LTCs.

Wilkes et al. (2014) used a modified Delphi research technique to attempt to define and validate the role of the community nurse in managing people with complex health needs realting to LTCs. They assert that while an effective multidisciplinary team working is required to provide quality care, it is important that the community nurse has clear role delineations (Wilkes et al., 2014). Their research identified six main domains that the community nurse is required to fulfil.

- Advocate
- Supporter
- Educator
- Coordinator
- Assessor
- Team member

Wilkes et al. (2014) state that clear role definition will aid the nurse to work within a multidisciplinary team more effectively and guide patient's expectations of what the nurse will provide in managing their complex and long term conditions.

As you can see from the above research summary, case management has a positive effect on people living with LTCs and their family and carers, particularly in relation to support and coordination of care.

> ### Activity 6.2   Reflection
>
> Reflecting on your recent clinical experience, identify a person living with LTCs who had complex care needs, and compile a map or diagram of the services involved in their care and management.
>
> Using the information provided in Table 6.1, apply the core elements to your chosen person and review how case management could have improved their care and management.
>
> *As the answers will be based on your own observations, there is no outline answer at the end of the chapter.*

Working through Activity 6.2 will demonstrate how, through ensuring that an appropriate and responsive plan of care is in place, case management can be used to improve the care and management of people living with LTCs. In your current role, you may not be actively involved in case management; however, using the information in Table 6.1 in your nursing practice will support you in your delivery of effective care to people living with LTCs.

Managing complex care

For some people living with LTCs, it is inevitable that as their condition deteriorates their health and social care needs will become increasingly more complex. One group of people who fall into this category, who have not been mentioned previously, are those living with frailty. It is generally recognised that the majority of LTCs affect a specific physiological system (e.g., cardiovascular, endocrine), or a specific organ (e.g., lung cancer, COPD), and that as the disease progresses, symptoms will increase, as will the level of care and management they require. Increasingly, alongside this more traditional view of LTCs, frailty is recognised as an LTC.

Frailty as an LTC

'Frailty' is a term that is often used to describe a group of people, such as those who are dependent on others for their activities of day living (ADLs), rather than being seen as a diagnosed medical condition. Like other LTCs, frailty is progressive, has a negative impact on health and well-being, and can result in people becoming acutely unwell if their condition is not managed carefully. It is estimated that approximately 14 per cent of the population have frailty (Gale et al., 2015). This rises to one in four of those over the age of 85 (RCN, 2018). Frailty is not an illness, but a syndrome that is related to the ageing process; in frailty, multiple body systems gradually lose their reserves. Its aetiology is not fully understood, but it is thought that changes in a person's immune system and a decline in musculoskeletal and endocrine systems are involved (Chen et al., 2014), resulting in a gradual decline in physical and cognitive function. Recognising frailty is not easy; older people may not see themselves as being frail. They may have made adjustments in their daily activities over time and are not aware of how frail they are. It may not be until an acute event, such as a fall or a chest infection, that a person's level of frailty is identified.

To support the identification, care and management of frailty, the NICE standard for *Multimorbidity: Clinical Assessment and Guidance* (2016) offer direction in which assessment tools to use in both community and hospital settings. NICE (2016c) suggest that all people with multimorbidity are considered for frailty, but recommend caution in assessment of the acutely unwell. Mulitimorbidity is defined as the presence of two or more LTCs, including physical and mental health conditions, ongoing learning disability and sensory impairments, as well as alcohol or substance misuse (NICE, 2016c).

The British Geriatric Society (BGS) in 2014 published *Fit for Frailty: Consensus Best Practice Guidance for the care of older people living with frailty in community and outpatient settings* to support healthcare professionals in managing frailty. The BGS (2014) identifies five syndromes that could indicate that a person has frailty. These are: falls, immobility, delirium, incontinence and susceptibility to the side effects of medication. If you are caring for a person presenting with any of these syndromes, this is an opportunity for you to identify if a person is frail. There is a range of tests that you can use, including the Timed Up and Go Test. This measures, in seconds, how long it takes a person to stand up from a standard chair, walk a distance of up to 3 metres, turn, walk back and sit down. The cut-off time for this test is 10 seconds (BGS, 2014). This test is easy to carry out and requires no specific equipment, making it ideal to carry out in a range of settings. Once a person has been diagnosed with frailty, it is important to manage this and maintain the person's overall health and well-being; some examples of this condition are provided in Table 6.2.

Clinical concern	Practical interventions
Poor nutrition	Refer to dietitian for assessment and nutritional support; provide education regarding what foods to eat – should include high-energy and high-protein foods. If the person is in a hospital setting, use of red tray system and provision of assistance at meal times.
Challenging behaviour (delirium)	Identify if there is an underlying cause: pain, constipation or urinary retention and investigate. Be alert to changes in the person's attitude that could indicate they are becoming agitated – e.g., facial expressions, verbal threats. Use of de-escalation techniques, such as asking open questions, listening and paying attention to the person.
Reduced mobility	Refer to physiotherapy for strengthening and balance exercises, ideally for two hours per week, to reduce the incidence of falls. Ensure that the environment is uncluttered with any trip hazards removed. Encourage correct use of mobility aids. Occupational therapy referral may also be appropriate.

Table 6.2   Interventions to manage aspects of frailty

As you can see from Table 6.2, there are some very practical steps that you can use to manage frailty, maintaining quality of life for the person. For those involved in caring for people with frailty and other LTCs, there are some useful resources available to support them in their delivery of person-centred care. Guidelines for assessing someone with frailty can be found in the NICE Guideline (NG56) (2016) *Multimorbidity: Clinical Assessment and Management.* Another such resource is integrated care pathways (ICPs). ICPs are also known as care pathways and maps of care, but for consistency the term 'integrated care pathway' will be used in this chapter.

Integrated care pathways and LTCs

An integrated care pathway is a framework that allows an interprofessional approach to care; its aim is to support a person with a specific condition, or set of symptoms, to move through health and social care services. The aim of ICPs is to improve both the coordination and consistency of care a person receives. They allow you to deliver the right care to the right person in the right place and at the right time. ICPs can be used in different ways.

They can be used to promote equity of care across a range of care settings by providing clear guidance and advice regarding the steps to be taken when providing care to a specific group of people. Examples are the integrated care pathways that detail the specific care of people with type 1 and type 2 diabetes – *NHS RightCare Pathway: Diabetes* (NHS, 2018). In relation to diabetes, they provide you with guidance from the point when a patient is identified as at risk from type 2 diabetes and preventative care, to structured education programmes and annual review of patients living with diabetes. The care pathway incorporates best evidence and national guidelines to support the care you provide (NHS, 2018). ICPs can also be used to provide a framework for the multidisciplinary team to use for specific health or approach, such as Age UK's integrated care pathway. This pathway brings together health, social care and voluntary organisations, putting the older person in control of their health, enabling them to maintain their independence and quality of life. The aim is to have services 'wrap around' the older person; the pathway is reviewed regularly with protocols put in place should the older person's situation change (Age UK, 2018).

In this instance, an ICP is used as the single document that all health and social care professionals use to document the clinical care. This single point of communication has the potential to lead to improved communication and coordination of care. Using an ICP can support you to deliver interprofessional and multi-agency working, and can empower patients and their carers to actively participate more in their care.

As the answers will be based on your own observations, there is no outline answer at the end of the chapter.

Activity 6.3   Reflection

Either on your own or with a colleague, reflect on the action plans, care plans and integrated care pathways you have used in your clinical practice and answer the following questions.

- How were they used to support patient care?
- Did they support interprofessional working? If so, how? If not, why?
- Did they support the delivery of person-centred care? If so, how? If not, why?
- Were they focused on a specific condition and intervention? If so, was the focus of this acute or long term social care situations, such as acute stroke?

You may have identified from Activity 6.3 that you have used a range of care planning strategies at different times and for different reasons. It is likely, however, that whichever tool you used, you planned care to take into consideration a person's physical, social, psychological and spiritual health, the impact this has on their symptoms and how they manage them.

It should be noted, however, that while ICPs form the template of the care to be delivered, the people receiving the care are individuals and will not all respond in the same way and follow the same pathway of care. It is necessary, therefore, that these individualities are accommodated within the ICP. These individualities are known as 'variances'. Variances allow for healthcare professionals to use their professional judgement in relation to the care being delivered, as well as promoting a person-centred approach to care. Recognising and managing variances requires you, as a student nurse, to be able to problem solve. Effective care planning, as discussed in Chapter 5, will support you in your ability to do this. When a variance is noted, the following should be recorded on the care pathway: what variance occurred and why, the action taken (personalised care plan) and the outcome of the action. The aim of the action taken in relation to a variance is to return the person to the ICP as soon as possible (Middleton *et al.*, 2001). Table 6.3 outlines how a care planning tool such as the nursing process can be applied to ICPs and managing variances in a person's care.

As you can see from Table 6.3, by providing you with a clear framework within which to work, both the nursing process and ICPs are useful resources to use to support your delivery of person-centred care.

The nursing process	Integrated care pathway	Application to practice
Assess	You are using an acute stroke ICP and are undertaking an initial assessment regarding the person's skin integrity.	You use a recognised risk assessment tool – e.g., the Waterlow pressure ulcer risk assessment tool – to assess the person's skin.
Systematic nursing diagnosis	This assessment gives you a risk score of 22, indicating that the person has a very high risk of developing a pressure ulcer.	

The nursing process	Integrated care pathway	Application to practice
Plan	You record the result of your assessment on the initial assessment sheet and as a variance, to ensure that all members of the healthcare team are aware of the results of your assessment. As you have recorded a variance, you compile a specific care plan to address the patient's high risk score.	You develop a care plan to maintain skin integrity; this should include what the patient can do and what the MD team will do, and should include clear aims and goals. You implement the use of pressure-relieving equipment and plan a range of nursing interventions and other healthcare measures.
Implement	In addition to using appropriate pressure-reducing equipment, working with the person, you implement a care plan and set goals that address the following aspects of nursing care: • general nursing care – regular positional changes; • liaise with physiotherapist regarding positioning and mobility assessment; • pain – any pain is being assessed and well controlled; • nutrition – a high protein nutritious diet is available; • person handling – the correct moving and lifting techniques are used; • skin care – good personal hygiene, ensuring that the skin in kept clean and dry. As care is provided, this is then recorded on the ICP; this may include how frequently specific aspects of care are to be delivered.	
Recheck	You record, on the ongoing assessment of the plan of care, the care planned. This will include any reassessment of the person's skin integrity using Waterlow. You record this change on the ongoing assessment of the plan of care. When providing care, you notice a change in skin integrity and record on the variance analysis sheet.	There is a change in skin colour on the right heel: the skin is intact; however, **non-blanching erythema** is present. As a grade one pressure ulcer is classed as a wound, you implement a care plan to address this. This includes: • regular positional changes; • ensuring that there is no pressure on the right heel; • applying a film or thin hydrocolloid dressing for protection.
Evaluate	Using the ICP and identified care plan to address the grade one pressure ulcer ensures that evaluation takes place as documented. This evaluation consists of: • ongoing pressure ulcer risk assessment; • ongoing review of the care plan.	

Table 6.3 Application of the nursing process and an integrated care pathway to your clinical practice

Activity 6.4   Evidence-based practice and research

During your next practice learning experience, with the support of your mentor, find the ICPs that are used to support care; these could be local or national. Considering the following questions, review a selection of these.

- Is there a clear evidence base presented for the ICP?
- Is there a regular review date?
- Is the ICP linked to other policy within the trust?
- Is there clear guidance on how to complete the ICP?
- Is the ICP easy to navigate: do you know where to document your initial assessment, ongoing care and variances?

You could include this activity as evidence in your portfolio in support of the NMC (2018) *Future nurse: Standards for proficiency for registered nurses*, especially in relation to Platform 5: Leading and managing nursing care and working in teams.

As the answers will be based on your own observations, there is no outline answer at the end of the chapter.

Undertaking Activity 6.4 will have identified that ICPs not only support the delivery of responsive person-centred care, they can also be used to support the delivery of evidence-based and cost-effective health and social care. NICE provides a range of online Pathways that map their guidance; these are quick and easy to use. NICE Pathways incorporate a range of conditions/situations, including acute heart failure to walking and cycling. The broad breadth of the NICE Pathways allows clinicians to access evidence-based pathways to support person-centred, holistic care for those with LTCs. Each Pathway is supported by an appropriate evidence base, including research and clinical guidelines; this ensures that the information provided is based on the best available evidence and is suitable for use throughout the UK. While the maps are not as detailed as an ICP, they provide information regarding treatment options and where care should be delivered – e.g., in primary or secondary care.

Case study: Joseph – using NICE Pathways

It is likely that NICE Pathways guided the care and management of Joseph's prostate cancer. For example, following his biopsy, once his **Gleason score** was known, the pathway would have indicated that Joseph's cancer was 'intermediate risk'. This result would have signposted the clinicians to offer radical treatment to Joseph, either prostatectomy or radiotherapy. Included in this pathway is how to manage any adverse effects of radical treatment – for example, incontinence, which Joseph is experiencing. This Pathway also includes what follow-up treatment Joseph should expect to receive.

As discussed above, the effective use of case management and care pathways improves the care and management for people living with LTCs, supporting independence and reducing unnecessary admission to secondary care. However it is recognised that it is not always possible to manage all acute exacerbations in primary care and that, at times, admission to hospital is necessary. For people living with LTCs and their carers, admission to secondary care can be a time of stress and anxiety, especially if the person has complex care needs. Hospital admission can place a person at risk of hospital-acquired infection; it can often result in a reduction in a person's functional ability, especially in older people and those with a cognitive impairment, and can increase a person's social isolation.

Research summary: Dementia and secondary care

For people with dementia, removal from their familiar surroundings where they may just be able to 'cope' to an unfamiliar setting where it is busy and there are lots of new faces, can be disorientating. It is known that up to 97 per cent of nurses in a secondary (or tertiary) care setting are responsible for caring for people with dementia (Alzheimer's Society, 2009). In a busy ward environment, people with dementia can be seen as being 'challenging' to nurses: they require more time to be spent with them, they may display unpredictable behaviour, they may wander and communication with them can be difficult. From the perspective of the carer, findings from the Alzheimer's Society's report (2016) noted that only 2 per cent of carers said that hospital staff understood the specific needs of people with dementia, 90 per cent of carers said that people with dementia became more confused in hospital and 92 per cent said that being admitted to hospital was a frightening experience for those with dementia. It is important, therefore, both for nurses and for those with dementia, that strategies are in place to support nurses to maximise care and to ensure that for those living with dementia, any deterioration in their condition is minimised. Strategies that have been identified include the following (Scerri et al., 2015).

- Improving orientation to the environment – this requires a committed approach from hospital management. Improving lighting, reducing noise and providing signposting, especially to toilets, can improve a person's orientation and reduce agitation (Waller, 2012). A homely, clean and safe environment

(Continued)

(Continued)

that is relaxed will support people wth dementia and their carers. These strategies can be simple, non-expensive and very effective in improving the hospital experience.

- Using a 'This is Me' guide and/or memory books (see Chapter 4) – these are simple and practical tools that provide an overview of the person with dementia. 'This is Me' addresses areas such as the person's ability to manage their activities of daily living, their likes and dislikes and what worries them.
- Learning from carers – as previously mentioned in this book, carers play an important role in supporting people living with an LTC, and it is important to use their knowledge of the person to inform the care you are providing. Acknowledging the carers as a source of information and assistance, as well as providing them with direct feedback about their family members' care, is much appreciated (Scerri et al., 2015).
- Improving communication – finding suitable ways of communication with people who have dementia will improve the quality of care given. Observing the person and talking to their carer will enable understanding of what different behaviours may mean. By speaking clearly with a calm and gentle voice, using the patient's own language and enhancing non-verbal communication such as smiling and use of touch, such as hand holding, can all help build an effective therapeutic relationship.

The strategies identified above, such as working with carers, improving communication, learning about the person and effective pain assessment and management (see Chapter 5, pages 101–109) have the potential to minimise the risk of challenging behaviours occurring. However, it is acknowledged that episodes of challenging behaviour may still occur, and using the ABC approach to assess challenging behaviour can support effective management (Heath et al., 2010).

- A – Antecedents/triggers: what was happening before the challenging behaviour occurred? Who was present and where did it happen?
- B – Behaviour: what challenging behaviour occurred? Has this happened before or is this behaviour new?
- C – Consequences: what happened as a result of this behaviour?

Using the strategies outlined above will improve the care delivered to those with dementia and their carers while in secondary care. By working to minimise any deterioration in a person's level of cognitive ability, and supporting and working with carers, appropriate and timely discharge can be achieved.

People living with LTCs who are admitted to hospital often have care packages at home that need to be reviewed or reinstated before discharge. For some people, they may not have had any input prior to admission, but because of a change in their health status, they require care on discharge. Therefore, it is important that any discharge is planned effectively and in a timely manner. Beginning to plan for discharge on admission has the potential to minimise a person's length of stay, maximising their function and minimising the risk of complications. When discharging a person with LTCs from hospital, it is important that this process is planned.

Discharge planning in LTCs

Discharge should not be seen as a discrete part of a patient's care; rather, it should be seen as an interactive process that starts on admission. However, in reality it often starts when a person is deemed 'medically fit for discharge', meaning that the process can be rushed and completed in a short space of time. A Cochrane Review by Gonçalves-Bradley et al. (2016) found that effective discharge planning reduced the overall length of stay and reduced readmission rates in older people. They also found that discharge planning increased patient and carer satisfaction. This update of a previous review found that personalised discharge plans could also have the positive impact of reducing average hospital admission by up to a day. However, it is recognised that there are many factors that influence when discharge planning starts and how effectively it is managed. In a busy acute setting, the priority might be on the person's acute presentation and managing that, rather than on starting discharge planning (Rhudy et al., 2009). The multidisciplinary nature of the care and management of people with complex care needs means that coordination of the discharge planning process can be problematic (Rhudy et al., 2009).

The important role that discharge planning plays has been recognised by NICE and the Social Care Institute for Excellence (SCIE) which published guidance in 2015 on supporting transition from acute care to community settings. The guidance has a focus on person-centred care and recommends use of the following principles to guide discharge planning.

- Patients are individuals and equal partners in the multidisciplinary team (MDT) who should be treated with dignity and respect.
- Identify and support those who may be less able to access services.
- Involve families/carers in discussions about care (provided the patient's consent has been obtained).
- If there is doubt about a patient's capacity to make a specific decision, follow the principles of the Mental Capacity Act, 2005.

With the development of bed managers and discharge coordinators, nurses can feel disengaged from the discharge planning process. The Queen's Nursing Institute (QNI) (2016) recognises the key role that nurses have in the discharge process, and in their report exploring the challenges and barriers to effective discharge planning in the UK identified three key areas of good practice.

- Improved communication, with patients and their carers, community nursing teams and the wider multidisciplinary team.
- Improved collaboration, in terms of sharing information, using shared IT systems and involving the whole team in care.
- Improved coordination, involving community teams early in the discharge process, using the same assessment tools and practical planning such as staffing levels out of hours and time of discharge, avoiding night-time discharges.

The report advocates that nurses from acute and community teams work in partnership together, and with patients and their families to promote a seamless health service from hospital to home. This document explains best practice in discharge planning and is a useful tool to guide your practice.

The Department of Health (2010) provides a ten-step framework to support effective, nurse-led discharge called *Ready to go? Planning the discharge and the transfer of patients from hospital to intermediate care.* The framework has been applied to one of the case studies below to show how these principles of effective discharge planning can be used in practice.

Case study: Linda (see Chapter 1 for further information)

Linda was admitted to hospital after being found lying on the floor by her son. He was concerned when she did not answer the phone and had called round to see if she was all right. When he found Linda, she was a bit confused and the left side of her face was drooping. Linda could not remember what had happened and was not sure how long she had been lying there for; she had tried to get herself up but was unable to do so. Her son phoned an ambulance and she was admitted to hospital; on admission, her blood glucose levels were found to be elevated (HbA1c was 50mmol/mol). Over the next 24 hours her confusion resolved, as did the drooping of the left side of her face. However, Linda's blood glucose levels remained elevated after admission; a diagnosis of type 2 diabetes was made and she was commenced on metformin 500mg twice a day (BD). Linda does not like being in hospital and is keen to return home to a familiar environment.

In Table 6.4, the DH ten-step framework has been applied to Linda's discharge planning.

Discharge planning is a crucial aspect of patient care; however, it is recognised that it does not always happen in a timely and organised manner. Take the time to complete Activity 6.5. This activity will allow you to examine your local discharge policy/protocol and explore some of the reasons why discharge planning is successful or not.

Step	Key points	Application to Linda
1. Start planning for discharge on or before admission	Start discharge planning before or on admission. Undertake a full assessment. Record any factors that may make discharge problematic. Ensure MD team are aware of their roles and responsibilities. Involve carers/family.	As Linda was an emergency admission, you will have to start this on admission. Carry out a full assessment, including medication and social situation. Linda lives alone and is socially isolated due to her anxiety. Liaise with the physiotherapist regarding mobility as Linda was admitted with a suspected fall at home. With Linda's consent, Linda's son should be informed about any plans for discharge.
2. Identify if the patient has simple or complex discharge planning needs	Simple discharge – person is likely to return to their own home and does not require complex ongoing care. Complex discharge – person requires complex ongoing health and/or social care input from an MD and/or interagency team.	While Linda has been diagnosed with having had a TIA and has been newly diagnosed with type 2 diabetes, she does not require complex ongoing care – therefore she has simple discharge planning needs.
3. Develop a clinical management plan within 24 hours of admission	This care plan should include treatment activities and goals, how these goals are going to be achieved and the estimated time frame. Diagnostic and investigative treatments should also be included.	Linda has been referred to the dietitian regarding her diabetes and for advice about her diet and how to make healthy changes. Due to Linda's anxiety she may require support from the MD team regarding confidence building to support her when she is home. There has been a change to Linda's medication, therefore medicines optimisation should take place with her to ensure that she understands her new medication. A date is set for Linda's discharge.
4. Coordinate the discharge through effective leadership and handover of responsibilities at ward level	Due to individual staff not being available every day, each day one person should take responsibility for coordinating the discharge planning process. Documentation should be kept up to date, both written and verbal (handover). For complex discharges, discharge coordinators may manage the process.	Keep Linda's case records up to date, document her progress and whether discharge planning is on track, liaise and coordinate the input of other members of the MD team.
5. Set an expected date of discharge within 24–48 hours of admission and discuss with the carer/family	This can be based on the patient's clinical picture: are they improving, staying the same or deteriorating? How long it will take for referrals, assessments and investigations to be carried out can also provide an estimated discharge date.	Review Linda's plan of care and clinical presentation, as her symptoms have resolved; then, once all her assessments are complete, she can be discharged. Keep Linda up to date with progress so that she can begin to plan for discharge.

Step	Key points	Application to Linda
6. Review the discharge plan each day with the patient and update progress towards discharge date	Review the patient's care plan daily to ensure that it is being met; discuss this with the patient. Take any necessary action to ensure that the care plan is being implemented and update the patient on discharge planning progress.	Discuss Linda's discharge with her each day, ensure that referrals have taken place, discuss with Linda any concerns she has about going home.
7. Involve patients and carers to make informed decisions about care to maximise independence	Involve the patient and carer throughout the discharge process. Using ICPs can support planning and delivery of care. If the person has complex discharge planning needs, liaise with community services and offer a carer assessment.	Keep Linda up to date with her discharge plans.
8. Plan discharges and transfers to take place over seven days	This approach promotes timely discharge and spreads the discharge load evenly across the week, avoiding peaks (Friday) and troughs (Monday).	Notify Linda that she may be discharged during the weekend; this might suit Linda better as her son will be available for a couple of days before returning to work on a Monday.
9. Use a discharge checklist 24–48 hours pre-discharge	Using a checklist allows for a record of all actions taken to be recorded; they can improve communication between the MD and the patient and family or carers. A checklist could include when aspects of care such as medication and transport have been ordered/received.	Complete Linda's discharge checklist, paying particular attention to medication. Discuss transport options with her.
10. Make decisions to discharge/ transfer each day	While the overall legal responsibility for a patient's care remains with the senior medical practitioner, nurses can take responsibility for initiating simple discharges. A key factor for this is the patient's 'clinical stability' and their need for 'hospital type' assessment and treatment.	Linda remains clinically stable with her condition improving. She understands her new medication and the need to adapt her diet.

Table 6.4 The DH ten-step framework applied to Linda's discharge planning

Activity 6.5 Evidence-based practice and research

During your next practice learning experience, locate your local discharge policy/protocol and associated documentation – for example, discharge checklist – and familiarise yourself with it. Then answer the following questions.

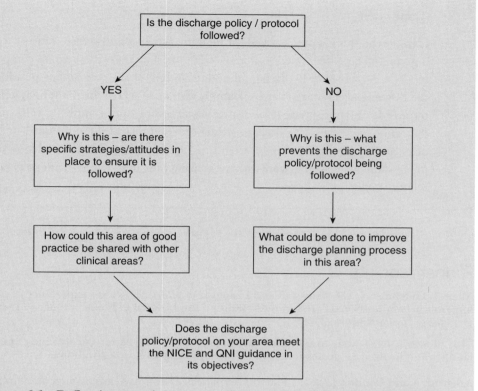

Figure 6.1 **Reflective questions to encourage effective discharge planning.**

As the answers will be based on your own observations, there is no outline answer at the end of the chapter.

Chapter summary

This chapter has provided you with an overview of complex care in LTCs and how it is managed. It has outlined the important role that case management plays in promoting proactive care and in increasing satisfaction in those living with an LTC, and applied this to your clinical practice. ICPs have been explored in relation to the care and management of those with LTCs; using ICPs ensures that an appropriate plan of care is provided. The importance of effective medicines optimisation has been acknowledged and the role of medicines review discussed. Discharge planning has been highlighted, with the emphasis being placed on the discharge planning process and the importance of this being a planned and timely event.

(Continued)

(Continued)

Having read this chapter, worked through the activities and accessed the further reading, you will have developed your knowledge and skills in relation to how complex care, in LTCs, is managed. By having an understanding of the role and responsibilities of the case manager you can liaise effectively with members of the multidisciplinary team to provide an appropriate level of care. By accessing and using ICPs, you can ensure that those living with LTCs receive evidence-based care at the right time, in the right place and by the right person. Recognising the importance of the discharge planning process will enable you to work with those living with an LTC and their carers to address relevant concerns and issues.

Further reading

Allen, J, Hutchinson, AM, Brown, R and Livingstone, PM (2017) User experience and care integration in transitional care for older people from hospital to home: a meta-synthesis. *Qualitative Health Research*, 27(1): 24–36.

This meta-synthesis aims to enhance understanding of the experience of older people, their families and healthcare professionals in the transition from hospital to home.

Askerud, A and Condor, J (2017) Patients' experiences of nurse case management in primary care: a meta-synthesis. *Australian Journal of Primary Health Care*, 23(5): 420–8.

This qualitative synthesis examines the findings of 15 studies looking at the perceptions of people living with LTCs care under a case manager.

Department of Health (2010) *Ready to Go? Planning the Discharge and Transfer of Patients from Hospital and Intermediate Care.* Leeds: Department of Health.

This guide explains the ten key steps to achieving a safe and timely discharge, and is aimed at both health and social care professionals.

Useful websites

http://pathways.nice.org.uk

This website provides information on a range of care pathways. They are easy to access and provide an up-to-date evidence-based resource for health and social care professionals

www.housinglin.org.uk/hospital2home_pack

This website provides useful information to support discharge planning and complements the DH ten-step framework.

www.institute.nhs.uk/building_capability/general/aims.html

The home page for High Impact Actions: The Essential Collection. It contains useful information and examples of case studies.

www.qni.org.uk/wp-content/uploads/2016/09/discharge_planning_report_2015.pdf

This is a link to the document by the Queen's Nursing Institute, Discharge planning: best practice in transitions of care, which explores some of the challenges to effective discharge planning and guidance for nurses.

Chapter 7 Palliative care in long term conditions

2   Evidence based, best practice approaches to communication for supporting people of all ages, their families and carers in preventing ill health and managing their care

    2.9   engage in difficult conversations, including breaking bad news and support people who are feeling emotionally or physically vulnerable or in distress, conveying compassion and sensitivity

NMC Annexe B:

Nursing procedures

At the point of registration, the registered nurse will be able to safely demonstrate the following procedures:

Part 2: Procedures for the planning, provision and management of person-centred nursing care

10   Use evidence based, best practice approaches for meeting needs for care and support at end of life, accurately assessing a person's capacity for independence and self-care and initiating appropriate interventions

    10.3   assess and review preferences and care priorities of the dying person and their family and carers

    10.4   understand and apply organ and tissue donation protocols, advance planning decision, living wills and health and lasting power of attorney for health

    10.5   understand and apply DNARCPR (do not attempt cardiopulmonary resuscitation) decisions and verification of expected death

11   Procedural competencies required for best practice, evidence based medicines administration and optimisation

    11.2   recognise the various procedural routes under which medicines can be prescribed, supplied, dispensed and administered; and the laws, policies, regulations and guidance that underpin them

Chapter aims

After reading this chapter, you will be able to:

* discuss and apply the principles of breaking bad news to the care and management of people living with an LTC;
* explain what palliative care is and its role in the management of LTCs;

(Continued)

(Continued)

- explain strategies to support palliative and end-of-life care and their relevance to people living with LTCs;
- recognise the importance of holistic assessment for palliative care in the management of LTCs.

Introduction

You matter to us because you are you, and you matter to the last moment of your life. We will do all we can not only to help you die peacefully, but also to live until you die.

(Dame Cicely Saunders, 1994)

As mentioned in Chapter 1, the incidence of LTCs is rising; there are many LTCs where the trajectory of the condition is such that there will come a time when all curative treatment options have been tried. Traditionally, this has meant that there was a specific point in a person's journey when their treatment and care moved from curative to palliative. Nowadays, it is generally accepted that supportive and palliative care should start at diagnosis of a life-threatening illness, or LTC, and form part of the care along with curative/active treatment. Initially, supportive and palliative care may be a small part of the care and management of LTCs, and will run alongside health promotion, self-care and symptom management. However, as the person's LTC progresses and symptom management becomes increasingly difficult as the disease burden increases, supportive and palliative care will play a larger role in their care and management. Whether the emphasis on supportive and palliative care, rather than curative treatment, comes early or late in a person's journey, it is important that they are provided with the knowledge to enable them to make informed decisions about their care, and that they are able to discuss their fears and desires with those caring for them.

Talking about death and dying is not something we are comfortable with, as it reminds us of our own mortality; however, effectively supporting people receiving palliative care requires you to become involved and empathise with the person and their situation. Utilising the knowledge and skills developed in Chapter 2 will enable you to recognise your own fears, as well as those of the people in your care, allowing you to effectively support both individuals living with LTCs and those who care for them.

As the above quote emphasises, palliative care is about focusing on the person and enabling them to carry on 'living' until they die. The point where a person's care becomes more palliative and less curative should not be seen as the end of the journey. Rather, it should be viewed as a time when support is provided to enable the person to remain as active and as involved in their life and community for as long as possible and to die a 'good' death. This chapter will help you to develop your knowledge about palliative care and related areas so that you can feel more confident about caring for people during this important time. It will help you to source the relevant skills and information so that you are better equipped to enable people in the end stages of their life to live and die in the place of their choice and in a manner appropriate for them.

Breaking bad news in long term conditions

Chapter 1 introduced you to the concept of physical and psychological 'noise' in your communication with people living with LTCs. The impact of 'noise' was discussed in relation to the delivery of a diagnosis of an LTC and its perception as being 'bad news'. Bad news is described as any news that implies the loss of something that an individual values, such as physical ability, or that is life-changing, affecting an individual's perception of themselves in a negative way. For many people living with an LTC, the fact that their treatment is now being described as 'palliative' rather than 'curative' can be seen as further bad news, and this is compounded by the fact that they are now faced with the realisation that their disease has worsened and they are entering the final stages of their journey. This may result in them asking challenging questions.

Activity 7.1 Reflection

Many healthcare professionals find it difficult to answer awkward questions. Either on your own or with a group of your peers, reflect on your clinical experience and identify awkward questions you have been asked which you did not feel comfortable answering. Now answer the following questions.

- What was it about the question that made it awkward?
- How did you respond to the person's question?
- Would you do it differently now?

As the answers will be based on your own observations, there is no outline answer at the end of the chapter.

Undertaking Activity 7.1 will have identified to you that there are many questions that healthcare professionals find it awkward to answer, some of which are listed below.

- Am I going to die?
- Is there anything else that can be done?
- How long do I have left?

Being asked questions like these reminds us of our own mortality. In addition, we are worried about saying the wrong thing or we do not know how to answer such a question, and we are unprepared for the reaction of the person. The following reflective questions may be useful for you to use when asked similar questions in the future.

- What makes you ask me this question?
- What do you already understand about your condition?
- Would it help you to know more about your condition?
- Would you like to have a member of your family with you when you find out more about your condition?

This approach will enable you to explore the person's concerns without having to give information that you may not feel capable or competent to deliver.

Although answering awkward questions and, by extension, breaking bad news can be difficult and unpleasant for both the person receiving the news and the healthcare professional, it is important. An audit of people living with cancer by Cox et al. (2006) identified that the majority of patients wanted to be provided with all relevant information about their prognosis, good or bad. Understanding their situation reduces uncertainty. People have a greater sense of control, are better able to make informed decisions and are less likely to undergo ineffective treatments (Hancock et al., 2007). With accurate information, people are able to plan appropriately for their future facilitating end-of-life care planning. Given the complexities of breaking bad news, some approaches have been developed to support and guide the process (Baile et al., 2000; Narayanan et al., 2010).

Approaches to use when breaking bad news in LTCs

Bad news should be delivered in a sensitive manner, allowing the person to feel that they have been listened to and understood. The person, their carer and family should leave knowing what the plan for their future care and treatment is. However, it should be recognised that this is the first point in a process of providing information to people and their families, rather than an isolated event.

To support healthcare professionals in breaking bad news, specific approaches have been developed. These include Baile et al.'s SPIKES six-step protocol (2000), Nardi and Keefe-Cooperman's PEWTER model (2006) and Narayanan et al.'s BREAKS protocol (2010). The following protocols were designed for different client groups.

- SPIKES – initially used in oncology care, particularly in relationship to a cancer recurrence or when palliative and/or hospice care was indicated.
- PEWTER – used primarily in acute mental health as a framework for difficult conversations – for example, suicide risk; additionally, it has been used by counsellors when explaining to parents that their child has a disability.
- BREAKS – devised to support doctors through enabling person-centred communication, addressing a person's feelings and responding with empathy.

While these protocols make the assumption that 'breaking bad news' can be planned for in the setting/background step, this is not always the case. As you may know from your clinical practice, and as reflected on in Activity 7.1, patients often ask questions on the spur of the moment. Whether you are able to plan for the conversation or not, you can use elements of these protocols to support sensitive, person-centred communication. Table 7.1 outlines Baile et al.'s SPIKES six-step protocol (2000), Nardi and Keefe-Cooperman's PEWTER model (2006) and Narayanan et al.'s BREAKS protocol (2010) and applies them to your practice.

SPIKES six-step protocol (Baile et al., 2000)	PEWTER (Nardi and Keefe-Cooperman, 2006)	BREAKS protocol (Narayanan et al., 2010)	Areas to consider
Setting	Prepare	Background	Know all the facts before the consultation, including patient's emotional state and support system, consider what language to use that will promote patient inclusion and understanding. Ensure privacy and comfort, switch off mobile phones and allow time for the meeting.
			If responding to 'spur of the moment' questions, try to ensure privacy. If in a hospital setting, pull curtains and, if possible, find a quiet room away from the ward area.
			Check that all the appropriate people are there; remember in some cultures it would be expected that the head of the family is present.
Perception	Evaluate	Rapport	Ask the person what they understand is happening: 'Do you know why we are meeting today?' and 'What is your main concern right now?' Use the response to this question to correct misinformation and consider possible solutions.
			Use open questions to develop a rapport; ask for a narrative of events from the person to determine their perception of the illness: 'Could you tell me . . . ' or 'How did it all start?' You could use one of the reflective questions listed after activity 7.1 to encourage the person to talk. Allow the person to complete their narrative before asking questions, listen to what they are saying and identify cues to explore further. Maintain a calm environment, observe non-verbal communication and be alert to yours, maintain an open body posture and attentive facial expression. Avoid making premature reassurances; explore the patient's (and family's) understanding of their condition and beliefs about their situation.
Invitation		Exploring	Obtain permission for the person for more information: 'Would you like me to explain a bit more?' Remember that for the person, it can be frightening asking for more information – how much do they want to know?

(Continued)

Table 7.1   (Continued)

SPIKES six-step protocol (Baile et al., 2000)	PEWTER (Nardi and Keefe-Cooperman, 2006)	BREAKS protocol (Narayanan et al., 2010)	Areas to consider
Knowledge	Warning and telling	Announce	Warn first about sharing bad news: 'I'm afraid this is rather serious' or 'The news is not what we had hoped for'. Allow a brief pause before going on to say what the news is, which allows the person to prepare psychologically for the news. Be aware of non-verbal communication; adopt an open body position. Denial is a natural coping mechanism. Allow the person to control how much information is given – for example, by asking 'How much would you like to know?' Narrow the information gap by providing information in simple language; ask them to summarise the information you have given them to check their understanding before continuing: 'Please explain back what you understand, I really want to make sure I was clear.' Try to 'chunk' information, providing no more than three pieces of information before checking understanding. Avoid being blunt, giving incomplete information or false hope. The detail may not be remembered, but how you gave the information will be.
Emotion	Emotional response	Kindling	This involves both your emotional response and the response of the recipients, including your non-verbal communication. People will respond in different ways; allow for expression of feelings. Some may want to get up and move around, others might respond with 'black' humour; allow time for this emotional outlet. Respond with empathy: 'What are your main concerns at the moment?' and address the person's concerns and emotions: 'This must be difficult for you.' Explore and validate the person's feelings: 'It is only natural that you feel this way.' For the person, this is the most important part in relation to their satisfaction with the meeting. Be alert to differential listening, when the patient only hears what they want to hear; conclude the meeting completely, clearly identifying areas to revisit at a later date.
Summary	Regrouping	Summarise	Review the information discussed and provide a summary, written if necessary. While the person may leave with information that is life-changing, answering questions, discussing options and putting together plans for future care can instil hope. Offer availability: some details may not be remembered; further support will be needed and they may need time to talk to the family. If the person is on their own, find out if there is someone that they would like to have contacted.

Table 7.1   Areas to consider when using Baile et al.'s SPIKES six-step protocol (2000), Nardi and Keefe-Cooperman's PEWTER model (2006), and Narayanan et al.'s BREAKS protocol (2010)

As the protocols discussed in Table 7.1 identify in the emotion/emotional, response/ kindling and summary/regrouping/summarise sections, breaking bad news should not be an isolated event. Rather, it is the first point in a process of providing information to people and their families (Tobin and Begley, 2008). People and their carer/families should be provided with a further opportunity to meet with healthcare staff to discuss their situation, and have any concerns and questions answered.

Activity 7.2   Evidence-based practice

Using a previous experience from your clinical practice when you have witnessed 'bad news' being broken, identify whether parts of Baile et al.'s SPIKES six-step protocol, Nardi and Keefe-Cooperman's PEWTER model or Narayanan et al.'s BREAKS were used and consider the following points.

- Identify what parts were used.
- If they were used, how effective were they?
- If they were not used, how would using this protocol have improved the situation?

As the answers will be based on your own observations, there is no outline answer at the end of the chapter.

When undertaking Activity 7.2, you may have identified that aspects of all three models were used or that you take aspects from one or more model, or you may find one mnemonic easier to remember. This is fine, as you are demonstrating your ability to apply theoretical models to your clinical practice and adapting these, if necessary, to suit your practice. Reflecting on your response to the activities in this section and using the approaches in Table 7.1 should help you to improve the process of breaking bad news, both for yourself, as the person delivering the bad news, and for the person receiving the bad news.

Breaking bad news to people with a learning disability

People with a learning disability (LD) have a higher mortality rate (Heslop and Glover, 2015) and die at a younger age (Public Health England, 2016) than those, in the general population, who do not have an LD. In addition, the life expectancy of people with an LD is increasing and with this, so is the incidence of them developing a life-threatening condition (Dunkley and Sales, 2014). Yet it is known that many people with an LD are not included in discussions about their diagnosis, prognosis and treatment options (Tuffrey-Wijne *et al.*, 2010). A systematic literature review carried out by Brownrigg (2018) explored the reasons why relative and healthcare professionals disclose, or not, bad news to people with an LD. Their review highlighted the complex nature of disclosing bad news to this group of patients. The themes identi-fied, in favour of disclosing, cited maintaining the rights and dignity of the person and healthcare professionals upholding their duty of care. The themes identified, in rela-tion to non-disclosure, included underestimating the resilience of the person with an LD to cope with the knowledge of their diagnosis and wanting to protect the person. The final theme relating to non-disclosure focused on understanding.

As with the PEWTER model of breaking bad news (Nardi and Keefe-Cooperman, 2006), Tuffrey-Wijne (2012) recognises that breaking bad news to people with an LD should be viewed as an ongoing process where knowledge is discussed in blocks and built on over time. This has been incorporated into new guidelines (Tuffrey-Wijne, 2012) in the following areas.

- Understanding – this focuses on the issue of capacity; to do this, it is important that you are aware of the legislation around capacity and how it applies to the individual person's situation. It is generally accepted that everyone is assumed to have capacity unless it can be proved otherwise. Having capacity means that a person has the ability to understand information, retain this and use it to make a specific decision. Knowing how much a person understands is important, as it will determine when and how bad news is broken.
- People – all people involved in the care of a person with an LD have a role to play in assisting the person to understand what has been said. Using a carer's knowledge of how a person communicates and their life history can support the person breaking the bad news to identify what blocks of information should be given and when. It is also important to take into consideration the views of the carer, although this should not focus on their 'wishes' – for example, they may not want the person to be told the bad news. However, everyone who has capacity has the right to be given information, unless they choose otherwise.
- Support – this includes support for the person with an LD and their family and carers; it should be recognised that in some cases formal carers may have been looking after the person for some time and will have developed a close therapeutic relationship with them. Ongoing support for the person with an LD will be needed; therefore, it is important that those caring for them are equipped with the knowledge and skills to do this.

Within these guidelines, it is recognised that capacity can change and that this should be reviewed at every interaction. However sensitively bad news is broken, the reaction of the person, and their family, to the news can be unpredictable. Knowing the person and how they have reacted to previous bad news will help you to support them during this stage.

Reactions to bad news

From your previous clinical and life experiences, you will be aware that people react to hearing bad news in a variety of ways. Their initial reactions may include denial ('I don't believe this'), numbness ('This can't be happening'), anger ('I knew there was something wrong – if only the tests had been carried out sooner') and grief. A person's reactions depend on the size of the loss and their usual coping mechanisms. How well they have coped with previous 'bad news' and changes in the status of their LTC will be an indicator as to how well they will cope with the news that their treatment is changing from curative to palliative. Many people put on a 'brave face' and, at the time of hearing the news, are able to conduct a rational dialogue, asking for further information and rechecking what has already been said. This is their way of confirming the reality of their situation as psychologically they struggle to come to terms with the news. However, as noted in Table 7.1, it is likely that they will not remember the details of the consultation and the information provided, so it is important to review their understanding at a later date. Early reactions to the news such as anger, guilt and sadness may also be present; anger may be expressed towards family and members of the healthcare team. You should remember that the person is not angry with you, but at the news that has been delivered. Once the initial reaction to the news has passed, some later reactions and coping mechanisms that people display include:

- fighting spirit – 'I will not let this beat me';
- stoical acceptance – 'This is how it is and I will just have to get on with it';
- denial – 'There is nothing wrong with me';
- resigned helplessness – 'What is the point in doing anything – the damage is already done?'.

Perhaps the most definitive work that researched people's responses to bad news is that of Elisabeth Kübler-Ross, who in 1969 completed a study that focused on people's reactions to their own dying and death. During this study, she interviewed over 200 people about their thoughts and feelings in relation to their dying and death. The result of this work was the five stages of dying: denial, anger, bargaining, depression and acceptance (Kübler-Ross, 2009). It should be noted that Kübler-Ross emphasised that these were the stages that people may go through and that they may not progress through them in a linear manner.

> *The stages have evolved since their introduction, and they have been very misunderstood over the past three decades. They were never meant to help tuck messy emotions into neat packages. They are responses to loss that many people have, but there is not a typical response to loss, as there is no typical loss. Our grief is as individual as our lives. Not everyone goes through all of them or in a prescribed order.*

(Kübler-Ross and Kessler, 2005, p7)

While Kübler-Ross does provide you with a framework, you should remember that it is not always easy to separate out the emotional (anger) and the cognitive (acceptance), and that these can be interdependent and displayed at the same time. Additionally, people may display other emotions such as disbelief and confusion in addition to anger and depression. Over time, the stages of dying have been applied to those who are grieving; however, their relevance to grieving has been questioned. Kübler-Ross stated that the bargaining stage was a time when the dying person makes a commitment to something and is rewarded for this by their death being postponed. It could be argued that, for a bereaved person, it is too late for bargaining, as the death has already occurred (Calderwood, 2011). To support you in your care of the bereaved, there are many available bereavement theories that are more suited for use with those who are bereaved. See the further reading list at the end of this chapter. At whatever point in the course of a person's illness bad news is broken, what is important is that their ongoing palliative care needs are met. However, for the progression of some LTCs (e.g., COPD, heart failure), it can be difficult to predict and many people will have lived through many exacerbations of their condition. It is essential, therefore, to ensure that the relevant care and management is in place early for these people, allowing for maximum symptom relief and quality of life.

Palliative care

Palliative care is an approach to a person's care that improves the quality of their life, and that of their carer and family, when they are living with an advanced and progressive illness. The term 'palliative' is derived from the Latin word *pallium*, which means 'cloak or cover'; in palliative care, a person's symptoms are not cured but 'cloaked' or minimised, through effective symptom management. The aim is to promote comfort, without cure, and to achieve a good quality of life: *May you be wrapped in tenderness, you my brother, as if in a cloak* (Qu'ran). Chapter 5 of this book discusses the use of effective care planning in symptom management; the same principles should be applied when managing symptoms in palliative care. Quality of life is improved through the early identification of problems, and the accurate assessment and treatment of them. Problems may be physical (e.g., pain), psychological (e.g., fear), social (e.g., stigma) and spiritual (e.g., loss of meaning). The WHO (2002, p84) states that palliative care:

- provides relief from pain and other distressing symptoms;
- affirms life and regards dying as a natural process;
- intends neither to hasten nor postpone death;
- integrates the psychosocial and spiritual aspects of patient care;
- offers a support system to help patients live as actively as possible until death;
- offers a support system to help the family cope during the patient's illness and in their own bereavement;
- uses a team approach to address the needs of patients and their families, including bereavement counselling, if indicated;
- will enhance quality of life, and may also positively influence the course of illness;
- is applicable early in the course of illness, in conjunction with other therapies that are intended to prolong life, such as chemotherapy or radiation therapy, and includes those investigations needed to better understand and manage distressing clinical complications.

Given that the disease progression of different LTCs varies – some people experience a sudden decline; others experience both a gradual decline and acute episodes; while others have a steady yet progressive decline – it is important to view palliative care as part of the continuum of care that people living with LTCs receive. As a person's LTC progresses and their symptoms increase, treatment that is aimed at modifying the LTC decreases, and at this point palliative care increases, providing support for the person and their carer and family before, during and after the person's death (see Figure 7.1).

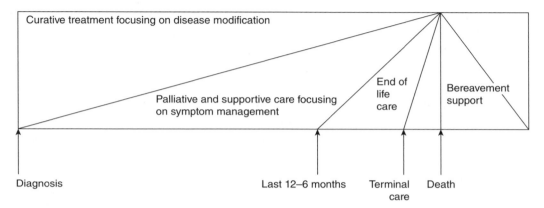

Figure 7.1   The need for care before, during and after a person's death

Activity 7.3   Reflection

Either on your own, or with a colleague, reflect on the care and management of a person living with an LTC and write down/discuss whether the diagram in Figure 7.1 represents how palliative care was used as part of the person's care and management, taking into consideration the following.

- Was this representation of palliative care used? If so, how?
- If it was not used, why was this? What difference might it have made to the person's care and management?

As the answers will be based on your own observations, there is no outline answer at the end of the chapter.

Hopefully, Activity 7.3 will have allowed you to see that palliative and end-of-life care are integral parts of a person's care and management. This approach means that palliative care is not delivered in a specific care setting; it can be delivered in a number of settings – e.g., a person's own home, acute hospital, nursing home or a hospice. Neither is it provided by one specific group of healthcare professionals: it is provided by many, including Macmillan nurses, district nurses, GPs and healthcare professionals working in secondary and tertiary care.

The Gold Standards Framework

The Gold Standards Framework (GSF) is a UK-wide evidence-based approach that can be used to support you to deliver effective palliative care in any setting. The GSF focuses on enabling people to live well in the last years, months or days of their life (Thomas, 2003). The main focus of the GSF is to enable you, as part of a healthcare team, to work collaboratively to maximise a person's continuity of care, identify their priorities for care, introduce advance care planning, promote symptom control and provide ongoing support. Through the use of GP practice-based palliative care registers, linked to the Quality Outcome Framework (see Chapter 1), those receiving palliative care are easily identified to all members of the team, improving communication and the care received. The GSF incorporates seven standards of care that relate to the effective delivery of holistic palliative care for people living with an LTC. Emphasis is placed on both direct care and management, and the management and coordination of the healthcare professionals delivering the care (Thomas, 2003). Table 7.2 outlines these standards and their aims.

GSF standards of care	Aim and areas to consider
Communication	The aim of this standard is to improve how information is communicated (written, verbal and electronic) and who is involved in any communication (person receiving palliative care, out-of-hours, family, etc.). A supportive care register allows a GP practice to record, monitor and review the care received by people in the last 6–12 months of their life. Through the use of monthly meetings, proactive care and management can be planned, with ACP being incorporated if required.
Coordination	The aim of this standard is to ensure that the care delivered to people requiring palliative care is well organised and coordinated with communication being maintained. Each PHCT should have a nominated palliative care coordinator – e.g., practice nurse, district nurse. The palliative care coordinator is responsible for maintaining relevant paperwork, including the supportive care register, arranging the monthly meetings and ensuring appropriate tools such as PEPSICOLA are used.
Control of symptoms	The aim of this standard is to promote effective symptom management through the use of appropriate assessment such as PEPSICOLA. Each person receiving palliative care is assured of having a holistic assessment with the results being discussed and an appropriate person-centred plan of care being devised.
Continuity	The aim of this standard is to ensure continuity of care during out-of-hours, ensuring that the person receiving palliative care is supported during out-of-hours. Using the protocol devised by Calderdale and Kirklees Health Authority (Thomas, 2003) will promote continuity of care. It addresses four key areas: • communication – between GP/district nurse and out-of-hours service; • carer support – does the carer know what to do in a crisis? is a night sitter required? • medical support – any anticipated management documented in handover form; • drugs/equipment – leave any anticipated medication in person's home.

GSF standards of care	Aim and areas to consider
Continued learning	The aim of this standard is to promote reflective learning or 'learning as you go' to further develop the care given to people receiving palliative care. Through the use of practice-based teaching, significant event analysis and other learning opportunities, the professional development of those caring for people requiring palliative care is enhanced. Learning should focus on all areas of palliative care: strategic (planning of resources/coordination of services), clinical (treatment/management options) and personal (communication skills).
Carer support	The aim of this standard is to improve carer support: carers are key in enabling people receiving palliative care to remain in their own home. Through the provision of emotional and practical support, carers are empowered to play as active a part as they would like to. Carer support does not stop when the person dies: bereavement support should be offered.
Care of the dying (terminal phase)	The aim of this standard is to promote suitable care in the last days of a person's life. Using such tools as the Liverpool Care Pathway for the Dying Patient will ensure that non-essential treatment is stopped, the person's symptoms are controlled, and psychological and religious/spiritual support is available.

Table 7.2 The 7Cs of the GSF (based on the work of Thomas, 2003)

As mentioned earlier in this chapter, palliative care should run alongside curative treatments. However, there will come a point at which conversations should take place about end-of-life care and specific requirements such as advance care planning. The General Medical Council (2013) states that people are approaching end of life if they are likely to die within 12 months. To support you to identify when people are nearing the end of their life and requiring additional supportive care, the Gold Standards Framework Proactive Identification Guidance (PIG) can be used. The GSF and PIG encourage you to 'Ask the Surprise Question': *Would you be surprised if the patient were to die in the next year, months, weeks, days?* If you would not be surprised, then it is time to begin the GSF process: identify, assess, plan. In addition to this, PIG also includes general and disease-specific indicators of decline that you can use to further identify and assess a person's level of need (Gold Standards Framework, 2016).

Preferred priorities for care

A systematic review on adult preferences for place of care at end of life or place of death carried out in 2013 (Gomes et al., 2013) identified that between 52 and 92 per cent of people not diagnosed with a 'life-threatening illness' would prefer to die at home. It could be said that asking this question to people who are not faced with the reality that they will die may not provide a true reflection of what actually occurs. This could be especially true if the lead up to a person's death is sudden or particularly challenging to manage. However, a narrative appraisal of people's preferences in relation to dying at home by Higginson et al. (2013) found that for the majority of people approaching the end of their life, home remains their preferred place of care and that this preference remains stable as their condition deteriorates. In addition, Higginson et al. (2017) explored the preferred place of care among older adults. In this population, home was the preferred place of death in 56 per cent of the participants, followed by inpatient hospice settings (22 percent), with hospital being the least preferred place of death. Currently, however, the majority of people do not die in their own home; 54 per cent of people die in hospital, meaning that approximately 60–70 per cent of people do not die in their preferred place (Royal College of General Practitioners, 2013). This is supported by research by Hunt et al. (2014) who carried out a post-bereavement survey exploring the place of death. Their research identified that only 49.3 per cent of bereaved people who had stated a preference to die at home managed to do so. Within this, those who died of cancer were more likely to die at home (62.4 per cent v. 29.7 per cent), while those who died of cardiovascular disease were least likely to die at home (12.8 per cent v. 26.7 per cent). To address this challenge, advance care planning was introduced, with the preferred priorities for care process being part of this.

The preferred priorities for care (PCC) is a voluntary process. Using the GSF framework, in particular PIG, can support healthcare professionals to identify people requiring palliative and end-of-life care. PPC, however, allows those receiving palliative and/or end-of-life care to prepare for their future. It provides the person receiving palliative care to consider, discuss and document their preferences and priorities for the care they receive at end of life. The completed document is kept by the person receiving palliative care, and the information on the PPC is shared with those planning and delivering their care. It documents aspects of their future care that is important to them, such as 'Where would you like to be cared for in the future?' and 'What are your priorities for your future care?', and focuses on the person's beliefs and values. You can then use this information to ensure that the care you deliver takes into account what is important to that person. Relevant information from the PPC can also be used in future care planning. This is particularly useful should a person receiving palliative care no longer be able to make decisions themselves – for example, a person with dementia or a degenerative neurological condition. It should not be used to record information relating to refusal of medical treatment, as the PPC is not a legally binding document. However, it is recognised that, under the Mental Capacity Act (2005), if a person has already completed a PPC and no longer has capacity to make decisions, the information recorded in their PPC should be taken into account. You should endeavour to ensure that a person keeps their PPC up to date as their wishes and views may change over time (Cancer Research UK, 2014). For those living with dementia or a degenerative neurological condition and who lack mental capacity, it may be necessary to discuss having a lasting power of attorney (LPA)/power of attorney (PoA). An LPA/PoA is a document that allows people living with LTCs to choose someone to make decisions on their behalf when they lack the mental capacity to do so themselves. Within the UK, there may be slight variations in law as it relates to LPA/PoA and mental capacity, so you will need to familiarise yourself with the law as it relates to mental capacity and LPA/PoA in the country where you work.

Advance care planning

Advanced care planning (ACP) is a voluntary process that allows for an open and structured discussion between the person receiving palliative care and those caring for them, including their family and carer. While these might have occurred informally, ACP allows for the person's preferences to be recorded and communicated between members of the health and social care team. ACP differs from traditional care planning, which addresses current areas of need, such as reduced nutritional intake and how they are to be managed. ACP addresses a person's anticipated deterioration and what their preferences for treatment would be; this is especially relevant should the person's ability to communicate reduce or their capacity to make decisions deteriorate (GSF, 2018). As such, ACP is recognised within the Mental Capacity Act (2005); ACP is a simple process, compiling the following five steps (GSF, 2018).

- Think – about your future and what is important to you, what would you like to happen, or not to happen, should you become unwell.
- Talk – to your family/friends/carer, ask someone to be your spokesperson or LPA/ PoA if you are not able to speak for yourself.
- Record – write down your thoughts, including who your spokesperson is and store this safely.
- Discuss – your plans with your health and social care team; this may include conversations about resuscitation or refusing further treatment.
- Share – this information with other people who need to know about you, through health records, and review it regularly.

It is important that any discussions you have are documented, reviewed regularly and communicated to appropriate people, including the person's carer and family, if required. Within the ACP framework there are two ways in which a person can state their preferences regarding their future care and management: (1) what you want to happen – an Advance Statement of preferences; and (2) what you do not want to happen – an Advance Decision to Refuse Treatment. Before discussing either of these options with a person in your care, it is essential that you have an understanding of mental capacity and its relevance to ACP. Within the UK, there may be slight variations in the law as it relates to ACP and mental capacity, so you will need to familiarise yourself with the law as it relates to mental capacity and ACP in the country where you work.

Advance statement of preferences

An Advance Statement of preferences (AS) allows the person living with an LTC, who is in the palliative stages of their illness, to either write down or verbally express and have documented their preferences in relation to future treatment. This may take the form of explaining their feelings, beliefs and values that influence how they make decisions. It may also include areas of a person's care such as where they would like to be cared for and what types of treatment they are prepared to have. While this is not a legally binding document, it does have legal standing as part of the Mental Capacity Act (MCA, 2005) and should be taken into account when deciding on a person's future treatment options.

Advance decision to refuse treatment

Some people living with LTCs may have strong feelings about specific treatments they would not want to have. In order to have this recognised, it is necessary for an advance decision to refuse treatment (an Advance Directive) to be made. An advance decision to refuse treatment is a legally binding document and is part of the MCA (2005) and should only be made under the guidance of a healthcare professional who understands the process. It only applies if the person making the decision is over the age of 18 and has the mental capacity to make the necessary decision and will only come into effect if the person loses their capacity to make decisions about their treatment. An advance decision to refuse treatment allows the person to specifically express and have documented the type of medical treatment they wish to refuse – e.g., being treated with antibiotics for a chest infection. It must relate to specific treatments and circumstances and will only come into effect at these times (National End of Life Care Programme and National Council for Palliative Care, 2013)).

ACP is a voluntary process that should be initiated by the person receiving the care. It should be handled sensitively and by a healthcare professional who has a clear understanding of the person's clinical condition, treatments options and side effects, and the legal and ethical issues involved. If you are uncertain about any of these, or lack the required knowledge, then ask a colleague who does to lead the discussions. To enable open and honest communication during palliative and end-of-life care, the importance of developing a therapeutic relationship cannot be underestimated. Discussions around palliative care should be carried out by those who have a rapport with the person and their family. The aspects of the GSF outlined above are there to support you in your delivery of appropriate and effective palliative care to people living with an LTC. Regardless of whether the person you are caring for has made explicit their preferences for care, ensuring that they are assessed correctly and that the care delivered meets their needs is your priority.

Activity 7.4 Advance Care Planning

Having read the information on the Gold Standards Framework and Advance Care Planning above, compile a strengths, weaknesses, concerns and expectations analysis regarding how competent you feel in having conversations about palliative and end-of-life care with people.

Identify one of your weaknesses or concerns and compile a learning plan to address this.

Identify learning need	Specify learning objective: what else will you learn by achieving this?	Identify the learning resources and strategies needed: what will help you to learn?	Provide evidence to demonstrate this has been met: how do I know and prove what I have learnt?	Evaluation of learning and the process of learning: did you learn what you set out to learn?

You might find the further reading and useful websites sections at the end of this chapter useful in compiling your learning plan.

As the answers will be based on your own observations, there is no outline answer at the end of the chapter.

When completing your learning plan in Activity 7.4, in the learning resources section you may have identified spending time working with other members of the healthcare team involved in delivering palliative care as a way to improve your competence; these could be both generalist and specialist professionals.

Holistic palliative care in long term conditions

Palliative care is delivered by a variety of healthcare professionals in a variety of settings and can be provided by both generalist and specialist healthcare professionals. Generalists should be able to provide the day-to-day care for people requiring palliative care, their carer and family through effective assessment, management and appropriate referral to specialist services. Specialists, such as palliative care consultants and clinical nurse specialists, are healthcare professionals with a high level of knowledge and skill in the field of palliative care who are responsible for directing a plan of care that allows for the integration of available resources and services. This may include providing care and management in the person's home or in a local hospice, and bereavement support.

Assessing for holistic palliative care

To enable both generalists and specialists to provide coordinated care to the person requiring palliative care and their family, it is important to fully assess the person and their needs. The GSF recommends the use of the PEPSICOLA approach. Table 7.3 provides an overview of this, with prompts for you to consider.

PEPSICOLA	Consider	Resources to access
P: physical	Assess symptoms and overall management plan, review medication and stop non-essential treatment. Identify the person's priorities: is there a specific concern and what effect is this having on their ADLs? Discuss options and explore any fears.	• Evidence-based assessment tools – e.g., pain • Specialist palliative care clinicians • Day services – e.g., day hospice • Members of the multidisciplinary team
E: emotional	Consider what the person knows about their condition, how they and their family are coping and what signifies deterioration for that person. What impact is this having on the person and their family, what have they done to manage their situation – e.g., relaxation – and what else could be done?	• Psychological assessment tool – e.g., distress thermometer • Refer for appropriate support
P: personal	Recognise cultural background, language, sexuality, spirituality and religious needs, and find out their beliefs and faith. Has their situation affected these? Identify any requirements for spiritual support. Does the person have any life goals they would like to achieve?	• Specific information for different populations – e.g., Marie Curie: caring for LGBT people at end of life • Local hospital/hospice switchboard • Hospital multi-faith centres
S: social support	Carry out a DS1500 assessment and carer assessment if not already completed. Where is the person's PPC? Identify what support the person is receiving and whether it needs reviewing.	• Social services • Citizens Advice Bureau • Community equipment services • Local support/ community groups
I: information and communication	Communication between the person and the healthcare team and vice versa. How will the healthcare team communicate with each other? Is the person aware of the plans and do they understand them? Is the mode of communication appropriate?	• Patient-held records • Macmillan, Marie Curie website • Patient information leaflets/sources
C: control and autonomy	Consider mental capacity and discuss treatment options, including, if required, PPC and ACP. Is there any conflict between the person and their family/carer?	• Single point of contact • Patient-held records • Advance Care Plan in place • GSF register
O: out-of-hours	Does the person know who to contact during out-of-hours and what carer support is available? Consider medication for use out-of-hours.	• Single point of contact • Patient held record • DNARCPR • Advance Care Plan in place

PEPSICOLA	Consider	Resources to access
L: living with your illness	Rehabilitation support, referral to other agencies and end-of-life planning (if appropriate). How are you managing daily tasks? Have you been able to discuss your future goals?	• Refer to members of the multidisciplinary team – e.g., physio • Self-support programmes • Intermediate/ rehabilitation services
A: after care	Planning for bereavement; consider post-bereavement support. Are there funeral arrangements? Do you require bereavement services information?	• Bereavement services information • Contact number for follow-up, if needed • Timely removal of equipment

Table 7.3 Areas to consider when completing an assessment using either PEPSICOLA (Thomas, 2003) or the holistic common assessment (NHS Improving Quality, 2010)

Case study: Andrew

Despite trying to improve both his levels of exercise and his nutritional intake, Andrew's condition has continued to deteriorate. He has continued to have recurrent chest infections that have reduced his appetite further, increased his level of dyspnoea and drastically reduced his exercise tolerance. Since his last chest infection he has required **long term oxygen therapy** (LTOT) at home due to reduced oxygen saturation levels. David (Andrew's community matron) has graded his dyspnoea at 4 on the Medical Research Council dyspnoea scale. This indicates that Andrew has to stop for breath after walking about 100 metres or after a few minutes on level ground. His most recent **spirometry** result stated that his FEV1 (forced expired volume) was 30 per cent, indicating end-stage COPD. Both Andrew's GP and David are concerned about his deteriorating condition and have asked each other the 'surprise' question: 'Would you be surprised if this person were to die in the next 6–12 months?' They both answered no to this question (RCGP, 2008).

With the consent of his GP, David has discussed the results of Andrew's spirometry with him and what this means for his future care, with the emphasis being on palliative care. Andrew has said that he would like to stay in his flat for as long as possible. However, he is now requiring homecare assistance in the morning and evening to assist him with his personal hygiene. He has a hot meal delivered three days a week; on the other days, his carers make and leave sandwiches for him. A neighbour in the sheltered housing accommodation cooks a hot meal for him at the weekend. He is finding the change in his situation rather lonely, as he is not able to get out and about. Recently, he has begun to talk about his wife Elizabeth.

Activity 7.5   Critical thinking

Drawing on the above information and the information in Chapter 6, use the PEPSICOLA/holistic common assessment framework to assess Andrew's needs in relation to his palliative care.

A brief outline answer is given at the end of the chapter.

Having used the PEPSICOLA/holistic common assessment framework to assess Andrew's needs (Activity 7.5) and using the nursing process, you are now able to plan and implement an appropriate plan of care that will address Andrew's ongoing health-care needs. Part of his plan may include anticipatory prescribing, which ensures that the necessary medications and means to administer them will be readily available to him, should he require them following an appropriate assessment. In many cases, anticipatory prescribing takes the form of a 'just-in-case box'. Just-in-case boxes are patient specific and should include written information about administration, such as algorithms. Additionally, medication should be checked regularly, both to check expiry dates and to ensure that nothing has been removed. Using just-in-case boxes has been linked to reducing admission to hospital for people at end of life, supporting a person to die in their preferred place of care.

Chapter summary

This chapter has provided you with an overview of breaking bad news, the components of the GSF and holistic patient assessment. These important areas are all key aspects of the care and management of people living with an LTC. It has outlined some approaches that can be used when breaking bad news and applied these to your clinical practice. The GSF has been been outlined in relation to providing appropriate care for people living with an LTC. Finally, the importance of undertaking a holistic assessment has been discussed and applied to your clinical practice.

Having read through this chapter and undertaken the activities, you will have developed your knowledge and skills in relation to the principles of breaking bad news, palliative care and how to assess a person's holistic palliative care needs. How you use the information in this chapter will depend on where you are working and your current roles and responsibilities. However, as a nurse, you can ensure that planning for palliative care becomes part of your overall care and management of people living with an LTC. By having an increased awareness of some of the approaches that can be used when breaking bad news, you will be better able to answer awkward questions and support those in your care. Increasing your knowledge of palliative care and the EoLC strategy will allow you to provide appropriate and relevant information to both the person living with an LTC and their carer, allowing them to make informed choices. Using frameworks such as PEPSICOLA will promote the delivery of person-centred holistic care that meets the ongoing needs of the person, their carer and family.

Activities: brief outline answers

Activity 7.5 Critical thinking (page 158)

P: physical	Review of Andrew's medication, use of bronchodilators and inhaled corticosteroids. Ongoing LTOT assessment and review: ensure that Andrew is aware of the health and safety issues. Comprehensive assessment regarding other possible symptoms – e.g., pain, nutritional intake.
E: emotional	Having spoken to his community matron, Andrew is aware that his condition has deteriorated. He is concerned about being on his own as he is no longer able to get out and about as much as he could. Andrew has started talking about his wife Elizabeth recently; this may mean that he is beginning to think about his own death. It is essential that Andrew knows who and how to contact people should his condition deteriorate. If he does not have one, then a pendant alarm would be appropriate.
P: personal	We don't know a lot about Andrew's personal beliefs; this is the time to begin to discuss these with him. It may be useful to find out what kind of funeral service he arranged for Elizabeth.
S: social support	Is Andrew claiming all the available benefits? Has a DS1500 been completed? Social isolation is a potential problem; Andrew enjoys company but may become increasingly isolated due to his dyspnoea. Does he have all the necessary aids at home to promote his independence? Andrew has indicated that he would like to stay in his flat for as long as possible; how to manage this and alternatives may have to be discussed.
I: information and communication	Does Andrew hold a copy of his case notes? Are they accessible to all relevant members of the PHCT? Andrew has a community matron. Does he know how to contact her? Andrew is aware that his condition is deteriorating and it may be appropriate to discuss issues such as his will with him.
C: control and autonomy	We do not know what Andrew's thoughts are on his future care, apart from the fact that he would like to stay in his flat for as long as possible. It is necessary to discuss preferred place of care and advance directives with him to ensure that his wishes are met.
O: out-of-hours	Communication between the community matron, GP and out-of-hours service should ensure that all know what to do in the case of a deterioration in Andrew's condition. Andrew should know who and how to contact the out-of-hours service.
L: late	Not yet applicable, though through effective communication and working in partnership with Andrew when the time comes, it should be possible to discuss end-of-life issues to ensure appropriate care.
A: after	This may not be discussed, though allowing Andrew time to talk about Elizabeth and her death may enable everyone involved to talk to Andrew about his own funeral.

Further reading

Brownrigg, S (2018) Breaking bad news to people with learning disabilities: a literature review. *British Journal of Learning Disabilities,* 46(4): 225–33.

Buglass, E (2010) Grief and bereavement theories. *Nursing Standard,* 24(41): 44–7.

Nicol, J and Nyatanga, B (2016) *Palliative and End of Life Care in Nursing.* London: Sage Publishing.

This book covers a range of topics relating to palliative and end-of-life care, and provides practical advice and support to enhance the knowledge and skills of carers of people who are receiving palliative and end-of-life care.

Warnock, C (2014) Breaking bad news: issues relating to nursing practice. *Nursing Standard,* 28(45): 51–8.

Useful websites

www.breakingbadnews.org

This website contains useful information about how to break bad news to people with a learning disability.

www.dyingmatters.org

This is the website for Dying Matters aimed at promoting public awareness of dying, death and bereavement. It has a range of useful information for health professionals and the public.

www.goldstandardsframework.org.uk

This is a UK-wide framework aimed at enabling generalists to maximise the care they deliver to people nearing the end of their life. This website provides information regarding all aspects of the GSF, including how to use it in a variety of settings – e.g., continuing care, secondary care, available research and the GSF toolkit.

www.ncpc.org.uk

The National Council for Palliative Care (NCPC) is an umbrella organisation for all those involved in providing, commissioning and using palliative care services in England, Wales and Northern Ireland. Its aim is to promote palliative care for all who need it. This site contains useful information on all aspects of palliative care, including publications.

www.palliativecarescotland.org.uk

This organisation has the same remit as the NCPC but in Scotland; it supports and contributes to the strategic direction of palliative care in Scotland. This site contains information on all aspects of their work, including publications.

Glossary

autonomy   when a person is able to make decisions about, and take responsibility for, their own situation.

comorbidity   the presence of one or more diseases and the effect of these diseases on the person.

concordance   agreement to participate in something – for example, concordance with medication regime, i.e., a person agreeing with the prescriber to take their prescribed medication as directed.

determinants of health   the factors that affect a person's health and include the person's social and economic environment, the person's physical environment and the person's individual characteristics and behaviour.

enabling   assisting a person to become able to do something, to make something possible.

Gleason score   a grading system used to help anticipate the prognosis of prostate cancer, using samples of tissue taken during a biopsy.

long term oxygen therapy (LTOT)   oxygen therapy that is usually delivered for a minimum of 15 hours per day, including overnight. Once this is started, it is likely that a person will be on this for the rest of their life.

multimorbidity   the presence of several diseases in the same person at the same time, and the combined effect of these diseases on the person.

non-blanching erythema   tissue redness that does not turn white when pressure is applied with a finger.

orthopnea   difficulty in breathing when lying down; it is usually relieved when the person sits or stands up.

polyneuropathy   a disorder that affects peripheral nerves, which can result in a person experiencing reduced sensation – for example, reduced ability to detect heat.

polypharmacy   multiple prescriptions, involving different drugs for a number of different conditions.

primary care   care delivered in or close to a person's home – for example, general practitioner practices, NHS walk-in centres and pharmacists.

respite care   short-term temporary care that is arranged to provide a break for those caring for people living with an LTC – for example, residential respite (where nursing or residential care is provided) or domiciliary respite (care is provided in the person's own home).

secondary care   medical services and hospital care, including elective and emergency care. Access is often via a referral from primary care.

self-efficacy   a person's belief that they can make a change to their current situation.

spirometry   a test that determines the breathing capacity of the lungs. It measures both the forced vital capacity (the volume of air expired until a person feels their lungs are empty) and the forced expired volume (the volume of air expired in the first second of expiration).

status asthmaticus   repeated asthma attacks, without relief, that do not respond to treatment.

syndrome   disease that has a distinct pattern of signs and symptoms – for example, dementia, Down's syndrome.

tertiary care   specialised care and treatment that is usually provided in specialist centres.

References

Achterberg, WP, Pieper, MJC, van Dalen-Kok, AH, de Waal, MWM, Husebo, BS, Lautenbacher, S, Kunz, M, Scherder, EJA and Corbett, A (2013) Pain management in people with dementia. *Clinical Interventions in Aging, 13*(8): 1471–87.

Adler, R, Rosenfeld, L and Towne, N (1989) *Interplay: The Process of Interpersonal Communication.* Orlando, FL: Rinehart & Winston.

Age UK (2018) *Blended Evaluation of Phase 2 of the Age UK Personalised Integrated Care Programme Final Evaluation Report.* London: Age UK.

Allen, D, Channon, S, Lowes, L, Atwell, C and Lane, C (2011) Behind the scenes: the changing role of parents in the transition from child to adult diabetes service. *Diabetic Medicine, 28*(8): 994–1000.

Alzheimer's Society (2009) *Counting the Cost: Caring for People with Dementia in Hospital Wards.* London: Alzheimer's Society.

Alzheimer's Society (2016) *Fix Dementia Care Hospitals.* London: Alzheimer's Society.

Askerud, A and Conder, J (2017) *Australian Journal of Primary Health,* 10/2017, *23*(5).

Bach, S and Grant, A (2018) *Communication and Interpersonal Skills in Nursing* (4th edn). London: Sage/Learning Matters.

Baile, WF, Buckman, R, Lenzi, R, Glober, G, Beale, EA and Kudelka, AP (2000) SPIKES – A six-step protocol for delivering bad news: application to the patient with cancer. *The Oncologist, 5*: 302–11.

Ball, J, Maben, J, Murrells, T, Day, T and Griffiths, P (2015) *12-hour shifts: prevalence, views and impact.* London: National Nursing Research Unit, King's College London.

Bandura, A (2004) Health promotion by social cognitive means. *Health Education and Behaviour, 31*(2): 143–64.

Barrett, D, Wilson, B and Woolands, A (2009) *Care Planning: A Guide for Nurses.* Harlow: Pearson Education.

Bee, PE, Barnes, P and Luker, KA (2008) A systematic review of informal caregivers' needs in providing home-based end-of-life care to people with cancer. *Journal of Clinical Nursing, 18*: 1379–93.

Bentley, A (2014) Case management and long-term conditions: the evolution of community matrons. *British Journal of Community Nursing, 19*(7): 340–5.

Bergman-Evans, B (2006) AIDES to improving medicines adherence in older adults. *Geriatric Nursing, 27*(30): 174–82.

Berkman, ND, Davis, TD and McCormack, L (2010) Health Literacy: What is it? *Journal of Health Communication 15* (52): 9–19.

Blunt, I (2013) *Focus on Preventable Admissions: Trends in Emergency Admissions for Ambulatory Care Sensitive Conditions, 2001 to 2013.* London: Health Foundation and Nuffield Trust.

Bramley, L and Matiti, M (2014) How does it really feel to be in my shoes? Patients' experiences of compassion within nursing care and their perceptions of developing compassionate nurses. *Journal of Clinical Nursing, 23*, 2790–9.

British Geriatric Society (2014) *Fit for Frailty: Consensus Best Practice Guidance for the Care of Older People Living with Frailty in Community and Outpatient Settings.* London: British Geriatric Society.

Brodaty, H and Donkin, M (2009) Family caregivers of people with dementia. *Dialogues in Clinical Neuroscience, 11*(2): 217–28.

Brownrigg, S (2018) Breaking bad news to people with learning disabilities: a literature review. *British Journal of Learning Disabilities, 46*(4): 225–33.

Calderwood, K (2011) Adapting the transtheoretical model of change to the bereavement process. *Social Work, 56*(2): 107–18.

Cancer Research UK (2015) *Prostate Cancer: Risks and Causes.* Available online at: www.cancerreasearchuk.org/about-cancer/prostate-cancer/risks-causes (accessed: 11/03/19).

Cancer Research UK (2014) *What Is the Preferred Priorities of Care (PCC) Document?* Available online at: www.cancerresearchuk.org/about-cancer/coping/dying-with-cancer/making-plans/care-planning/preferred-priorities-for-care (accessed: 11/03/19).

Carers UK (2014a) *Facts about Carers.* Available online: www.carersuk.org/for professionals/policy/policy-library/facts-about-carers-2014 (accessed: 11/03/19).

Carers UK (2014b) *Carers Manifesto.* London: Carers UK.

Carers UK (2015) *Facts and Figures.* Available online at: www.carersuk.org/news-and-campaigns/press-releases/facts-and-figures(accessed: 19/03/19).

Carmichael, F and Hulme, C (2008) Are the needs of carers being met by government policy? *Journal of Community Nursing. 22*: 4–12.

Carrier, J (2015) *Managing Long-term Conditions and Chronic Illness in Primary Care: A Guide to Good Practice* (2nd edn). Abingdon: Routledge.

Chan, MF, Ng, SE, Tien, A, Man Ho, RC and Thayala, J (2013) *A randomised controlled study to explore the effect of life story review on depression in older Chinese. Singapore Health & Social Care in the Community, 21*(5): 545–53.

Chen, X, Mao, G and Leng, SX (2014) Frailty syndrome: an overview. *Clinical Interventions in Aging, 9*. 433–41.

Cherniss, C (1998) *Emotional Intelligence: What It Is and Why It Matters.* Available online at: www.eiconsortium.org/pdf/what_is_emotional_intelligence.pdf (accessed: 11/03/19).

Chilton, S, Melling, K, Drew, D and Clarridge, A (2004) *Nursing in the Community: An Essential Guide to Practice.* London: Hodder Arnold.

Chronic Pain Policy Coalition (2011) *Putting Pain on the Agenda: The Report of the First English Pain Summit.* London: Chronic Pain Policy Coalition.

CKS (Clinical Knowledge Summaries) (2014) *CVD Risk Assessment and Management.* Available online at: http://cks.nice.org.uk/cvd-risk-assessment-and-management#!topicsummary (accessed: 11/03/19).

CKS (2015) *Depression.* Available online at: https://cks.nice.org.uk/depression#!topicSummary (accessed: 27/03/19).

CKS (2017a) *Heart Failure: Chronic.* Available online at: https://cks.nice.org.uk/heart-failure-chronic (accessed: 27/03/19).

CKS (2017b) *Dementia.* Available online at: https://cks.nice.org.uk/dementia#!topicSummary (accessed: 27/03/19).

CKS (2017c) *Diabetes – type 2.* Available online at: https://cks.nice.org.uk/diabetes-type-2#!diagnosisSub (accessed: 27/03/19).

CKS (2018) *Asthma.* Available online at: https://cks.nice.org.uk/asthma (accessed: 13/06/18).

Clark, D (2002) Between hope and acceptance: the medicalization of dying. *British Medical Journal, 324* (7342): 905–7.

Codling, M (2015) Helping service users to take control of their health. *Learning Disability Practice, 18*(3): 26–9.

Cooper, S.-A. et al. (2018) Management and prevalence of long-term conditions in primary health care for adults with intellectual disabilities compared with the general population: a population-based cohort study. *Journal of Applied Research in Intellectual Disabilities, 31*(S1): 68–81.

Corbin, J and Strauss, A (1985) Managing chronic illness at home: three lines of work. *Qualitative Sociology, 8*(3), 224–47.

Coulter, A, Roberts, S and Dixon, A (2013) *Delivering Better Services for People with Long-term Conditions.* Available online at: www.kingsfund.org.uk/sites/default/files/field/field_publication_file/delivering-better-services-for-people-with-long-term-conditions.pdf (accessed: 27/07/18).

Coulter A, Entwhistle V, Eccles, A, Ryan, S, Shepperd, S and Perera, R (2015) Personalised care planning for adults with chronic or long-term conditions. *The Cochrane Database of Systematic Reviews, 3.*

Cox, A, Jenkins, V, Catt, S, Langridge, C and Fallowfield, L (2006) Information needs and experiences: an audit of UK cancer patients. *European Journal of Oncology Nursing, 10,* 263–72.

CQC (Care Quality Commission) (2014) *From the Pond in to the Sea: Children's Transition to Adult Health Services.* Gallowgate: Care Quality Commission.

Dahlgren, G and Whitehead, M (1991) *Policies and Strategies to Promote Social Equity in Health.* Stockholm, Sweden: Institute for Future Studies.

Dahlgren, G and Whitehead, M (2007) *European Strategies for Tackling Social Inequalities in Health: Levelling Up, Part 2.* Copenhagen: World Health Organization.

Davis, N (2011) Reflection: Looking Backwards, Moving Forwards, in Davis, N and Clark, AC, *Learning Skills for Nursing Students.* Exeter: Learning Matters, pp173–92.

De Silva, D (2011) *Helping People Help Themselves: A Review of the Evidence Considering Whether It Is Worthwhile to Support Self-Management.* London: The Health Foundation.

Delgado, C, Upton, D, Ranse, K, Furness, T and Foster, K (2017) Nurses' resilience and the emotional labour of nursing work: an integrative review of empirical literature. *International Journal of Nursing Studies, 70:* 71–88.

DH (Department of Health) (2006) *Transition: Getting It Right for Young People. Improving the Transition of Young People with Long Term Conditions from Children's to Adult Health Services.* London: Department of Health.

DH (2008a) *Transition: Moving on Well.* 8651. London: Department of Health.

DH (2008b) *Raising the profile of Long Term Conditions Care: A Compendium of Information.* London: Department of Health.

DH (2009) *Living Well with Dementia: A National Dementia Strategy.* London: Department of Health.

DH (2010) *Ready to Go? Planning the Discharge and the Transfer of Patients from Hospital and Intermediate Care.* Leeds: Department of Health.

DH (2012) *Long Term Conditions Compendium of Information* (3rd edn). London: Department of Health.

DH (2015) *Prime Minister's Challenge on Dementia.* Available online at: www.dementiaendoflife.co.uk/wp-content/uploads/2015/09/Prime-ministers-challenge-on-dementia-2020.pdf (accessed: 07/09/18).

Department of Health and NHS Commissioning Board (2012) *Compassion in Practice.* London: Department of Health.

DHSSPS (Department of Health, Social Services and Public Safety) (2012) *Living With Long Term Conditions: A Policy Framework.* Available online at: https://www.health-ni.gov.uk/publications/living-long-term-conditions-policy-framework (accessed: 11/03/19).

DiClemente, CC (2007) The transtheoretical model of intentional behaviour change. *Drugs and Alcohol Today, 7*(1): 29–32.

Dixon, A (2008) *Motivation and Confidence: What Does It Take to Change Behaviour?* London: King's Fund.

DiZazzo-Miller, R, Samuel, PS, Barnas, JM and Welker, KM (2014) Addressing everyday challenges: feasibility of a family caregiver training program for people with dementia. *American Journal of Occupational Therapy, 68*(2): 212–20.

Driscoll, J (1994) Reflective practice for practice. *Senior Nurse, 14*(1): 47–50.

Dunkley, S and Sales, R (2014) The challenges of providing palliative care for people with intellectual disabilities: a literature review. *International Journal of Palliative Nursing,* *20*(6): 279–85.

Endacott, R, Jevon, P and Cooper, S (eds) (2009) *Clinical Nursing Skills: Core and Advanced.* Oxford: Oxford University Press.

Feast, A, Orrell, M, Charlesworth, G, Melunsky, N, Poland, F and Moniz-Book, E (2016) Behavioural and psychological symptoms in dementia and the challenges for family carers: systematic review. *The British Journal of Psychiatry, 208*(5): 429–34.

Forbes, A and While, A (2009) The nursing contribution to chronic disease management: a discussion paper. *International Journal of Nursing Studies, 46*(1): 120–31.

Gale, CR, Cooper, C and Sayer, AA (2015) Prevalence of frailty and disability: findings from the English Longitudinal Study of Ageing. *Age and Ageing, 44*(1): 162–5.

Gardner, H (1983; 1993) *Frames of Mind: The Multiple Intelligences.* New York: Basic Books (2nd edn published in Britain by Fontana Press).

Gardner, H (1999) *Intelligence Reframed: Multiple Intelligences for the 21st Century.* New York: Basic Books.

George, J and Martin, F (2016) *Briefing Paper: Living with Long Term Conditions.* London: British Medical Association.

Gibson, G, Newton, L, Pritchard, G, Finch, T, Brittain, K and Robinson, L (2014) The provision of assistive technology services for people with dementia. *Dementia, 2014*: 1–21.

GMC (General Medical Council) (2013) *Good Medical Practice.* Available online at: www. gmc-uk.org/ethical-guidance/ethical-guidance-for-doctors/good-medical-practice.asp (accessed: 11/03/19).

Gomes, B, Calanzini, N, Gysels, M, Hall, S and Higginson, J (2013) Heterogeneity and changes in preferences for dying at home: a systematic review. *BNC Palliative Care, 12*(7).

Gonçalves-Bradley, D, Lannin, NA, Clemson, LM, Cameron, ID and Shepperd, S (2016) *Discharge planning in hospital. Cochrane Review.*

GSF (Gold Standards Framework) (2016) *Proactive Identification Guide (PIG).* Available online at: www.goldstandardsframework.org.uk/PIG (accessed:06/02/19).

GSF (2018) *Advance Care Planning.* Available online at: www.goldstandardsframework. org.uk/advance-care-planning (accessed: 13/12/18).

Haddad, M (2010) Caring for patients with long-term conditions and depression. *Nursing Standard, 24*(24): 40–9.

Halldorsdottir, S (2008) The dynamics of the nurse–patient relationship: introduction of a synthesised theory from the patient's perspective. *Scandinavian Journal of Caring Sciences, 22*: 643–52.

Hancock, K, Clayton, JM, Parker, SM, Walder, S, Butow, PN, Carrick, S, Currow, D, Ghersi, D, Glare, P, Hagerty, R and Tattersall, MHN (2007) Truth telling in discussing prognosis in advanced life-limiting illnesses: a systematic review. *Palliative Medicine, 21*(6): 507–17.

Heath, H, Sturdy, D and Wilcock, G (2010) *Improving Quality of Care for People with Dementia in General Hospitals.* London: RCN Publishing.

HEE (Health Education England) (2017) *Health Literacy.* Available online at: www.hee.nhs.uk/our-work/health-literacy (accessed 07/09/18).

Heslop, P and Glover, G (2015) Mortality of people with intellectual disabilities in England: a comparison of data from existing sources. *Journal of Applied Research in Intellectual Disabilities, 28*(5): 414–22.

Hibbard, J and Gilburt, H (2014) *Supporting People to Manage their Health: An Introduction to Patient Activation.* Available online at: www.kingsfund.org.uk/sites/default/files/field/field_publication_file/supporting-people-manage-health-patient-activation-may14.pdf (accessed: 06/02/19).

Hibbard, JH, Mahoney, ER, Stockard, J and Tusler, M (2005) Development and testing of a short form of the patient activation measure. *Journal of Health Services Research, 40*(6): 1918–30.

Hibbard, JH, Mahoney, ER, Stockard, J and Tusler, M (2007) Do increases in patient activation result in improved self-management behaviours? *HSR: Health Services Research, 42*(4): 1443–63.

Higginson, IJ, Sarmento, VP, Calanzani, N, Benalia, H and Gomes, B (2013) Dying at home – is it better: a narrative appraisal of the state of the science. *Palliative Medicine, 27*(10): 918–24.

Higginson, IJ, Daveson, BA, Morrison, RS, Yi, D, Meier, D, Smith, M, Ryan, K, McQuillan, R, Johnson, BM and Normand, C (2017) Social and clinical determinants of preferences and their achievement at the end of life: prospective cohort study of older adults receiving palliative care in three countries. *BMC Geriatrics, 17*: 271.

Huang, SL, Li, CM, Yang, CY and Chen, JJJ (2009) Application of reminiscence treatment on older people with dementia: a case study in Pingtung, Taiwan. *Journal of Nursing Research, 17*(2): 112–18.

Hunt, KJ, Shlomo, N and Addington-Hall, J (2014) End of life care and achieving preferences for place of death in England: results of a population-based survey using the VOICES-SF questionnaire. *Palliative Medicine, 28*(5): 412–21.

Janata, P (2012) Effects of widespread and frequent personalised music programming on agitation and depression in assisted living facility residents with Alzheimer-type dementia. *Music and Medicine, 4*(1):8–15.

Katbamna, S, Manning, L, Mistri, A, Johnson, M and Robinson, T (2017) Balancing satisfaction and stress: carer burden among white and British Asian: indian carers of stroke survivors. *Ethinicity and Health, 22*(4): 425–41.

Kaufman, G (2014) Polypharmacy, medicines optimisation and concordance. *Nurse Prescribing, 12*(4): 197–201.

Kellett, U, Moyle, W, McAllister, M et al. (2010) Life stories and biography: a means of connecting family and staff to people with dementia. *Journal of Clinical Nursing, 19*: 11–12, 1707–15.

King's Fund (2017) *What is Social Prescribing?* Available online at: www.kingsfund.org.uk/publications/social-prescribing (accessed 24/09/18).

Kingston, A, Robinson, L, Booth, H. Knapp, M and Jagger, C (2018) Projections of multi-morbidity in the older population in England to 2035: estimates from the Population Ageing and Care Simulation (PACSim) model. *Age and Ageing, 47*(3): 374–80.

Kivimäki, M, Hammer, M, Batty, GD, Geddes, JR, Tabak, AG, Pentti, A, Virtanen, M and Vahtera, J (2010) Antidepressant medication use, weight gain, and risk of type 2 diabetes. *Diabetes Care, 33*(12): 2611–16. Available online at: http://care.diabetesjournals.org/content/33/12/2611 (accessed: 11/03/19).

Knight, T, Skouteris, H, Townsend, M and Hooley, M (2017) The act of giving: a pilot and feasibility study of the My Life Story programme designed to foster positive mental health and well-being in adolescents and older adults. *International Journal of Adolescence and Youth, 22*(2): 165–78.

Kübler-Ross, E (2009) *On Death and Dying: What the Dying Have to Teach Doctors, Nurses, Clergy and Their Own Family* (40th anniversary edn). Abingdon: Routledge.

Kübler-Ross, E and Kessler, D (2005) *On Grief and Grieving: Finding the Meaning of Grief Through the Five Stages of Loss.* London: Simon & Schuster.

Lalkhen, AG, Bedrod, JP and Dwuer, AD (2012) Pain associated with multiple sclerosis: epidemiology, classification and management. *British Journal of Neuroscience Nursing, 8*(5): 267–74.

Lewis, V, Bauer, M, Winbolt, M, Chenco, C and Hanley, F (2015) A study of the effectiveness of MP3 players to support family carers of people living with dementia at home. *International Psychogeriatrics, 27*(3): 471–9.

Lorig, KR and Holmann, H (2003) Self-management education: history, definition, outcomes and mechanisms. *Annals of Behavioural Medicine, 26*(1): 1–7.

Lorig, K, Holman, H, Sobel, D, Laurent, D, Gonzales, V and Minor, M (2006) *Living a Healthy Life with Chronic Conditions: Self-Management of Heart Disease, Arthritis, Diabetes, Asthma, Bronchitis, Emphysema and Others.* Boulder, CO: Bull Publishing.

Lorig, K, Laurent, DD, Plant, K, Krishnan, E and Ritter, PL (2014) The components of action planning and their association with behaviour and health outcomes. *Chronic Illness, 10*(1): 50–9.

Mafuba, K and Gates, B (2015) An investigation into the public health roles of community learning disability nurses. *British Journal of Learning Disabilities, 43*(1): 1–7.

Matthews, J (2014) Voices from the heart: the use of digital storytelling in education. *Community Practitioner, 87*(1): 28–30.

McCarron, RM, Vanderlip, ER and Rado, J (2016) Depression. *Annals of Internal Medicine, 165*(7): ITC49–64.

McDonald, C (2014) Patients in Control: Why People with Long-Term Conditions Must be Empowered. London: Institute for Public Policy Research.

McGrath, A and Yeowart, C (2009) Rights of Passage: Supporting Disabled Young People Through the Transition to Adulthood. London: New Philanthropy Capital.

McKeown, J, Clarke, A, Ingleton, C et al. (2010) The use of life story work with people with dementia to enhance person-centred care. *International Journal of Older People Nursing*, 5(2): 148–58.

McKinney, A (2017) The values of life story work for staff, people with dementia and family members. *Nursing Older People*, 29(5): 25–9.

Mental Capacity Act (2005) Available online at: www.legislation.gov.uk/ukpga/2005/9/contents (accessed: 20/05/15).

Mezuk, B, Eaton, WW, Albrecht, S and Golden, SH (2008) Depression and type 2 diabetes over the lifespan: a meta analysis. *Diabetes Care*, 31(12): 2383–90.

Mid Staffordshire NHS Foundation Trust Public Inquiry (2013) *Report of the Mid Staffordshire NHS Foundation Trust Public Inquiry: Executive Summary*. London: The Stationery Office.

Middleton, S, Barnett, J and Reeves, D (2001) *What Is an Integrated Care Pathway?* Available online at: bandolier.org.uk/painres/download/whatis/What_is_an_ICP (accessed: 11/03/19).

Miller, WR and Rollnick, S (2012) *Motivational Interviewing Helping People Change* (3rd edn). New York: Guilford.

Muralitharan, M and Peate, I (2013) *Fundamentals of Applied Pathophysiology: An Essential Guide for Nursing and Healthcare Students*. Singapore: Wiley-Blackwell.

Murphy, J and Oliver, T (2013) The use of Talking Mats to support people with dementia and their carers to make decisions together. *Health and Social Care in the Community*, 21(2): 171–80.

Murphy, J, Tester, S, Hubbard, G, Downs, M and MacDonald, C (2004) Enabling frail older people with a communication difficulty to express their views: the use of Talking Mats as an interview tool. *Health and Social Care in the Community*, 13(2): 95–107.

Naidoo, J and Wills, J (2016) *Foundations for Health Promotion (Public Health and Health Promotion)* (3rd edn). China: Bailliere Tindall, Elsevier.

Narayanan, V, Bista, B and Koshy, C (2010) 'BREAKS' protocol for breaking bad news. *Indian Journal of Palliative Care*, 16(2): 61–5.

Nardi, TJ and Keefe-Cooperman, K (2006) Communicating bad news: a model for emergency mental health helpers. *International Journal of Emergency Mental Health*, 8: 203–7.

National End of Life Care Programme and National Council for Palliative Care (2013) *Advance Decisions to Refuse Treatment: A Guide for Health and Social Care Professionals*. Available online at: www.ncpc.org.uk/sites/default/files/ADRT%20books.pdf (accessed 13/12/18).

National Health Service Improving Quality (2010) *Holistic Common Assessment of Supporting and Palliative Care Needs for Adults Requiring End of Life Care*. London: NHS Improving Quality.

National Voices (2018) *Priorities for the plan: the long term NHS plan and beyond; views from leaders of in charities and voice organisations*. London: National Voices.

NHS (2016) *Compassion in Practice: Evidencing the Impact*. London: NHS

NHS (National Health Service) (2018) *NHS RightCare pathway: diabetes NHS prevention programme*. London: NHS.

NHS Digital (2017) *Quality Outcomes Framework.* Available online at: https://qof.digital. nhs.uk (accessed: 13/06/18).

NHS England (2013) *House of Care: A Framework for Long Term Condition Care* Available online at: www.england.nhs.uk/ourwork/ltc-op-eolc/ltc-eolc/house-of-care/ (accessed: 12/06/18).

NHS England (2017) *Next Steps on the Five Year Forward View.* Available online at: www. england.nhs.uk/wp-content/uploads/2017/03/NEXT-STEPS-ON-THE-NHS-FIVE-YEAR-FORWARD-VIEW.pdf (accessed: 12/06/18).

NHS Scotland (2010) *Long Term Conditions Collaborative: Improving Care Pathways.* Available online at: www.gov.scot/publications/long-term-conditions-collaborative-improving-care-pathways/ (accessed: 11/03/19).

NICE (2009) *Depression in Adults with a Chronic Physical Health Problem: Treatment and Management.* London: NICE.

NICE (2015a) *Depression Clinical Knowledge Summary.* Available online at: https://cks. nice.org.uk/depression#!topicsummary (accessed: 13/06/18).

NICE (2015b) *Leg Ulcers: Venous.* Available online at: https://cks.nice.org.uk/leg-ulcer-venous#!topicsummary (accessed: 13/06/18).

NICE (2015c) *Medicines Optimisation: The Safe and Effective Use of Medicines to Enable the Best Possible Outcomes.* Available online at: www.nice.org.uk/guidance/ng5 (accessed: 06/02/19).

NICE (2016a) *Motor Neurone Disease.* Available online at: www.nice.org.uk/guidance/ qs126 (accessed: 13/06/18).

NICE (2016b) *Transition from Children's to Adult's Services for Young People Using Health and Social Care Services NG43.* Available online at: www.nice.org.uk/guidance/ng43/chapter/ Recommendations#transition-planning (accessed: 13/06/18).

NICE (2016c) *Multimorbidity: Assessment and Management.* Guideline (NG56). London: NICE.

NICE (2017) *Diabetes – type 2 Clinical Knowledge Summary.* Available online at: https://cks. nice.org.uk/diabetes-type-2#!topicsummary (accessed: 13/06/18).

NICE (2018) *Multimorbidity and Polypharmacy.* Available online at: www.nice.org.uk/ advice/ktt18 (accessed 24/09/18).

Nicholson, A, Kuper, H and Hemingway, H (2006) Depression as an aetiologic and prognostic factor in coronary heart disease: a meta-analysis of 6362 events among 146 538 participants in 54 observational studies. *European Heart Journal,* 27(23): 2763–74.

NMC (2015) *The Code: Professional Standards of Practice and Behaviour for Nurses and Midwives.* London: Nursing and Midwifery Council.

NMC (2018) *Future Nurse: Standards of Proficiency for Registered Nurses* Available online at: www. nmc.org.uk/globalassets/sitedocuments/education-standards/future-nurse-proficiencies. pdf (accessed: 13/06/18).

Offredy, M, Bunn, F and Morgan, J (2009) Case management in long term conditions: an inconsistent journey? *British Journal of Community Nursing, 14*(6): 252–7.

ONS (Office for National Statistics) (2014) *Life Expectancy at Birth and at Age 65 for Local Area in the United Kingdom, 2006–08 to 2010–12.* Available online at: https://webarchive.nationalarchives.gov.uk/20160107151042/http://www.ons.gov.uk/ons/dcp171778_360047.pdf (accessed: 15/02/19).

ONS (2017a) *National Life Tables: UK 2014–2016.* Available online at: www.ons.gov.uk/peoplepopulationandcommunity/birthsdeathsandmarriages/lifeexpectancies/bulletins/nationallifetablesunitedkingdom/2014to2016 (accessed: 12/06/18).

ONS (2017b) *Overview of the UK Population: July 2017.* Available online at: www.ons.gov.uk/peoplepopulationandcommunity/populationandmigration/populationestimates/articles/overviewoftheukpopulation/july2017 (accessed: 12/06/18).

Pallant, JF and Reid, C (2013) Measuring the positive and negative aspects of the caring role in community versus aged care setting, *Australasian Journal of Aging. 33*(4): 244–9.

Park, C and Park, E (2018) Factors influencing patient-perceived satisfaction with community-based case management services. *Western Journal of Nursing Research, 40*(11): 1598–613.

Porth, CM and Matfin, G (2014) *Essentials of Pathophysiology: Concepts of Altered Health Status* (4th international edition). Philadelphia, PA: Wolters Kluwer Health/Lippincott Williams & Wilkins.

Public Health England (2016) *Learning Disabilities Observatory: People with Learning Disabilities in England 2015: Main Report.* Available online at: https://assets.publishing.service.gov.uk/government/uploads/system/uploads/attachment_data/file/613182/PWLDIE_2015_main_report_NB090517.pdf (accessed: 13/12/18).

QNI (Queens Nursing Institute) (2016) Discharge planning, best practice in transitions of care. London: Queens Nursing Institute.

RCGP (Royal College of General Practitioners) (2013) *Matters of Life and Death: Helping People to Live Well Until They Die.* London: Royal College of General Practitioners.

RCN (Royal College of Nursing) (2014) *Defining Nursing.* London: Royal College of Nursing.

RCN (2014) *RCN fact sheet: nurse prescribing in the UK.* London: Royal College of Nursing.

RCN (2018) *Frailty in Older People.* Available online at: www.rcn.org.uk/clinical-topics/older-people/frailty (accessed 15/02/19).

Reitz, C and Dalemans, R (2016) The use of Talking Mats by persons with Alzheimer in the Netherlands: increasing shared decision making by using a low tech communication aid. *Journal of Social Inclusion, 7*(2): 35–46.

Rhudy, L, Holland, D and Bowels, K (2009) Illuminating hospital discharge planning: staff nurse decision making. *Applied Nursing Research, 23*: 198–206.

Robinson, M, Hanna, E, Raine, G and Robertson, S (2017) Extending the comfort zone: building resilience in older people with long-term conditions. *Journal of Applied Gerontology, 1*–25.

Royal College of Physicians (2010) *Passive Smoking and Children: A Report by the Tobacco Advisory Group of the Royal College of Physicians.* London: Royal College of Physicians.

Royal Commission on Long Term Care (1999) *With Respect to Old Age: Long Term Care – Rights and Responsibilities.* London: The Stationery Office.

Royal Pharmaceutical Society (2016) *A Competency Framework for Prescribers.* London: Royal Pharmaceutical Society. Available online at: www.rpharms.com/Portals/0/RPS%20document%20library/Open%20access/Professional%20standards/Prescribing%20competency%20framework/prescribing-competency-framework.pdf (accessed: 11/03/19).

Salovey, P and Mayer, JD (1990) *Emotional Intelligence.* Available online at: http://ei.yale.edu/wp-content/uploads/2014/06/pub153_SaloveyMayerICP1990_OCR.pdf (accessed: 11/03/19).

Saunders, C (1994) The medicalization of death. *European Journal of Cancer Care (Engl),* *3*(4): 148.

Scerri, A, Innes, A and Scerri, C (2015) Discovering what works well: exploring quality dementia care in hospital wards using an appreciative inquiry approach. *Journal of Clinical Nursing, 24*: 13–14.

Schulman-Green, D, Jaser, M, Martin, F, Alonzo, A, Grey, M, McCorkle, R, Redeker, NS and Whittlemore, R (2012) Processes of self management in chronic illness. *Journal of Nursing Scholarship, 44*(2): 136–44.

Self Care Forum (2018) *What do we mean by self care and why is it good for people?* Available online at: www.selfcareforum.org/about-us/what-do-we-mean-by-self-care-and-why-is-good-for-people/ (accessed 27/07/18).

Shamaskin-Garroway, AM, Lageman, SK and Rybarczyk, B (2016) The roles of resilience and nonmotor symptoms in adjustment to Parkinson's disease. *Journal of Health Psychology, 21*(12): 3004–15.

Simon, C, Everitt, H, van Dorp, F and Burkes, M (2014) *Oxford Handbook of General Practice* (4th edn). Oxford: Oxford University Press.

Sutherland, D and Hayter, M (2009) Structured review: evaluating the effectiveness of nurse case managers in improving health outcomes for three major chronic diseases. *Journal of Clinical Nursing, 18*(21): 2978–92.

Sykes, S, Wills, J, Rowlands, G and Popple, K (2013) Understanding critical health literacy: a concept analysis. *BMC Public Health, 13*: 150.

Taverner, T (2014) Neuropathic pain: an overview. *British Journal of Neuroscience Nursing, 10*(3): 116–23.

Tebes, JK, Irish, JT, Puglisi-Vasquez, MJ and Perkins, DV (2004) Cognitive transformation as a marker of resilience. *Substance Use and Misuse, 39*: 769–88.

Telford, K, Kralik, D and Koch, T (2006) Acceptance and denial: implications for people adapting to chronic illness: a literature review. *Journal of Advanced Nursing, 55*(4): 457–64.

Terry, L, Newham, R, Hahessy, S, Atherley, S, Babenko-Mould, Y, Evans, M, Ferguson, K, Carr, G and Cedar, SH (2017) A research-based mantra for compassionate caring. *Nurse Education Today, 58*: 1–11.

Thomas, K (2003) *Caring for the Dying at Home: Companions on the Journey.* Abingdon: Radcliffe Medical Press.

Tobin, G and Begley, C (2008) Receiving bad news: a phenomenological exploration of the lived experience of receiving a cancer diagnosis. *Cancer Nursing, 31*(5): E31–9.

Tuffrey-Wijne, I (2012) A new model for breaking bad news to people with intellectual disabilities. *Palliative Medicine, 27*(1): 5–12.

Tuffrey-Wijne, I., Bernal, J., Hubert, J., Butler, G. and Hollins, S. (2010) Exploring the lived experience of people with learning disabilities who are dying of cancer. *Nursing Times, 106*(19): 15–19.

Wales Audit Office (2014) *The Management of Chronic Conditions in Wales: An Update.* Available online at: http://audit.wales/publication/management-chronic-conditions-wales-update (accessed: 11/03/19).

Waller, S (2012) Redesigning wards to support people with dementia in hospital. *Nursing Older People, 24* (2): 16–21.

Washington, KT, Meadows, SE, Elliot, SG and Koopman, RJ (2011) Information needs of informal carers of older adults with chronic health conditions. *Patient Education and Counselling, 83,* 37–44.

WHO (World Health Organization) (1997) *WHOQOL: Measuring Quality of Life.* Geneva: WHO.

WHO (2002) *National Cancer Control Programmes: Policies and Managerial Guidelines.* Geneva: World Health Organization.

WHO (2010) *The Determinants of Health.* Available online at: www.who.int/hia/evidence/doh/en (accessed: 11/03/19).

WHO (2013) *Noncommunicable Diseases.* Geneva: WHO. Available online at: www.who.int/mediacentre/factsheets/fs355/en/ (accessed: 11/03/19).

WHO (2016) *What is Health Promotion?* Geneva: WHO. Available online at: www.who.int/features/qa/health-promotion/en/ (accessed 06/09/18).

WHO (2017) *Promoting Health: Guide to National Implementaion of the Shanghai Declaration.* Geneva: World Health Organization.

Wilkes, L, Cioffi, J, Cummings, J, Warne, B and Harrison, K (2014) Clients with chronic conditions: community nurse role in a multidisciplinary team. *Journal of Clinical Nursing, 23*(5–6): 844–55.

Wilmot, J (2002) Palliative Care of Non-malignant Conditions, in Charlton, R (ed.) *Primary Palliative Care: Dying Death and Bereavement in the Community.* Abingdon: Radcliffe Medical Press.

Wood-Allum, CA (2014) Unanswered questions and barriers to research in the palliative care of motor neurone disease patients. *Journal of Palliative Care, 30*(4): 302–6.

Index

Added to a page number 'f' denotes a figure and 't' denotes a table.

earth

This book is on loan from
Library Services for Schools

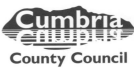
County Council

LONDON, NEW YORK,
MELBOURNE, MUNICH, and DELHI

Senior Art Editor Tory Gordon-Harris
Senior Editors Elinor Greenwood and Elizabeth Haldane

Editors Lorrie Mack, Zahavit Shalev, Penny Smith, Fleur Star
Designers Clare Harris, Karen Hood, Poppy Joslin,
Laura Roberts-Jensen, Clare Shedden

Writers
Introduction and Temperate forests: Dr Lynn Dicks
Polar regions: Chris Woodford
Tropical forests and Mountains: Michael Scott
Deserts and Grasslands: Dr Kim Dennis-Bryan
Freshwater and Oceans: Dr Frances Dipper

Science consultant Dr Lynn Dicks

Publishing Manager Susan Leonard
Category Publisher Mary Ling
Picture Researcher Liz Moore
Production Controller Claire Pearson
Production Editor Siu Chan
Jacket Designers Sophia Tampakopoulos and Natalie Godwin

First published in Great Britain in 2008
This paperback edition published in 2011 by
Dorling Kindersley Limited,
80 Strand, London, WC2R 0RL

2 4 6 8 10 9 7 5 3 1
TD304 – 12/10

A CIP catalogue record for this book
is available from the British Library

Hardback ISBN 978-1-40531-888-4
Paperback ISBN 978-1-40536-506-2

Colour reproduction by MDP, UK
Printed and bound by Toppan, China

Jacket images: *Front:* Corbis: Momatiuk - Eastcott.
Back: Alamy Images: Seb Rogers tc; Konrad Wothe
/ LOOK Die Bildagentur der Fotografen GmbH tr.
Corbis: Yann Arthus-Bertrand clb. Getty Images:
National Geographic / Tim Laman bc, bl; Stone
/ Bob Elsdale tl; Nobuaki Sumida / Sebun Photo
cra. SeaPics.com: crb. stevebloom.com: br.

Discover more at
www.dk.com

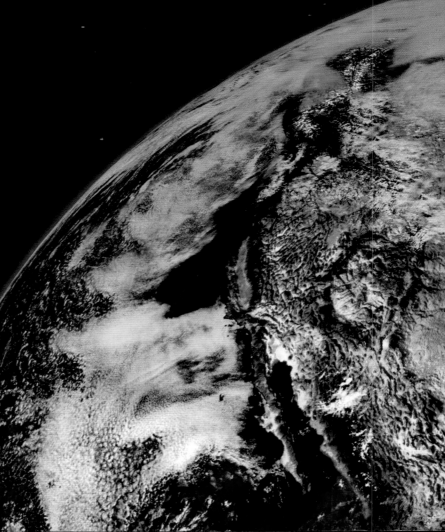

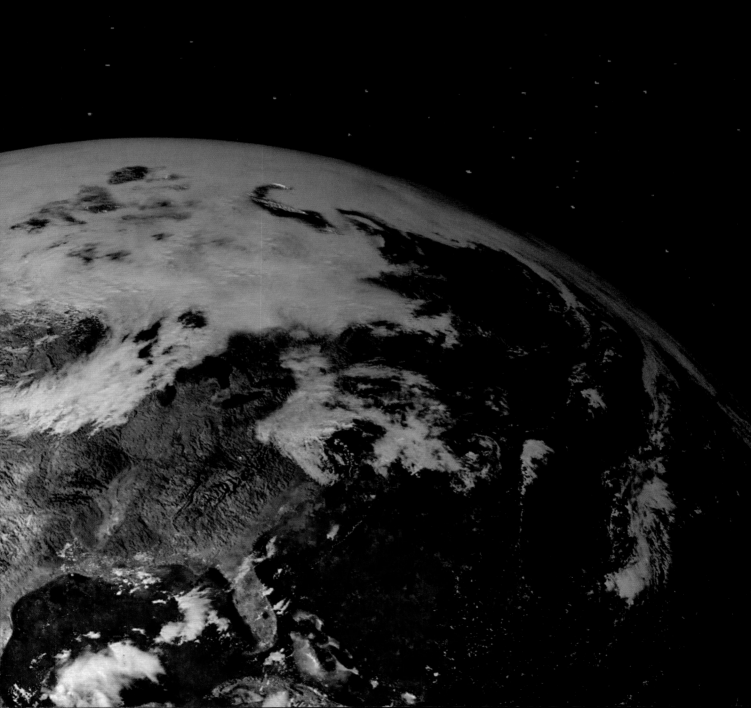

EARTH
matters

contents

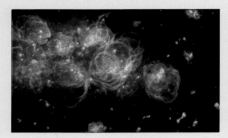
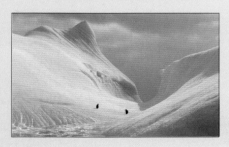
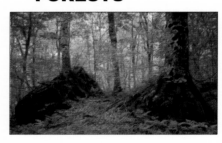
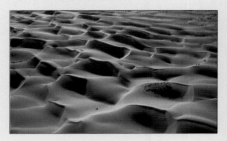
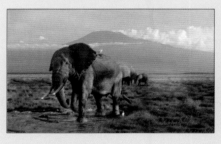

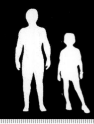
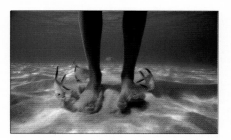

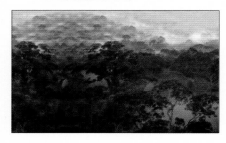
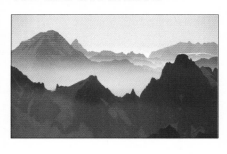
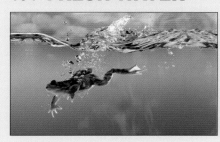

foreword

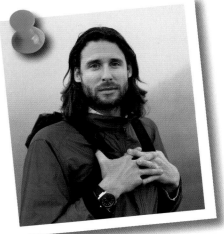

David de Rothschild

Protecting our planet has never been more important or urgent. On my adventures to the poles of the Earth – extreme, spectacular, and dangerous locations – I have seen for myself the shrinking glaciers, melting ice sheets, and struggling polar bears.

If you're anything like me, the scale and **complexity** of the problems we face sometimes seem overwhelming and rather frightening. With *clear evidence* now showing that it's our everyday actions driving climate change, it only requires a little more **understanding**, **commitment**, and **motivation** in order for us to create the solutions our planet craves.

Inside *Earth Matters,* you will find everything you will ever want to know about Earth's ecology. From the top of the tallest mountain to the bottom of the deepest sea, from the polar wilderness to the teeming jungle, each page is crammed with easy-to-understand facts and figures, specially commissioned maps, and outstanding photography.

Bell heather

King penguin

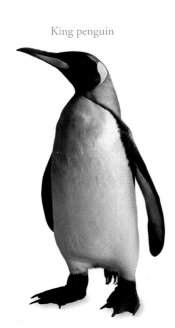

Our home planet is **beautiful**, miraculous, and possibly *unique* in the Universe... **Earth matters.** That's for sure.

Angel fish

The *Plastiki* Adventure My aim is to publicize the problems facing our planet using the romance of adventure and the power of the internet. My next adventure is to sail a boat made entirely out of recycled plastic bottles from the USA to Australia via the Great Pacific Garbage Patch – huge, floating "clouds" of plastic trash caught in a swirling vortex of ocean currents.

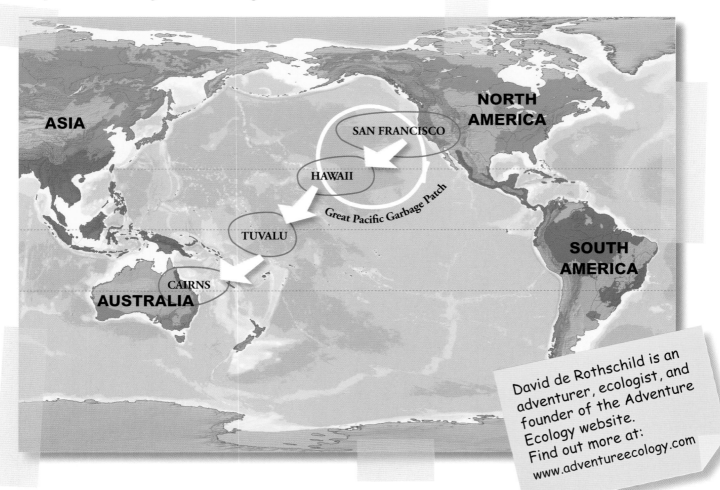

ASIA

NORTH AMERICA

SAN FRANCISCO

HAWAII

Great Pacific Garbage Patch

TUVALU

CAIRNS

AUSTRALIA

SOUTH AMERICA

David de Rothschild is an adventurer, ecologist, and founder of the Adventure Ecology website. Find out more at: www.adventureecology.com

one person can make

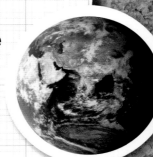

"One person can make all the difference in the world. For the first time in recorded human history, we have the fate of the whole planet in our hands."

Chrissie Hynde (b. 1951), musician

"I'd put my money on the Sun and solar energy. What a source of power! I hope we don't have to wait 'til oil and coal run out before we tackle that!"

Thomas Edison (1847–1931), inventor

"We have a very small number of years left to fail or to succeed in providing a sustainable future to our species."

Jacques Cousteau (1910–1997), explorer and marine conservationist

We do not inherit the land from our ancestors, we borrow it from our children.

Native American proverb

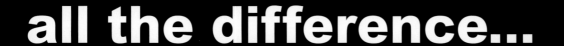

all the difference...

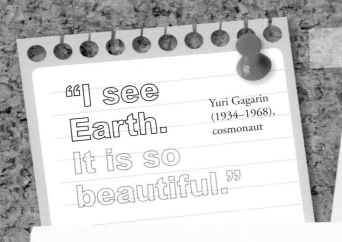

"I see Earth. It is so beautiful."

Yuri Gagarin (1934–1968), cosmonaut

"The more I studied about ecology, the more I cared and wanted to do something, to help in some way even if it's a small way."

Woody Harrelson (b. 1961), actor

$1

"YOU MUST BE THE CHANGE YOU WISH TO SEE IN THE WORLD."

Mahatma Gandhi (1869–1948), spiritual and political leader

If you want one year of prosperity, plant corn.
If you want ten years of prosperity, plant trees.
If you want one hundred years of prosperity, educate people.

Chinese proverb

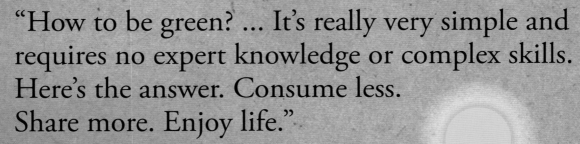

"How to be green? ... It's really very simple and requires no expert knowledge or complex skills. Here's the answer. Consume less. Share more. Enjoy life."

Dr Derek Wall, Green politician and lecturer

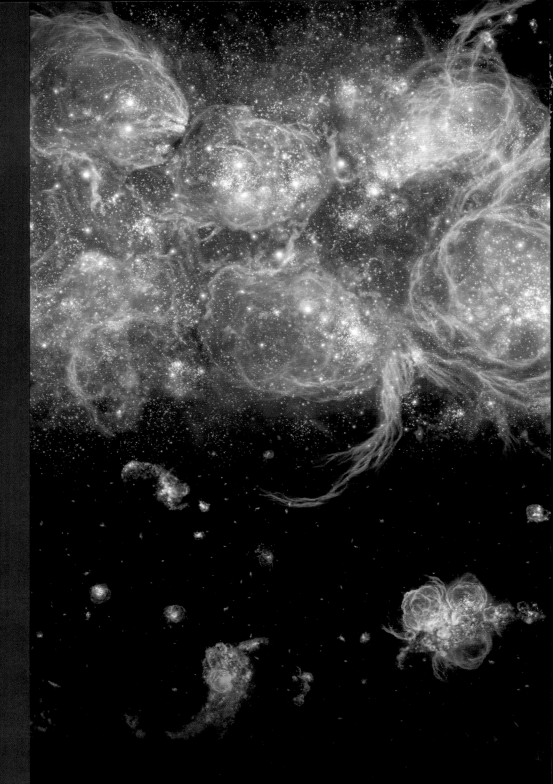

INTRODUCTION

Once upon a time, a long time ago (13.7 billion years ago), there was a bang and the *Universe began.*

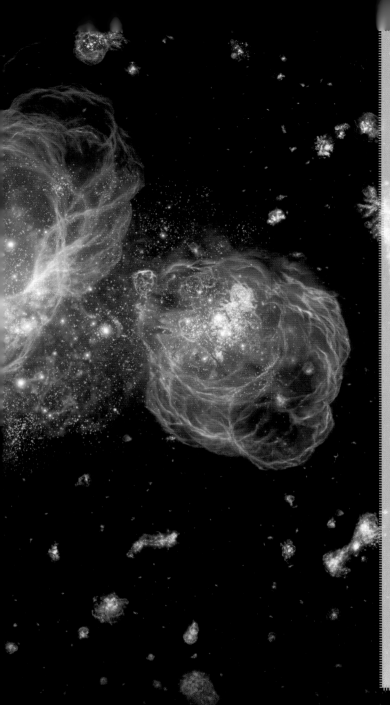

INTRODUCTION

Some call it the "Big Bang", and it seems our universe did start
with a massive, mind-bendingly huge explosion. The result was
the birth of a billion stars and from this our tiny planet emerged –

what is the **universe?**

The Universe is everything that exists: all the stars, planets, rocks, dust, and gas, and all the space in between them. Each star is a sun. Many are far larger and hotter than our own Sun. Stars are grouped into galaxies – huge spirals or whirlpools full of stars. With telescopes, we can see billions of galaxies, and each one contains billions of stars. But the more we know, the more questions are thrown up, and the more mysteries emerge. We are still discovering new things about our Universe all the time.

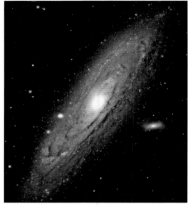

This is a spiral galaxy similar to the Milky Way called Andromeda.

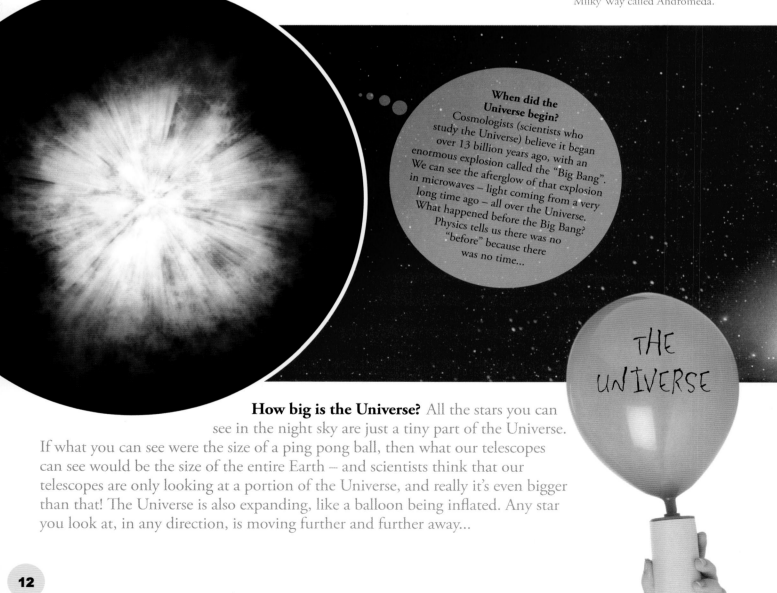

When did the Universe begin? Cosmologists (scientists who study the Universe) believe it began over 13 billion years ago, with an enormous explosion called the "Big Bang". We can see the afterglow of that explosion in microwaves – light coming from a very long time ago – all over the Universe. What happened before the Big Bang? Physics tells us there was no "before" because there was no time...

THE UNIVERSE

How big is the Universe? All the stars you can see in the night sky are just a tiny part of the Universe. If what you can see were the size of a ping pong ball, then what our telescopes can see would be the size of the entire Earth -- and scientists think that our telescopes are only looking at a portion of the Universe, and really it's even bigger than that! The Universe is also expanding, like a balloon being inflated. Any star you look at, in any direction, is moving further and further away...

our place in space

Earth is a tiny speck of rock in the vastness of the Universe. In our solar system, it is one of eight planets that circle around a star – the Sun.

Our Sun is one of several hundred billion stars grouped together in a spiral galaxy called the Milky Way. On a clear night you can see one of its arms as a streak of white across the sky. The brightest part is the centre of the galaxy. The Milky Way is just one of the billions of galaxies scattered through space. All together, they form the Universe.

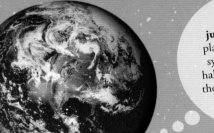

Earth is just one of eight planets in our solar system, which lies halfway along one of the spiral arms of the Milky Way.

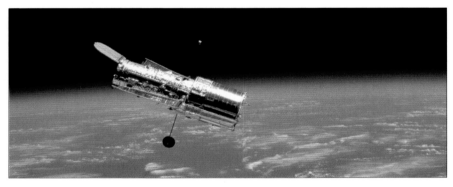

This is the Milky Way!

The Hubble Space Telescope was launched in 1990 and can view huge distances because it is outside the haze of the Earth's atmosphere. It can see 12 billion light years away (one light year is about 5.880 trillion miles), making it the most powerful telescope ever. Without it we would know far less about our universe.

13

just right for life

Earth is the only place in our solar system that sustains any known form of life – we haven't found life anywhere else in the Universe. Yet our planet contains millions of different life forms, all perfectly adapted to their environments – from tiny ants to chimpanzees, jewel beetles to humankind itself, living in teeming seas, lush forests, and barren deserts. Here are the ingredients that make our Earth the perfect place to be.

1 Just the right SIZED SUN

Big stars burn out faster than small ones, and really massive stars burn out so fast that life doesn't have time to develop on any of their planets. Small stars aren't suitable either because they're prone to surface storms that can destroy life on nearby planets. Our Sun is an ideal middle-sized star that will burn for about 10 billion years.

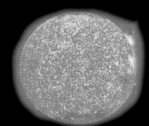

The SUN is
1.4 million km
(865,000 miles) in diameter
(distance across)

By comparison, Earth
is so small that you
can barely see it.

2 Just the right SIZED PLANET

The size of a planet controls the strength of its gravity. Jupiter is much larger than Earth, and its atmosphere is under a great deal of pressure – it would crush a spaceship like a paper cup. Mars, on the other hand, is just over half the size of Earth, and its thin atmosphere is under much, *much* less pressure. If you stood on Mars, the water in your cells would evaporate, turning to gas. Since you are 60 per cent water, you would probably explode. Earth has *just* enough gravity to hold on to its atmosphere, which protects us from the Sun's harmful rays and keeps us warm (see pages 24–25).

Jupiter

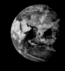

EARTH is
12, 756 km
(7, 926 miles)
in diameter

Mars

30 million different species thrive on Earth.

Earth is called a "Goldilocks planet". This is a scientific term that refers to a planet that is neither too hot nor too cold, too big nor too small, too near its star nor too far away, to support life as we know it. It's *just right*.

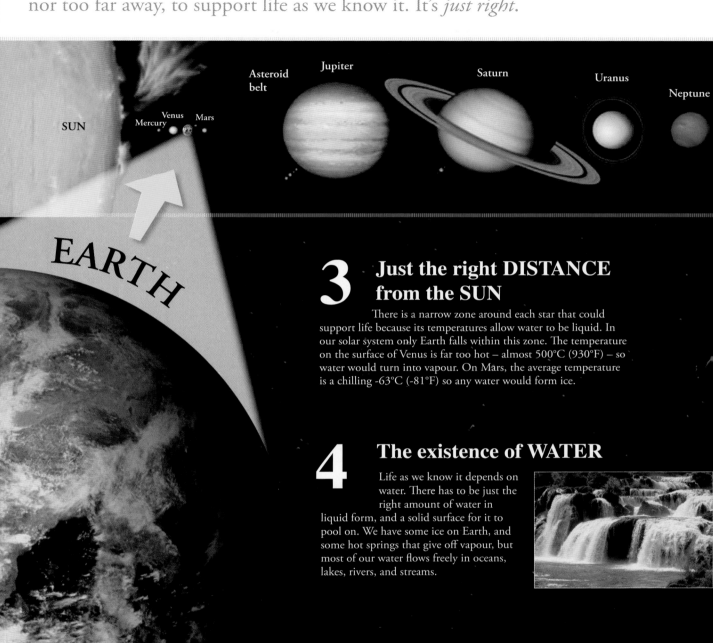

SUN
Mercury
Venus
Mars
Asteroid belt
Jupiter
Saturn
Uranus
Neptune

EARTH

3 Just the right DISTANCE from the SUN

There is a narrow zone around each star that could support life because its temperatures allow water to be liquid. In our solar system only Earth falls within this zone. The temperature on the surface of Venus is far too hot – almost 500°C (930°F) – so water would turn into vapour. On Mars, the average temperature is a chilling -63°C (-81°F) so any water would form ice.

4 The existence of WATER

Life as we know it depends on water. There has to be just the right amount of water in liquid form, and a solid surface for it to pool on. We have some ice on Earth, and some hot springs that give off vapour, but most of our water flows freely in oceans, lakes, rivers, and streams.

5 A little help from JUPITER

Without giant planets, Earth-sized planets would suffer lots of damaging collisions from asteroids and comets. Jupiter, 11 times the size of Earth (with much stronger gravity), mops up lots of rubble in the inner solar system. The comet Shoemaker-Levy 9 was drawn in by Jupiter's gravity in 1994. The collision with the planet caused huge fireballs and scarred its surface badly. We're lucky we avoided that particular collision!

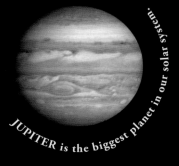

JUPITER is the biggest planet in our solar system.

life begins

The Earth finished forming more than four and a half billion years ago. For the first half a billion years, its rock was slowly cooling, forming a solid crust. Over time, **volcanoes** spat gases out from the Earth's core, forming an atmosphere of carbon dioxide, nitrogen, and water vapour. As Earth continued to cool, the water vapour turned to rain, which filled the seas. Rock fragments found in Greenland (see below) reveal that the earliest of all life forms was a type of green bacteria that started growing in these oceans three and a half billion years ago – almost as soon as the oceans were formed.

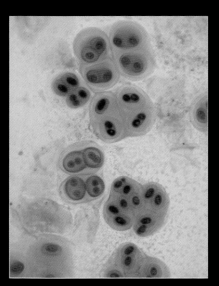

How did it start?

The oldest existing fragments of Earth's surface were found in Greenland. Dating from 3.85 billion years ago, they don't contain any fossils, but the chemicals inside them prove that life, in the form of green bacteria, already existed when the rocks were formed. Early Earth was pounded by asteroids, deadly ultraviolet radiation, and cosmic rays – there was no ozone layer then and the Earth itself was more radioactive than it is now. There are four main theories about how this harsh environment first produced life.

What is life? Living things (things that can grow and reproduce) are made of cells – each one is a fatty-membrane sac full of chemicals. For the first three billion years of Earth's existence, all living things had only one cell. In your body, there are at least 10 trillion cells.

Key to life

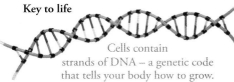

Cells contain strands of DNA – a genetic code that tells your body how to grow.

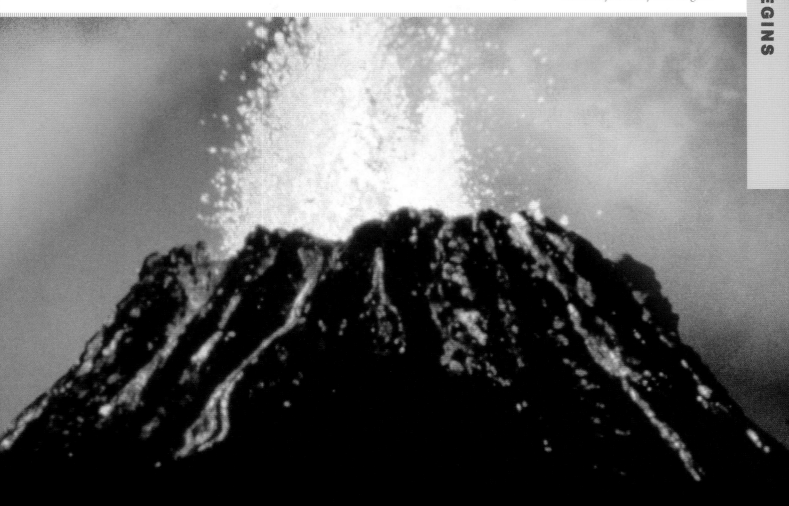

1. PRIMORDIAL SOUP

Life may have begun spontaneously, from reactions between the atmosphere and early oceans. Bolts of electricity from the atmosphere hitting the sloshy mixture that contained the elements of early Earth could have produced fats, proteins, and sugars – the building blocks of living cells.

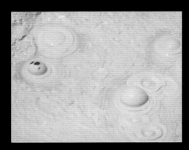

2. DEEP-SEA VENTS

Deep beneath the oceans are "hydrothermal vents", where hot volcanic gases bubble up from the Earth's core. Some bacteria, instead of needing sunlight or food, can survive here on energy from sulphur. Early life forms may have developed in this unique habitat, where they were also safe from asteroid attacks.

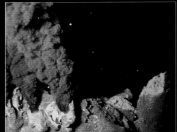

3. LIFE FROM SPACE

The basic chemicals of life may have come from outer space. Some meteorites contain amino acids – organic molecules that are the building blocks of living cells. Several thousand tonnes of these molecules land on Earth every year, and these may have resulted in the first sparks of life.

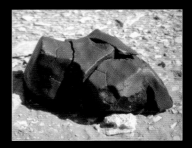

4. ONE BIG EXPERIMENT

Maybe life was sent to Earth by aliens. But could anything living survive a journey through space, with no air or water, and so cold that atoms stop vibrating? It's just possible a microorganism could make it inside a meteorite. After all, bacteria have survived for 25 million years inside the stomach of a fossilized bee.

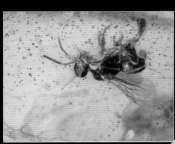

the story of life

Primitive life arrived on Earth nearly **4 billion years** ago, but it took another *3 billion years* for animals as we know them to form from groups of cells. These time scales are almost *impossible* to imagine, so think of them as one 24-hour day.

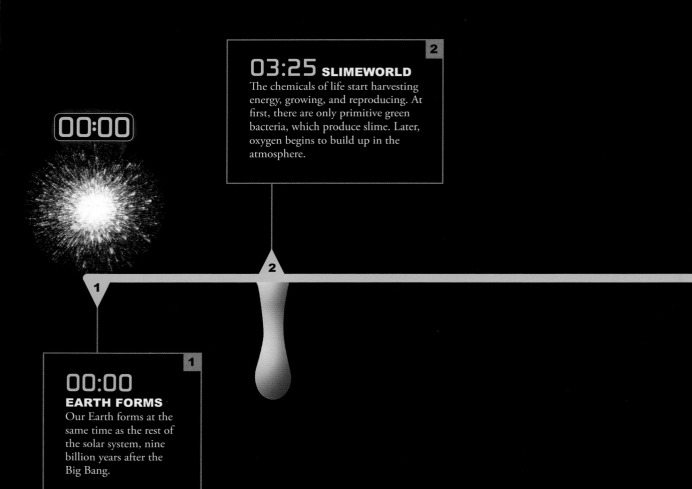

03:25 SLIMEWORLD 2
The chemicals of life start harvesting energy, growing, and reproducing. At first, there are only primitive green bacteria, which produce slime. Later, oxygen begins to build up in the atmosphere.

00:00

00:00
EARTH FORMS 1
Our Earth forms at the same time as the rest of the solar system, nine billion years after the Big Bang.

Until mid afternoon, bacteria are the only living things.

How does our 24-hour history of life on Earth work? Imagine the world formed at midnight and we have just reached the next midnight. On this time scale every second represents 52,662 years, and each minute represents over three million years.

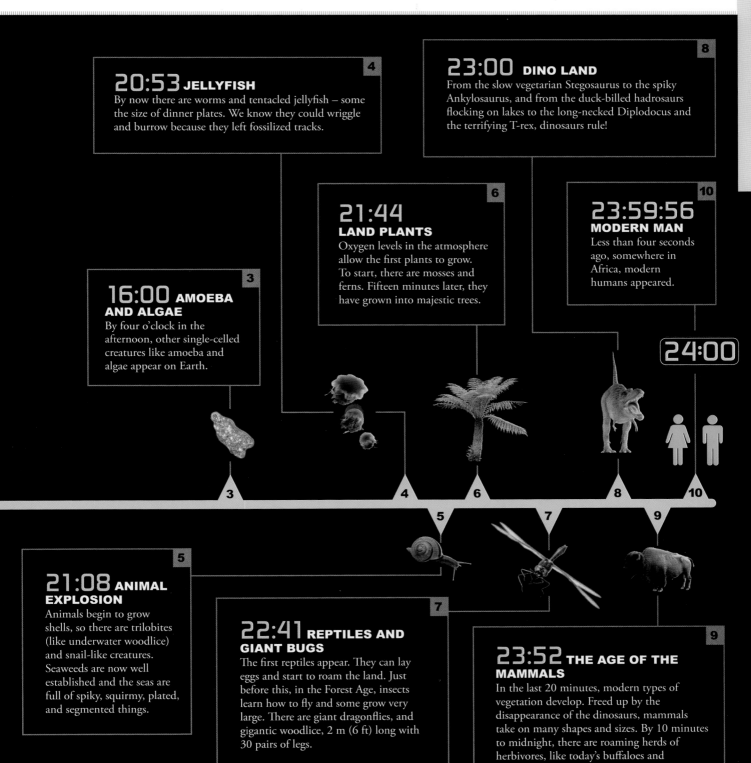

20:53 JELLYFISH [4]
By now there are worms and tentacled jellyfish – some the size of dinner plates. We know they could wriggle and burrow because they left fossilized tracks.

23:00 DINO LAND [8]
From the slow vegetarian Stegosaurus to the spiky Ankylosaurus, and from the duck-billed hadrosaurs flocking on lakes to the long-necked Diplodocus and the terrifying T-rex, dinosaurs rule!

21:44 LAND PLANTS [6]
Oxygen levels in the atmosphere allow the first plants to grow. To start, there are mosses and ferns. Fifteen minutes later, they have grown into majestic trees.

23:59:56 MODERN MAN [10]
Less than four seconds ago, somewhere in Africa, modern humans appeared.

16:00 AMOEBA AND ALGAE [3]
By four o'clock in the afternoon, other single-celled creatures like amoeba and algae appear on Earth.

24:00

21:08 ANIMAL EXPLOSION [5]
Animals begin to grow shells, so there are trilobites (like underwater woodlice) and snail-like creatures. Seaweeds are now well established and the seas are full of spiky, squirmy, plated, and segmented things.

22:41 REPTILES AND GIANT BUGS [7]
The first reptiles appear. They can lay eggs and start to roam the land. Just before this, in the Forest Age, insects learn how to fly and some grow very large. There are giant dragonflies, and gigantic woodlice, 2 m (6 ft) long with 30 pairs of legs.

23:52 THE AGE OF THE MAMMALS [9]
In the last 20 minutes, modern types of vegetation develop. Freed up by the disappearance of the dinosaurs, mammals take on many shapes and sizes. By 10 minutes to midnight, there are roaming herds of herbivores, like today's buffaloes and kangaroos. Animals looking like rabbits, rhinos, elephants, camels, pigs, moles, dogs, and cats have all arrived. Warm-blooded whales and dolphins, evolved from hippos, have taken to the seas.

a changing world

The Earth has **changed** dramatically over time. Its temperature has veered between tropical and icy. Its surface is constantly shifting, moving continents and creating mountains. And Earth's species have changed too, none with such drastic consequences as the development of humankind.

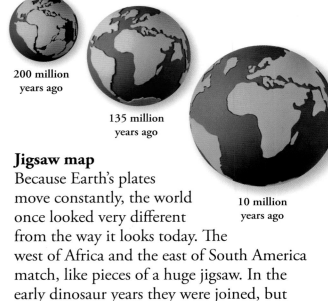

200 million years ago

135 million years ago

10 million years ago

Jigsaw map
Because Earth's plates move constantly, the world once looked very different from the way it looks today. The west of Africa and the east of South America match, like pieces of a huge jigsaw. In the early dinosaur years they were joined, but they started to separate over 150 million years ago and they've been drifting apart ever since.

Humans arrive Humans belong to a species of ape called *Homo sapiens*. Our direct ancestors first appeared just under two million years ago. As they spread across the Earth's surface, the changes they brought were immense. They learned how to hunt and eat big mammals and they tamed wild animals. They also began to live in colonies and farm the land, thereby changing the face of the world forever.

Many species, like the woolly mammoth, became extinct after coming into contact with humans – clever pack-hunting predators with dogs and spears.

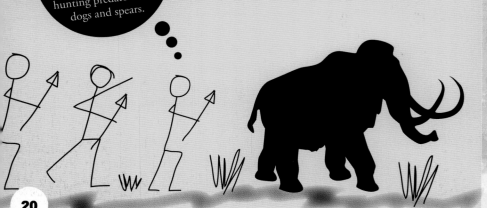

The world map – as it was

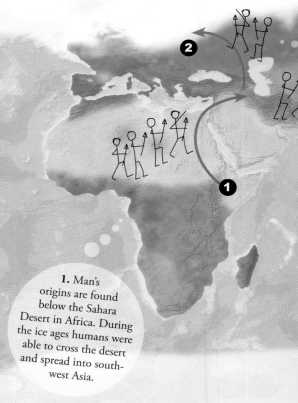

1. Man's origins are found below the Sahara Desert in Africa. During the ice ages humans were able to cross the desert and spread into south-west Asia.

Flickering thermostat We live in somewhat chilly times, with huge ice sheets at the Poles, but Earth, during its history, has been much colder than it is now – and much hotter too. For the last 2½ million years, it's as if someone has been turning the planet's thermostat up, then down, then up again, about every 100,000 years.

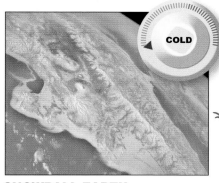

SNOWBALL EARTH
Between 900 and 600 million years ago, the Earth was probably covered in ice four separate times. Because volcanoes pumped carbon dioxide into the atmosphere, things slowly warmed up.

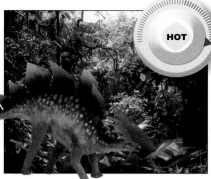

HOT DINOS
Carbon dioxide in the atmosphere traps the Sun's heat. In dinosaur times, there was much more than there is now. The planet was so warm there was no ice at the poles.

Tectonic plates There are seven major tectonic plates and 23 smaller ones – and they are moving all the time, some more than 8 cm (3 in) a year. Earthquakes happen along fault lines where two plates are moving in opposite directions. Big valleys form where two plates are moving apart.

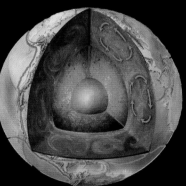

The crusty surface of the Earth floats on the soft mantle beneath. The closer to the centre of the Earth you go, the hotter it becomes. In the centre there is a core of molten iron.

when humans were advancing

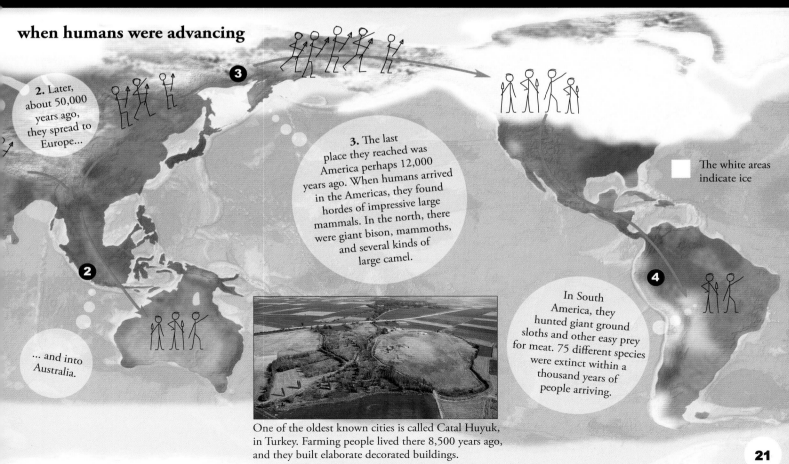

2. Later, about 50,000 years ago, they spread to Europe…

… and into Australia.

3. The last place they reached was America perhaps 12,000 years ago. When humans arrived in the Americas, they found hordes of impressive large mammals. In the north, there were giant bison, mammoths, and several kinds of large camel.

The white areas indicate ice

In South America, they hunted giant ground sloths and other easy prey for meat. 75 different species were extinct within a thousand years of people arriving.

One of the oldest known cities is called Catal Huyuk, in Turkey. Farming people lived there 8,500 years ago, and they built elaborate decorated buildings.

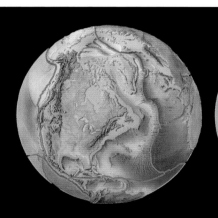

21

our crowded world

Homo sapiens has been the most **successful** of species – mankind has literally **taken over** the Earth. The world population reached *6 billion* in **October 1999**. By **summer 2005**, it had reached *6.5 billion*. **In 2006,** we added more than 90 million people to the planet.

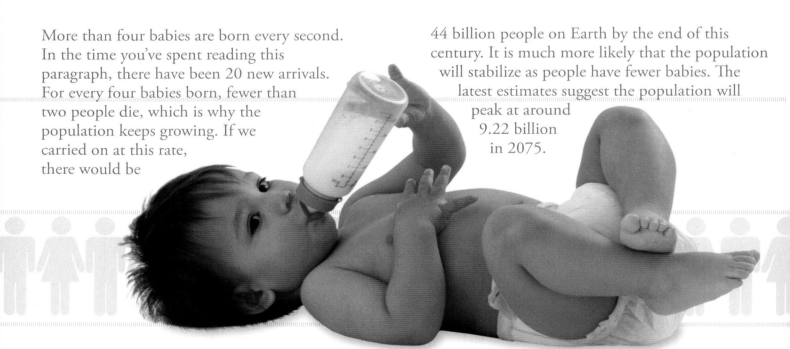

More than four babies are born every second. In the time you've spent reading this paragraph, there have been 20 new arrivals. For every four babies born, fewer than two people die, which is why the population keeps growing. If we carried on at this rate, there would be

44 billion people on Earth by the end of this century. It is much more likely that the population will stabilize as people have fewer babies. The latest estimates suggest the population will peak at around 9.22 billion in 2075.

DATE   **1100**   **1200**   **1300**   **1400**   **1500**

The latest estimates suggest the population

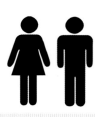

China has the most people There are over 1.3 billion Chinese people. India has over 1.1 billion and is expected to have more people than China in the next few decades. Between them, China and India have a third of all the people on Earth. The next most populous country is the US, which has around 300 million.

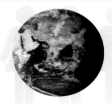

Where do they all live? In 2007, for the first time ever, half the people on Earth live in cities. The number of people living in urban areas will have grown from 309 million in 1950 to 3.9 billion by 2030. More people need more housing and sanitation, which produces more pollution, more concrete, and fewer green spaces.

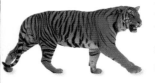

Biodiversity is threatened All these people are having a serious impact on the rest of Earth's inhabitants. Many species are being lost forever, because we are making such great changes to the places they live. There are between 10 and 30 million species on Earth but thousands, like the tiger, are in danger.

The sixth mass extinction...

Scientists think we are losing 30,000 species a year. That's three distinct species lost forever, every hour. There have been five previous episodes of mass extinction in the history of life. Each happened because of major geological events, like the asteroid that brought the end of the dinosaurs. There is no doubt we are in the middle of the sixth mass extinction. Almost a quarter of all the world's mammal species, and one in eight bird species, are likely to be extinct in the next 25 years. But the cause is different this time. There is no major geological event — just one species on Earth damaging habitats and altering the atmosphere.

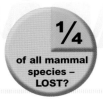

Cockroaches and rats are flourishing, however.

1/4 of all mammal species – LOST?

Population in billions

7

6

5

4

3

2

1

0

OUR CROWDED WORLD

1600   1700   1800   1900   2000

will peak at around 9.22 billion in 2075.

our atmosphere

Our atmosphere floats above our heads, like an unseen blanket round the world. Its existence is why our planet is such a lively place to be! It keeps Earth at the right temperature for plants to thrive and produce the life-giving gas – oxygen.

Energy from the Sun arrives on Earth in "short" waves called "solar radiation".

THE ATMOSPHERE HAS FOUR LAYERS

500 km (310 miles)

Satellite

Shuttle

THERMOSPHERE

Northern lights

85 km (50 miles)

MESOSPHERE

Meteors

50 km (30 miles)

STRATOSPHERE

Weather balloon

ozone layer

0-10 km (about 6 miles)

TROPOSPHERE

Jumbo jet

Mount Everest

AIR THAT WE BREATH
It's remarkable that there is so much oxygen in the Earth's atmosphere. For one thing, oxygen is unusually reactive, so it binds easily with lots of other elements to form life-giving compounds like water. Also, it's the one gas that all animal life on Earth needs to survive. So how does so much free oxygen get into the atmosphere? It's only there because plants and microbes continually create it.

78% Nitrogen

21% Oxygen

0.9% Argon

0.1% Other gases (carbon dioxide, methane, water vapour, helium, neon, hydrogen)

Layers of air The atmosphere has four layers. The air we breathe is in the troposphere. In fact, 80–90% of Earth's air is in the troposphere, held there by gravity. Almost all the rest of the air is in the stratosphere, above the clouds, where aircraft fly. Outside a plane window, the air is too thin to breathe. Higher up, in the mesosphere, it becomes very cold, dropping to a shivery -90°C (-130°F). Then, in the thermosphere, it gets hotter and hotter the higher up you go. It can be up to 1,500°C (2,730°F) up there. There is no sharp edge to the atmosphere – it gradually thins out and becomes space.

6%

6% of solar radiation is reflected straight back to space by molecules in the atmosphere.

Without the atmosphere, Earth's average temperature would be -6°C (21°F).

84% of solar radiation is absorbed by the rocks, soil, and water on Earth, where it changes into "long" waves – the type of heat picked up by an infra-red camera. Some of these waves are stopped from dispersing into space by the atmosphere.

10%

10% of solar radiation bounces off the Earth's surface and back to space.

84%

and the greenhouse effect

The greenhouse effect Water vapour, carbon dioxide, methane, and some other gases in the atmosphere absorb long-wave heat radiation, and send it back to Earth again. It's like what happens when you wrap yourself in a duvet. The heat from your body doesn't escape, but some is absorbed by the duvet. Some of it goes back to your body, and gradually you warm up, but you don't keep getting hotter and hotter because some of the duvet's warmth escapes into the air.

94% of the Sun's heat enters through the atmosphere.

Some heat escapes out of the atmosphere. But most is reflected back by greenhouse gases.

What's gone wrong? Greenhouse gases are increasing because we have upset the balance of the atmosphere by burning fossil fuels, and through other activities that produce greenhouse gases like carbon dioxide and methane. These keep more heat inside the atmosphere, which means the Earth warms up.

the ozone layer

What does it do? Ozone is a highly reactive molecule that exists in a 7 km (4.3 miles) thick layer in the stratosphere. The ozone layer absorbs most of the harmful ultraviolet radiation from the Sun, preventing it from reaching Earth. Without it, sunlight would be very damaging to our bodies, causing sunburn, skin cancer, and eye cataracts.

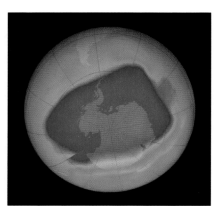

In 1985, British scientists found that almost half the ozone over Antarctica had disappeared. This shocked the world. It was because gases called chlorofluorocarbons (CFCs) had been building up in the stratosphere and these continually destroy ozone for 100 years.

CFCs were used in aerosols and to cool fridges. Now, they are hardly used at all. The rapid phase-out of CFCs shows that all the countries in the world can work together to change things quickly, if necessary.

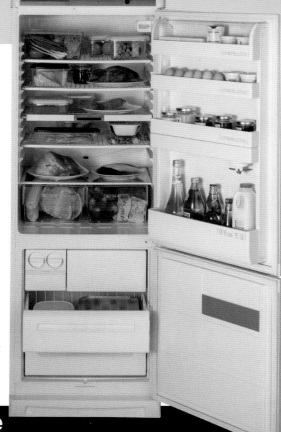

Good news: the hole in the ozone layer is mending and will return to normal by 2050.

the **carbon**

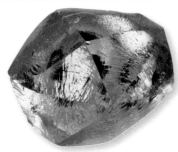

A diamond crystal is 100% pure carbon.

There is a lot of talk about carbon. But what is it? And where does it come from? Carbon is a natural substance, and one of the chemical elements. In its pure form, it mainly exists as a black solid (coal) or an extremely hard transparent crystal (diamond). Carbon forms only a small part of the Earth itself – less than one per cent – but it's a vital element in our bodies. All the chemicals in

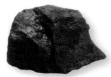

A lump of coal is 95% carbon.

PENCIL "LEAD" IS NOT LEAD AT ALL. IT'S MOSTLY GRAPHITE, A SOFT FORM OF PURE CARBON.

Carbon atoms move in a natural cycle between land, water, and the atmosphere. But humans have upset the balance...

IN WATER

Carbon dioxide dissolves in water and moves from the atmosphere into the ocean. Some (usually less) also moves from the ocean to the atmosphere by a process called "diffusion".

THE ATMOSPHERE

absorption

diffusion

Like land plants, ocean plants use carbon dioxide from the water for a process called "photosynthesis" (using light to help make food). They also store carbon.

Finally, water containing carbon moves from the ocean depths to the surface. Some of the ocean's carbon then moves from the surface to the atmosphere.

diffusion

photosynthesis

respiration

When the plants and animals die, they rot in the water, dissolving or sinking to the ocean floor. There they are buried and crushed by the pressure of water above. Eventually, they turn into rocks or fossil fuels.

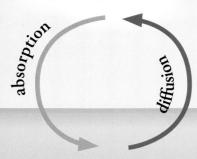

Ocean animals eat ocean plants and absorb the carbon they store. Both plants and animals release carbon dioxide back into the water through respiration (breathing).

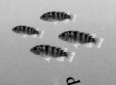

Some sea creatures can take carbon out of the water and use it to make their shells. When these creatures die, their carbon-rich shells dissolve or settle on the ocean floor. Then they too get compacted and gradually turn into fossil fuel, limestone, or chalk.

decay

compaction

cycle

living things have an underlying structure of carbon. It also joins with oxygen to form an important gas in Earth's atmosphere – carbon dioxide. Carbon moves around on Earth more than any other element in something called the "carbon cycle".

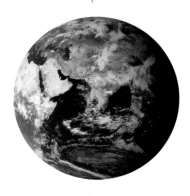

The Earth is less than 1% carbon

... but our bodies are 18% carbon

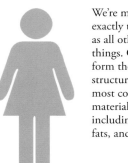

We're made from exactly the same stuff as all other living things. Carbon chains form the basic structure of all the most complex materials inside us, including proteins, fats, and even bone.

Carbon is the basis of life on Earth.

ON LAND

All plants take carbon dioxide from the atmosphere through photosynthesis. Trees store carbon in their wood as they grow. Cutting down lots of trees all over the world slows the removal of carbon dioxide from the air.

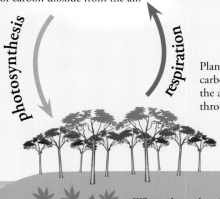

photosynthesis

respiration

Plants also release carbon into the atmosphere through respiration.

When plants die, they rot and become part of the soil. After a long time, some of this soil gets packed down and becomes fossil fuels like coal and oil.

compaction

WHAT PEOPLE DO

Humans have a big influence on the carbon cycle. When we take fossil fuels out of the ground and burn them for energy, the carbon in them turns into carbon dioxide and enters the atmosphere. But this carbon has been out of circulation for hundreds of millions of years. Rapidly adding it to the air is upsetting the balance.

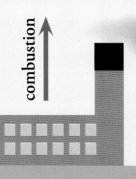

combustion

combustion

Burning trees also puts carbon dioxide into the air. This process doesn't normally upset the balance because the carbon was only just taken out of the air, by the trees themselves, as they grew.

extraction

Both the burning of fossil fuels and deforestation move carbon stored in fuel and trees to the atmosphere.

trees and plants turn into compacted soil

FOSSIL FUELS

fuels are taken from the ground

global WARMING

The carbon cycle Because people on Earth are burning so much fossil fuel and cutting down so many forests, the carbon cycle is off-balance. There is more carbon going into the atmosphere through burning than leaving it through photosynthesis.

GLOBAL WARMING FACTS AND STATS

The rise in world temperatures is called global warming. This is due in part to the amount of methane and carbon dioxide (CO_2) in the atmosphere (shown to the right). The increase in carbon dioxide comes from four main sectors (shown below).

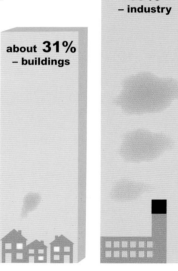

more than **40%** – industry

about **31%** – buildings

about **22%** – transport

about **4%** – agriculture

Source: IPCC 2001 report

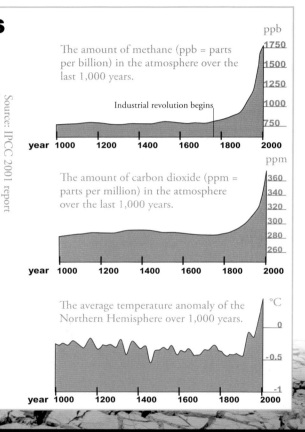

The amount of methane (ppb = parts per billion) in the atmosphere over the last 1,000 years.

ppb

Industrial revolution begins

The amount of carbon dioxide (ppm = parts per million) in the atmosphere over the last 1,000 years.

ppm

The average temperature anomaly of the Northern Hemisphere over 1,000 years.

°C

So far, the world has warmed

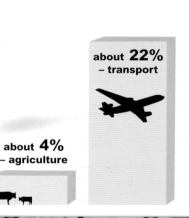

The danger from cows' bottoms
Methane is increasing too and each molecule is eight times better at warming the Earth than carbon dioxide! Methane comes from rotting waste and wet paddy fields. It is also burped out – from both ends – in huge quantities by grass-eating animals such as cows. The more people there are on Earth eating meat, rice, and throwing out rubbish, the more methane we produce.

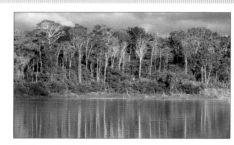

MOPPING UP
Earth's seas and vegetation are absorbing some of the extra CO_2. Plants are growing more lushly. Oceans are becoming more acidic because of it. Perhaps the oceans and plants are reaching the peak of their ability to absorb extra gases.

11 of the 12 years from 1995 to 2006 are

The amount of greenhouse gases (methane and carbon dioxide) being released into the atmosphere has gone up dramatically, and so have world temperatures. This is because more greenhouse gases in the atmosphere trap more heat.

Q How do we know global warming is caused by us?

A There is plenty of uncertainty about the science of global warming: how much will it warm up? Where will there be more rain? or less? and so on. But most of the world's scientists agree, without doubt, that **human greenhouse gas emissions** are responsible...

... whether they come from our factories, the boilers in our houses, our cars, power stations, or farms.

by 0.76°C (1.37°F) since 1900.

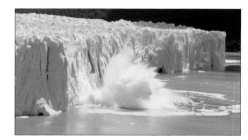

WARMING WORLD
Already, there is less snow and ice in the world. The great ice sheets in Antarctica (in the south) and Greenland (in the north) are melting, adding an estimated 20 billion tonnes of water each year to the sea.

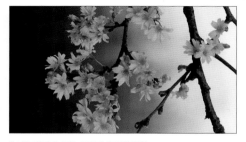

NATURE'S RHYTHMS
The growing season has lengthened across much of the northern hemisphere. Japan's famous cherry blossom now blooms five days earlier on average in Tokyo than it did 50 years ago.

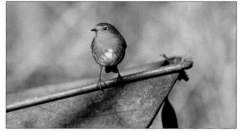

BIRD WATCHING
Animals and birds are entering new territories and higher altitudes because of increasing warmth. Inuits in the Canadian Arctic have spotted previously unseen birds such as robins. But, like many animals in this book, not all fauna can keep up with the changes.

in the top 12 warmest years ever recorded.

the search for **energy**

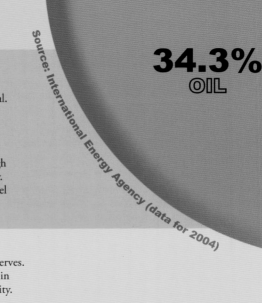

Energy flows so easily into our daily lives, we hardly notice it. Every time you drive in a car, take a hot shower, switch on a light, or watch TV, you use power that has travelled around the world. What's more, everything you use, including what you eat and the clothes you wear, has taken lots of energy to grow or to make, and find its way to you.

FOSSIL FUELS Once the remains of living things, fossil fuels such as coal, oil, and natural gas come from underground. They are fairly cheap, so people use their energy to do things they could do just as well by themselves, like travelling short distances in a car. But fossil fuels won't last forever, and burning them is harming our atmosphere – they are responsible for over 80 per cent of carbon dioxide emissions caused by humans. If we carry on burning them until they run out, the world's temperature could rise by more than 4°C (7.2°F). We urgently need to reduce energy use, and find new sources.

Where does OUR

25.1%
COAL

34.3%
OIL

Source: International Energy Agency (data for 2004)

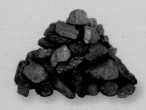

COAL
Coal is burned to create heat or, in power stations, to drive steam turbines that generate electricity.

HOW MUCH IS LEFT? There is enough coal in the ground to power the world for more than 1,000 years. Even now, developing industrial countries like China and India are busy building new coal-fired power stations.

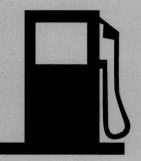

OIL
Large reserves of oil were first discovered in the early 20th century. Because it's a liquid, oil is easier to work with than coal. It can be refined into fuels like petrol and diesel to run cars, trucks, aeroplanes, and heating systems. It's also used to make products like plastics, medicines, and washing powders.

HOW MUCH IS LEFT? Some experts think there is still enough oil underground to power the world for the rest of this century. Others believe that world oil production is close to its peak level now, and will soon decrease.

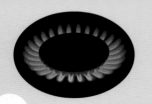

NATURAL GAS
Natural gas is actually methane that has collected above oil reserves. It's the last fossil fuel to be exploited and was first used widely in the 1930s and 1940s. Like coal, it's burned for heat or electricity.

HOW MUCH IS LEFT? Experts believe there is enough natural gas to last out the century, but beyond that, it's likely to become very expensive and difficult to extract.

Until about 150 years ago, humans burned wood for heating and cooking, and used animals for moving things around. But since fossil fuels became widely available, world energy use has shot up, and demand is still rising fast.

NUCLEAR ENERGY Nuclear reactors generate electricity using energy from inside atoms. Here, uranium atoms are split apart, releasing masses of energy. The first nuclear power plant opened in the United States of America in 1960, and there are now 435 similar plants around the world – 104 of them in the USA. Some countries rely more on nuclear power than others – it provides half of Sweden's electricity, and a huge 78 per cent of France's electricity.

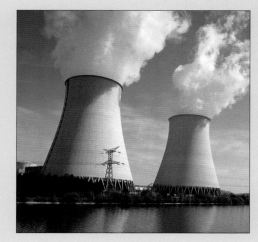

energy come from?

20.9% NATURAL GAS

6.5% NUCLEAR

13.2% RENEWABLES

RENEWABLE ENERGY Unlike fossil fuels, renewable energy sources will never be used up – the energy just keeps on coming. Among the natural sources that can generate electricity or make fuels are sunlight (collected in solar panels), wind (powering tall turbines, below), water (harnessed to make hydroelectricity from waterfalls and dams), ocean waves, Earth's heat trapped under the ground, and growing plants.

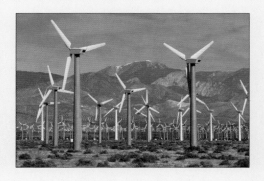

Renewable energy breakdown

- 10.6% burning biomass or waste
- 2.2% hydroelectric (water) power
- 0.4% all other renewables

SAVING ENERGY Because fossil fuels are cheap, our buildings, our transport, and even our power generators waste a great deal of it. For each unit of electrical power that arrives at your house, two units have been lost along the way, mostly in the form of heat. Experts have worked out that, by 2020, we could cut world greenhouse gas emissions in half – just by saving energy and doing things more efficiently.

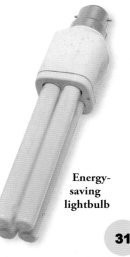

Energy-saving lightbulb

water of life

People need water for drinking, growing food, and keeping clean, and we also require large amounts for industry. The amount of water being used is increasing all the time – while Earth's population trebled in the 20th century, its water use increased six-fold. As standards of living rise, people want cleaner surroundings, and they eat a wider variety of food (leading to increasingly intensive farming). These conditions require even more water. We are already taking half the water in rivers, lakes, and streams for our own use, but wild animals and plants need it too.

ONLY 1% OF THE WORLD'S WATER IS DRINKABLE

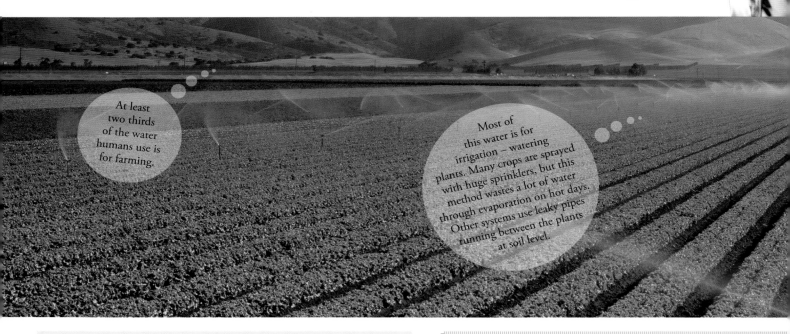

At least two thirds of the water humans use is for farming.

Most of this water is for irrigation – watering plants. Many crops are sprayed with huge sprinklers, but this method wastes a lot of water through evaporation on hot days. Other systems use leaky pipes running between the plants at soil level.

TO HAVE...
In rich countries, most people have an unlimited supply of fresh clean water that flows out of taps in their kitchen and bathroom.

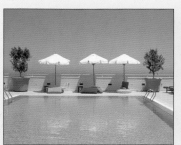

... AND HAVE NOT
But in many countries, people have little access to clean water. Some women in rural Africa spend a quarter of their time carrying water.

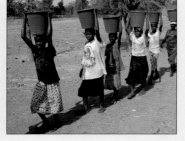

WATER FACTS AND STATS

ONLY THREE PER CENT OF THE WORLD'S WATER IS FRESH WATER. OF THIS...

... 68.7%
is in glaciers and ice-caps

... 31%
is groundwater

... 0.3%
is surface water (lakes, rivers, and streams)

THE WATER CYCLE

Water evaporates from the surface of the sea and enters the atmosphere as a gas. Some of it condenses into tiny droplets that we see as clouds. These then fall as rain or snow. Some rainwater is taken up by plants, some runs into long-term storage underground (becoming "groundwater"), and some flows into rivers and streams. This last source is where humans get most of their water.

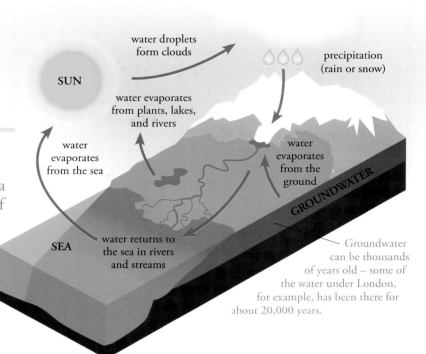

water droplets form clouds

precipitation (rain or snow)

SUN

water evaporates from plants, lakes, and rivers

water evaporates from the sea

water evaporates from the ground

GROUNDWATER

SEA

water returns to the sea in rivers and streams

Groundwater can be thousands of years old – some of the water under London, for example, has been there for about 20,000 years.

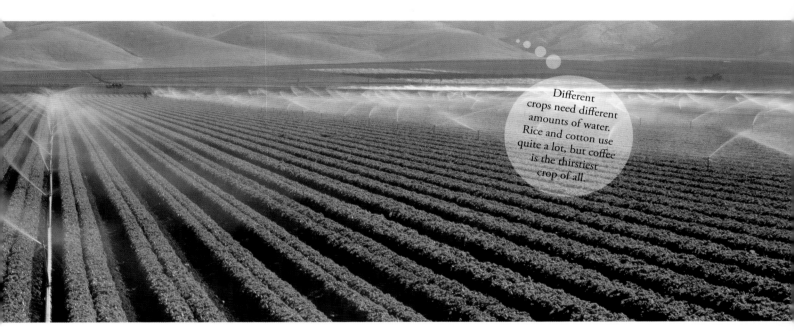

Different crops need different amounts of water. Rice and cotton use quite a lot, but coffee is the thirstiest crop of all.

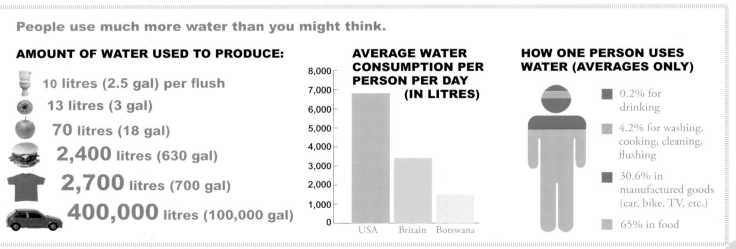

People use much more water than you might think.

AMOUNT OF WATER USED TO PRODUCE:

10 litres (2.5 gal) per flush

13 litres (3 gal)

70 litres (18 gal)

2,400 litres (630 gal)

2,700 litres (700 gal)

400,000 litres (100,000 gal)

AVERAGE WATER CONSUMPTION PER PERSON PER DAY (IN LITRES)

8,000
7,000
6,000
5,000
4,000
3,000
2,000
1,000
0

USA   Britain   Botswana

HOW ONE PERSON USES WATER (AVERAGES ONLY)

0.2% for drinking

4.2% for washing, cooking, cleaning, flushing

30.6% in manufactured goods (car, bike, TV, etc.)

65% in food

high-waste society

Hundreds of thousands of tonnes of plastic, glass, metal, and even electronics, are thrown away every day. A hundred years ago, this kind of waste *hardly existed*. People re-used things at home. They burned or

In rich countries each person produces *five to ten times* their own BODY WEIGHT in rubbish each year.

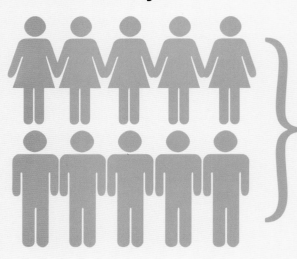

So what happens to all the rubbish?

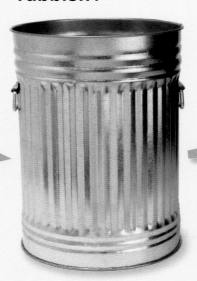

It's recycled

60% of what you throw away can be recycled or composted. Glass, paper, cardboard, metals, and plastics can be crushed, pulped, or melted, and used again. This fleece, for example, is made from recycled bottles.

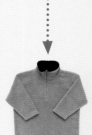

So what about industrial waste?

Only 10 per cent of waste is household. Factories also produce waste, but because this often consists of one material (such as broken-up concrete or ash) another use can sometimes be found for it.

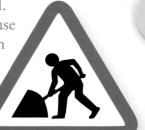

As landfill sites fill up fast, we need to re-think our approach to rubbish.
Reduce – buy less stuff.
Re-use – think of other uses for things before throwing them out.
Recycle – separate out rubbish into things that can be recycled, and things that can't.
See this website for lots of handy tips: www.wasteonline.org.uk/

composted waste paper, food, and garden cuttings. They didn't buy large quantities of packaged goods. We need to go back to how we used to be and **reduce, re-use,** and **recycle**.

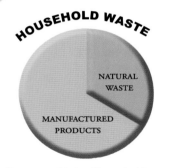

HOUSEHOLD WASTE

NATURAL WASTE

MANUFACTURED PRODUCTS

About two thirds of household waste comes from manufactured products, the rest from our food or garden.

It's composted

Composting is nature's way of dealing with waste. Food and garden waste ("green waste") are easily broken down by bacteria and other microbes. Paper, card, and board ("brown waste") can be composted too. Left in a pile in the corner of the garden, green waste will slowly change into dark compost that can improve the soil. Add worms to the mix and fertilizer is made even more quickly.

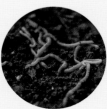

It's burnt

Household waste can be burnt, or heated in a big furnace without air in a process called "pyrolysis". This gets rid of much of the waste, and the heat can be used to generate electricity by heating water to drive a steam turbine.

The difficult wastes

The toughest wastes to deal with are hazardous wastes, such as batteries and computer parts, that contain toxic substances. These should be disposed of carefully, but in reality, they often end up in ordinary landfill sites.

It's dumped in landfill

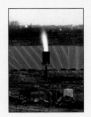

Landfill sites are often old holes in the ground where rock has been quarried. The rubbish going into them contains lots of food, paper, and garden waste, which rots and creates methane, a greenhouse gas. What remains after the rotting is a foul liquid that can seep into groundwater, carrying with it toxic chemicals from hazardous wastes. Space in landfills is running out fast.

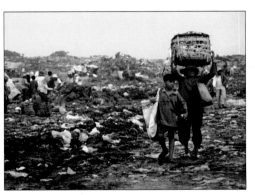

EXPORTING WASTE

Many rich countries export hundreds of thousands of tonnes of waste a year to countries where it can be handled more cheaply. Much of it ends up in China, which buys large quantities of waste plastic, paper, and cardboard, as well as electronic waste. The huge freight ships that carry manufactured goods from China to Europe and America often return to China filled with lightweight waste.

sustainable life

Planet Earth provides all the resources we need to live – air to breathe, water to drink, soil to grow crops in, fuels to burn, and materials, like metals, to build things. Most of the Earth's resources are constantly being made on Earth. Some are made quickly like wood when trees grow, or fresh water when rain falls. Some take thousands of years to form, like soil. And some are limited, like land.

Land use Land is a very basic resource, because it is needed to grow plants, which are used for food, fuel, and materials. The world's land is not divided fairly at the moment – people in industrialised countries use far more than their fair share to support their lifestyle. If people in developing countries like India and China start consuming as much fuel and food, the world will not be able to support us all.

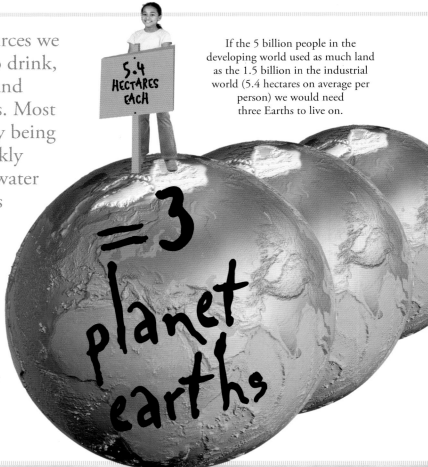

5.4 HECTARES EACH

=3 planet earths

If the 5 billion people in the developing world used as much land as the 1.5 billion in the industrial world (5.4 hectares on average per person) we would need three Earths to live on.

What is your **eco** footprint?

Your footprints on Earth One way of seeing how sustainable your activities are is to measure your ecological footprint. This is not a foot-shaped mark in the ground! It is a number that tells you how much of the Earth's resources you use. An ecological footprint is the amount of land that would be needed to grow all the food, fuel, and materials you use. It is measured in hectares. (One hectare equals 0.01 sq km or 2½ acres.)

USA
9.7 hectares of land needed for each person

UK
5.6

World average
2.2

Brazil
2.1

Sustainable average
1.8

China
1.6

India
0.7

Already, the average ecological footprint for the whole world is 2.2 hectares, higher than the sustainable level of 1.8 hectares each.

1.8 hectares per person is a sustainable footprint for today's population.

SUSTAINABLE VS UNSUSTAINABLE

Going on forever The word "sustain" means to keep going – if something is "sustainable", it can be carried on forever. We can only sustain the Earth's resources by consuming them at the same rate – or more slowly – than they are being produced.

SEAWEED Seaweed is harvested in many countries. Farmers have long used it as a fertilizer. Now it's also used as a food supplement, and chemicals from it are used to thicken cosmetics and food. In France, the harvest is strictly managed by law. Removing the "holdfasts", where the seaweeds attach to the rock, is prohibited. And each area that is cut must be left to regrow.

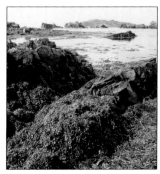

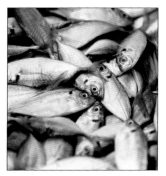

FISHING The worst case of humans overusing a natural resource at the moment is sea fishing. So many fish are being caught that wild fish populations have collapsed in many places. The fish cannot reproduce fast enough to replace the fish that are eaten. Fish species many of us eat regularly, like cod and tuna, may never recover.

ORGANIC FARMERS Organic farmers are very careful to protect their soil, so that over time it builds up and improves, rather than being blown or washed away. Unlike ordinary farmers, they seldom leave bare soil exposed over winter. They leave crop stubbles or plant a cover crop to protect the soil. They also add compost to the soil and plant hedges as windbreaks.

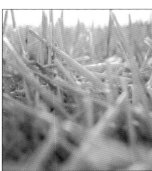

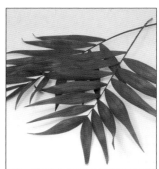

PALM HARVEST Some resources are over-harvested for surprising purposes. American and Canadian churches import 30 million palm fronds for Palm Sunday. They come from Mexico and Guatemala, and rainforest conservation groups say many are taken from wild rainforests. More palm plants are taken than the forest can regrow.

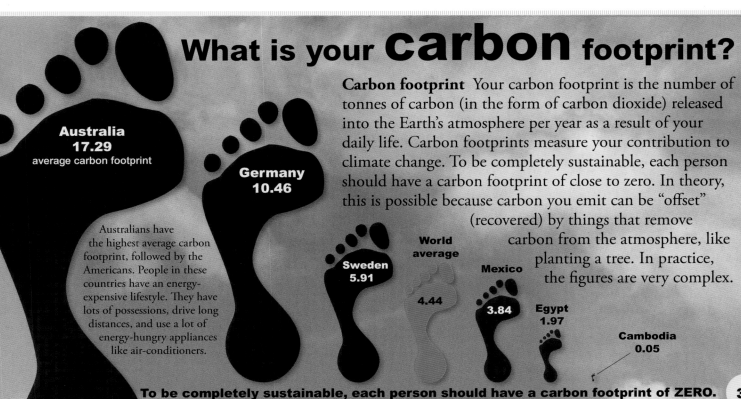

What is your **carbon** footprint?

Carbon footprint Your carbon footprint is the number of tonnes of carbon (in the form of carbon dioxide) released into the Earth's atmosphere per year as a result of your daily life. Carbon footprints measure your contribution to climate change. To be completely sustainable, each person should have a carbon footprint of close to zero. In theory, this is possible because carbon you emit can be "offset" (recovered) by things that remove carbon from the atmosphere, like planting a tree. In practice, the figures are very complex.

Australia 17.29 average carbon footprint

Germany 10.46

Sweden 5.91

World average 4.44

Mexico 3.84

Egypt 1.97

Cambodia 0.05

Australians have the highest average carbon footprint, followed by the Americans. People in these countries have an energy-expensive lifestyle. They have lots of possessions, drive long distances, and use a lot of energy-hungry appliances like air-conditioners.

To be completely sustainable, each person should have a carbon footprint of ZERO.

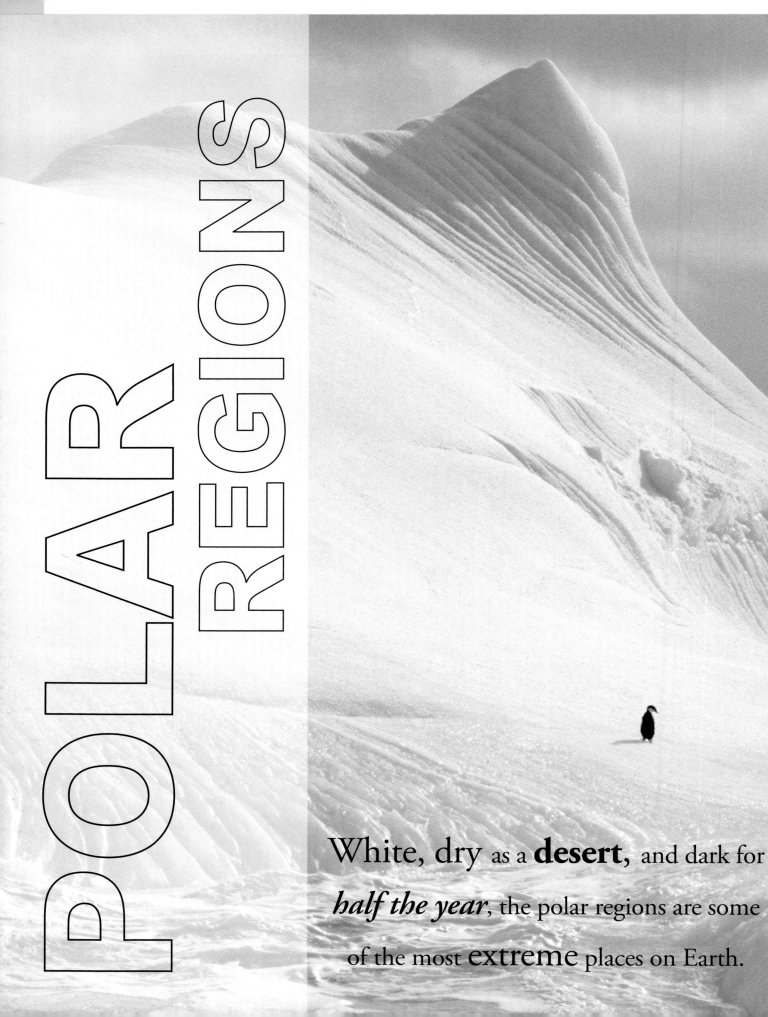

POLAR REGIONS

White, dry as a **desert,** and dark for *half the year*, the polar regions are some of the most **extreme** places on Earth.

POLAR REGIONS

And they are also the most fragile, warming twice as fast as the Tropics. In these vulnerable places, changing climate is affecting the plants, animals, and people that live there. These areas are of special importance to the world and we need to do all we can to protect them.

where on earth...?

With months of endless darkness, hurricane winds, and freezing temperatures, the poles really are vast, frozen wildernesses. Yet plants and animals thrive here and have become so good at living in the "freezer" that they probably could not survive anywhere else. They like it cold!

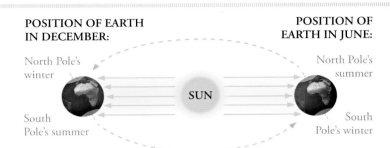

POSITION OF EARTH IN DECEMBER:

North Pole's winter

SUN

South Pole's summer

POSITION OF EARTH IN JUNE:

North Pole's summer

South Pole's winter

The Arctic and Antarctic have seasons at opposite times of the year. From this diagram you can see that during both places' winters, they receive no sunlight at all.

THE ARCTIC
– frozen sea surrounded by land at the top of the Earth

Six countries own different parts of the Arctic – Greenland, Russian Federation, Norway, Finland, Canada, and the United States. The US bought a part of the Arctic (Alaska) from Russia in 1867 for $7.2 million (approximately $135 million in today's money), and it became a US state in 1959.

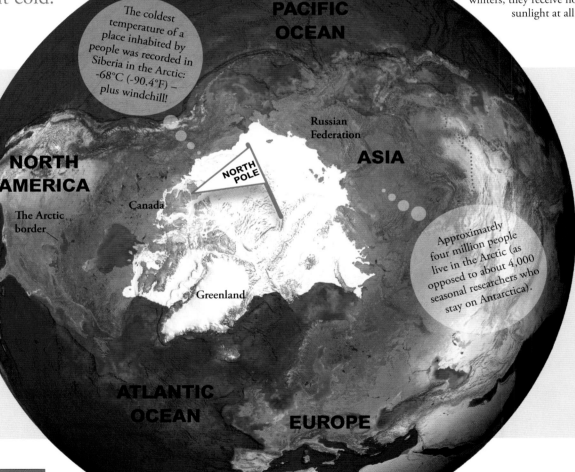

The coldest temperature of a place inhabited by people was recorded in Siberia in the Arctic: -68°C (-90.4°F) – plus windchill!

PACIFIC OCEAN

Russian Federation

ASIA

NORTH AMERICA

NORTH POLE

Canada

The Arctic border

Greenland

ATLANTIC OCEAN

EUROPE

Approximately four million people live in the Arctic (as opposed to about 4,000 seasonal researchers who stay on Antarctica).

What is the Arctic? Most of the Arctic is taken up by the frozen Arctic Ocean. The central part, around the North Pole, is frozen solid all year round, but the outer edges thaw and break up in summer. The Arctic also includes land, at the edges of which is a treeless landscape called tundra.

WHY SO COLD?

Because Earth has a curved surface, the poles receive 20 per cent less sunlight than the tropics at the Equator. While the Sun shines overhead at the tropics, it is always low in the sky at the poles. At such a shallow angle, its rays have to cut across more of Earth's atmosphere, so less energy gets through. As well as this, fierce, freezing gales make heat disappear more quickly: "windchill", as this is known, makes -48°C (-54°F) feel like -69°C (-93°F). The centre of Antarctica is on average much colder than the Arctic for two reasons: it's higher with more mountains, and it's further from the warming waters of the oceans.

THE ARCTIC

Average summer temperature: **1.5°C (35°F)**

Average year-round temperature: **-14°C (7°F)**

Average winter temperature: **-29°C (-20°F)**

THE ANTARCTIC

Average summer temperature: **2°C (35.6°F)**

Average year-round temperature: **-48°C (-54°F)**

Average winter temperature: **-79°C (-110°F)**

CHALLENGING CLIMATE

Life at the poles is a fight for survival. At both poles, the meagre sunlight means there is little energy for plants to grow and little food for animals. There is not enough energy to make trees grow and, without them, there is no shelter from blistering winds. In this harsh environment, animals rush to breed in the brief respite of summer. For everything else, the pace of life is more relaxed. In the slow-motion Arctic, some caterpillars take 14 years to become moths.

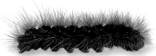

Arctic caterpillar, Alaska

AFRICA

ATLANTIC OCEAN

INDIAN OCEAN

SOUTH AMERICA

PACIFIC OCEAN

SOUTH POLE

Antarctica is the world's driest desert; in some places it has not rained or snowed for centuries.

What time is it? This is a tricky question in Antarctica where all time zones meet. So people there use New Zealand time.

New Zealand

The coldest temperature recorded was -89.2°C (-128.6°F) in 1983.

AUSTRALIA

ANTARCTICA
– frozen land surrounded by sea at the bottom of the Earth

Antarctica is the only continent on Earth dedicated to peaceful scientific cooperation, "for the benefit of all mankind," by virtue of the Antarctic Treaty, signed in December 1959. The continent is not "owned" by any country.

What is Antarctica? The region around the South Pole, Antarctica, is the coldest place on Earth. While the Arctic is a flat, frozen ocean surrounded by land, Antarctica is the opposite, a frozen mountainous continent, surrounded by ocean. The only land animals in this freezing desert are penguins and seals.

the high arctic

The Arctic has two very different ecosystems. At the extreme north, there is a world of sea ice dominated by a few marine mammals, such as polar bears, whales, walruses, and seals. This is known as the "high Arctic". Further south, the warmer, sunnier tundra has a richer ecosystem and is home to many more species of animals, birds, insects, and plants. Although most Arctic species are adapted for life on either the ice cap or the tundra, some – including polar bears – will range between both.

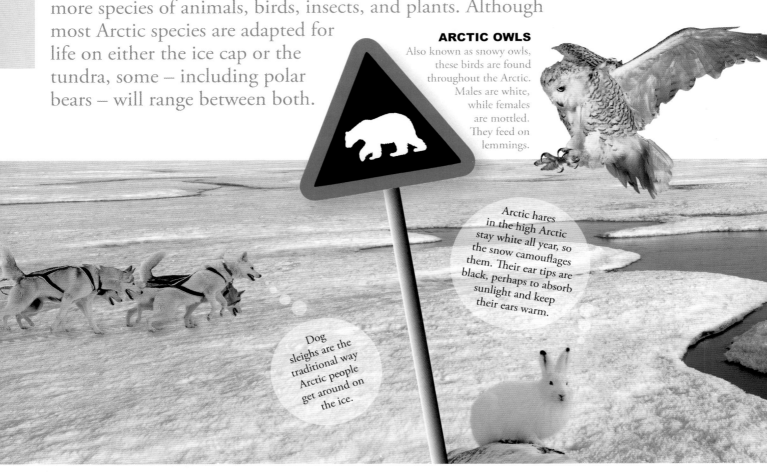

ARCTIC OWLS
Also known as snowy owls, these birds are found throughout the Arctic. Males are white, while females are mottled. They feed on lemmings.

Arctic hares in the high Arctic stay white all year, so the snow camouflages them. Their ear tips are black, perhaps to absorb sunlight and keep their ears warm.

Dog sleighs are the traditional way Arctic people get around on the ice.

Close to nature In the Arctic, humans are closely linked to the ecosystem and the animals that live there. They only thrive if the Arctic animals are thriving.

Watch out for polar bears! Signs like this in the inhabited part of the Arctic warn people that there could be polar bears about.

ICE FOX
The Arctic fox lives farther north than any other fox. It also has the warmest fur of any mammal, including the polar bear. These foxes hunt lemmings, but will eat any leftovers they find as well.

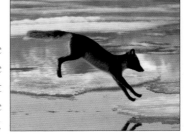

A world of ice Ice dominates the Arctic. During winter, the North Pole sees no sunlight at all for six months, which is why a large area round the Pole remains permanently frozen. Further south, there is more sunlight and it is warmer. Here, the ice is frozen in winter, but thinner and more broken-up (or completely melted) in summer.

The Arctic food web The ocean is a vital part of the Arctic, creating the marine food web on which its ecosystem depends. The food web is fuelled by energy harnessed from the Sun by tiny microscopic creatures. The energy is carried right up to the polar bears, and the top predator – man.

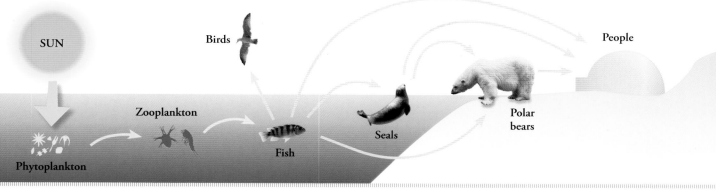

SUN

Birds

People

Zooplankton

Seals

Polar bears

Fish

Phytoplankton

PRODUCERS
At the base of the web, microscopic algae called phytoplankton turn sunlight into food energy.

PRIMARY CONSUMERS
Microscopic ocean creatures known as zooplankton feed on the phytoplankton.

SECONDARY CONSUMERS
Then fish such as cod and Arctic charr eat the zooplankton.

SECONDARY CONSUMERS
Seabirds and seals feed on the fish.

TOP CARNIVORES
Polar bears will feed on almost anything lower down the web – from seals to small walruses and even whales.

PEOPLE
Arctic people like the Inuit eat fish, and hunt polar bears and seals for their meat and skins.

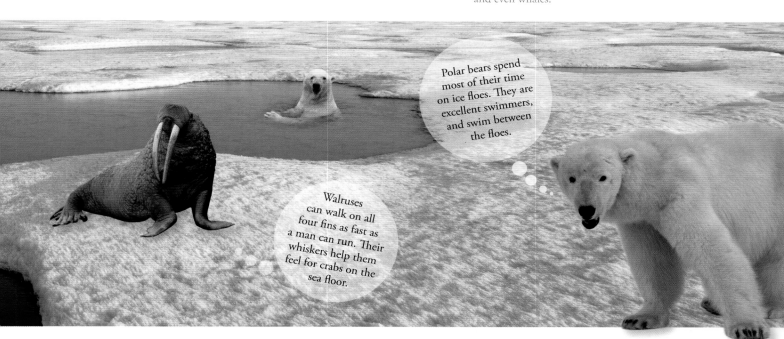

Polar bears spend most of their time on ice floes. They are excellent swimmers, and swim between the floes.

Walruses can walk on all four fins as fast as a man can run. Their whiskers help them feel for crabs on the sea floor.

ARCTIC "RABBITS"
Lemmings live in Northern Canada and are an important part of the food chain there. They make burrows in the snow where they are safe from the cold and wind.

HOLE MAINTENANCE
In autumn and early winter, holes in the ice start freezing over, so seals create breathing holes. They keep the holes open with their strong claws, and by pushing their noses through.

SUMMER VEGETATION
It is hard for plants to grow in the Arctic. Even in the summer it is cold and windy. Yet many types of plants have adapted to Arctic life by growing low to the ground.

FUR COATS
In the high Arctic, people still live by hunting seals for food and clothing. Some still use traditional sledges pulled by dogs, but most now use snowmobiles (snow motorbikes).

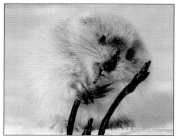
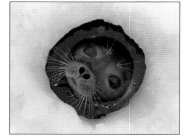
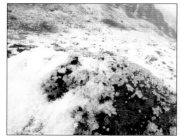
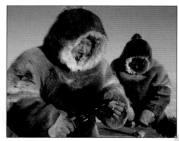

melting arctic

People are worried about global warming everywhere on Earth, but the poles are giving most cause for concern. The Arctic is warming *twice as quickly* as the world average and both the ice cap and the tundra further south are beginning to melt. Scientists think the Arctic may **lose** almost all its **summer sea ice** within decades.

1979

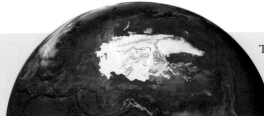

The area of Arctic sea ice has been shrinking by about 0.7% each year for several decades.

2007

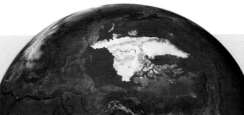

By 2007, the area of Arctic sea ice had plummeted to a 29-year low.

These images show the yearly minimum area of ice, which occurs each year in summer, between September and October.

Sea levels could rise by 1 m (3 ft) by 2100,

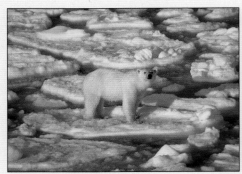

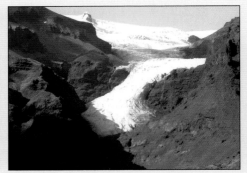

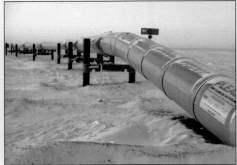

Threatened animals An Arctic with less ice would be a different place. Polar bears hunt on the pack ice and use ice floes as stepping stones to move around. Seals and walruses give birth on ice and rest there when they are not in the water. In a warmer Arctic, these animals could become extinct.

Glaciers Apart from the ice cap, there are huge glaciers in the continents further south: frozen rivers of ice that snake down through mountains in places such as Greenland and Norway. When the Arctic heats up, the glaciers will also start to melt and drain into the sea, further adding to the problem.

Industry The gas and oil industry in the Arctic causes pollution and has brought new settlers to the Arctic, turning native people into small minorities in their traditional areas. Reduced sea ice could increase marine transport and access to natural resources, making oil spills more likely.

Local changes, global effects Sea-level rises caused by melting polar ice will cause more flooding in coastal areas around the world. Extreme floods currently happen in low-lying New York City once a century. But if sea levels were 1 m (3 ft) higher, floods could happen every three years. The melting Arctic will bring a worrying change. Currently, the icy white poles reflect most sunlight back into space, keeping the planet cooler. But as the ice disappears, more of the Sun's heat will be absorbed instead. Earth will warm more quickly – and climate change may accelerate.

80% of the Sun's heat is reflected off ice

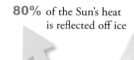

SUN

10% of the Sun's heat is reflected off water

Low-lying islands, like the Maldives, are already threatened by rising sea levels.

20% of the Sun's heat is absorbed into ice

90% of the Sun's heat is absorbed into the sea

 Over 80 per cent of Greenland is covered by a gigantic layer of ice called the Greenland Ice Sheet. If the whole thing melted, the world's sea levels could rise by over 7 m (24 ft). This huge rise is not an immediate risk, however: scientists think it could take hundreds of years for the ice sheet to melt completely.

Greenland

partly due to Greenland ice starting to melt.

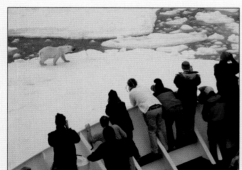

Tourism Tourist cruises are gaining better access to the frozen north, bringing disturbance, litter, and pollution with them. But the wilderness they come to see may have long gone.

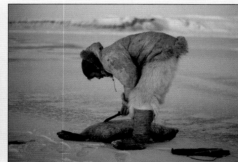

Native people If seals disappear, what would happen to the Inuit hunters who depend on them for food? To hunt, catch, and share ringed seals is their way of life.

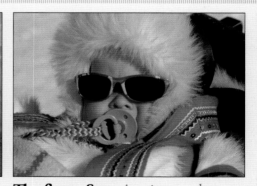

The fierce Sun Arctic people have noticed that the Sun's heat feels "stronger, stinging, and sharp". Sunburn and strange skin rashes never experienced before are becoming common. This is due to too much ultraviolet radiation from the Sun penetrating the thin ozone layer over the Arctic.

 With the sea ice and permafrost melting, the Inuit of the Arctic face an uncertain future. Find out more about their lives and culture at: www.athropolis.com/links/inuit.htm

the polar bear

THESE ULTIMATE ARCTIC WARRIORS, FOUND AS FAR NORTH AS THE POLE ITSELF, ARE THREATENED BY THE MELTING ICE CAP

Ice is vital for polar bears. They hunt seals on it, eat on it, and use it like a bridge to move from one part of the frozen ocean to another. But now the Arctic ice is threatened by global warming, polar bears are threatened too. Summer comes sooner, so the ice melts earlier and the bears have less time to feed. They put on less weight for the winter and therefore have less chance of survival. Already polar bears are being seen in poor condition and the average weight and number of cubs has declined. Now there is less ice and more water, the bears are having to swim further. An Arctic without polar bears seems unthinkable, but there are fewer than 25,000 bears left worldwide. They are becoming a threatened species and may disappear entirely if global warming trends continue.

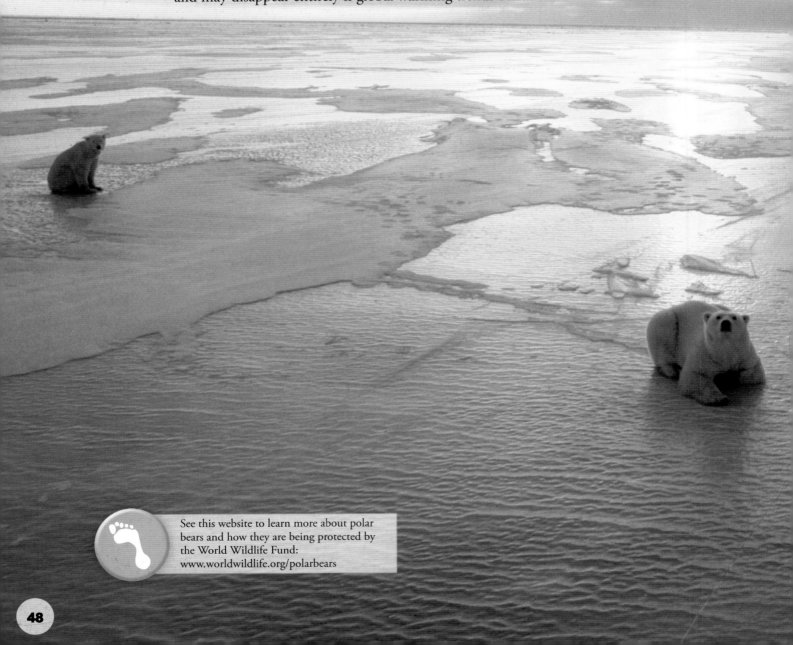

See this website to learn more about polar bears and how they are being protected by the World Wildlife Fund:
www.worldwildlife.org/polarbears

Polar bears live in the Arctic and the very north of Canada. The effects of global warming can be seen in the declining number of cubs being born.

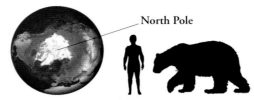

North Pole

Polar bears hunt ice-living ringed seals. The seals have also been affected by the rise in temperatures as the snow caves in which they rear pups are melting earlier. Fewer seals means less food for the bears.

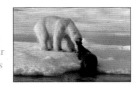

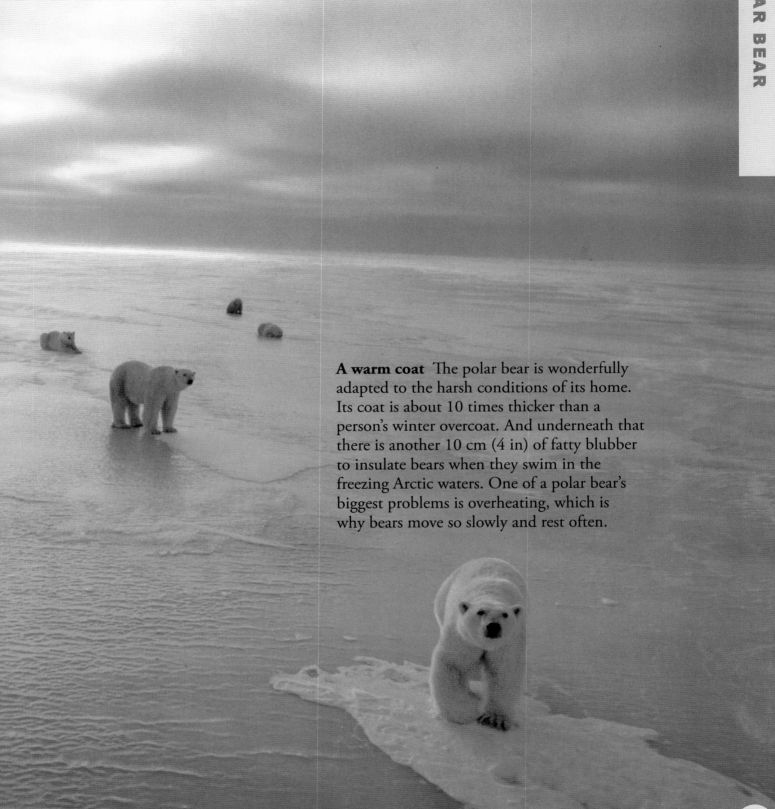

A warm coat The polar bear is wonderfully adapted to the harsh conditions of its home. Its coat is about 10 times thicker than a person's winter overcoat. And underneath that there is another 10 cm (4 in) of fatty blubber to insulate bears when they swim in the freezing Arctic waters. One of a polar bear's biggest problems is overheating, which is why bears move so slowly and rest often.

tundra ecosystem

Between the icy wastelands

of the Arctic north and the forest biomes further south there is a swathe of in-between territory called tundra. Tundra is too cold for trees to grow apart from a few dwarf species at its southern edges. Tundra covers four per cent of the Earth's surface.

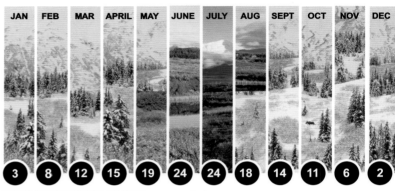

JAN	FEB	MAR	APRIL	MAY	JUNE	JULY	AUG	SEPT	OCT	NOV	DEC
3	8	12	15	19	24	24	18	14	11	6	2

HOURS OF DAYLIGHT IN LAPLAND (average per day)
During most of the year the tundra is bitingly cold and windy. The winter is long and dark with only a few hours of light each day. In the brief warm summer, when it is daylight almost continuously, life takes off.

TO THE NORTH
Arctic ice cap

N

S

TO THE SOUTH
boreal forests

What is permafrost?

Tundra is built on frozen soil called permafrost, which lies 50 cm (21 in) beneath the surface. Above it is an active layer of soil that thaws in summer and freezes in winter.

Bright buttercups, poppies, and sedges, as well as mosses and grasses, cover the tundra in summer.

SUNBATHING

Sulphur butterflies almost always stand with their folded wings side-on to the Sun so they can absorb the maximum amount of solar energy.

How the animals cope The tundra is a biome with a very cold climate, hardly any rain, and a short growing season. Plants are low-growing to escape the wind, and flowers turn their faces to track the Sun. Animals are adapted to long, cold winters and breed and raise young quickly in the short summer. Many birds are migrants that come to breed and then fly somewhere warmer.

Tundra food web Food is more limited at the poles than anywhere else on Earth. Creatures compete to survive, but the fate of each one depends on all the others.

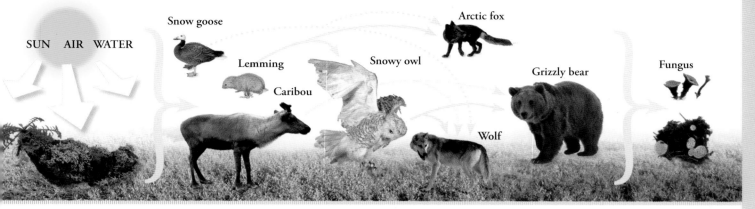

SUN AIR WATER

Snow goose · Lemming · Caribou · Snowy owl · Arctic fox · Wolf · Grizzly bear · Fungus

PRODUCERS
Plants use sunlight to turn air, water, and nutrients into food, ultimately fuelling everything else on the tundra.

PRIMARY CONSUMERS
The next link in the chain are herbivores, which eat plants. They include caribou, geese, lemmings, and grouse.

SECONDARY CONSUMERS
Secondary consumers are carnivores, living off primary consumers. They include wolves, foxes, owls, and insect-eating animals.

TOP CARNIVORES
Grizzly bears eat plants and berries in season. They will also eat whatever meat is available including moose, caribou, hare, and fish.

DECOMPOSERS
Fungi and miscroscopic organisms break down dead matter and waste, returning it to the soil so the cycle can begin again.

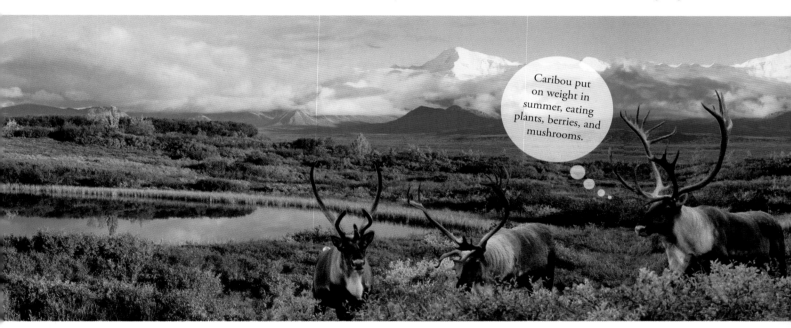

Caribou put on weight in summer, eating plants, berries, and mushrooms.

FUR AND FLEECE
An ice-age survivor, the musk ox has the ultimate fur coat and can stay out all winter. It's the only animal that never needs shelter. Reintroductions to the wild have boosted numbers.

MOSQUITO BITES
Huge swarms of mosquitoes thrive in the shallow lakes of the tundra. They come out in early summer and bite animals and birds. Caribou are particular favourites.

SUMMER HOLIDAY
The Arctic tern visits the tundra in summer to breed and then flies south to catch another summer in Antarctica. It sees more daylight than any other animal on Earth.

CARIBOU FOOD
Lichens, made up of fungi living with algae, are an important part of the tundra vegetation. Caribou are able to eat lichen because they produce a special enzyme that helps them digest it.

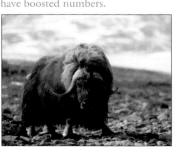
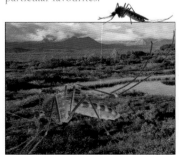
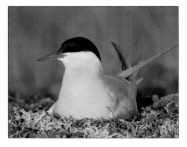
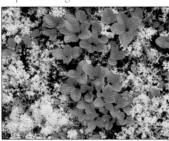

warming **tundra**

Some areas of tundra have **warmed faster** than almost **anywhere else** on Earth, with an average temperature increase of 3°C (5.4°F) in the last 40 years. This is thought to be caused by a combination of man-made *climate change* and melting ice exposing more bare ground, which warms up more quickly than **snow** and **ice**.

SOURCE: Arctic Council ACIA

Current permafrost area

Projected permafrost area (2100)

Current sea ice

Projected change in Arctic permafrost by 2100

A thawing permafrost not only affects the

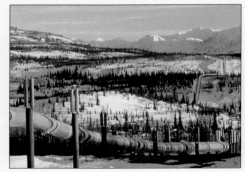

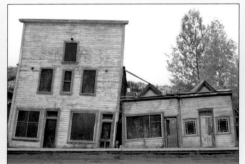

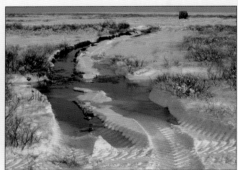

Keeping it cool The Trans-Alaska pipeline was raised above the ground for 640 km (400 miles) of its length to stop it transferring heat onto the ground and thawing the permafrost. It is likely that as the ground becomes more unstable, maintenance costs will rise.

Cracking up The thawing permafrost also causes problems to buildings. This house in Canada was built on hard, frozen ground, but as it melts, the building moves. The same problem occurs to railway tracks, runways, and other infrastructure in the far north.

End of the road As the permafrost thaws, the number of days each year that ice roads and tundra are frozen solid enough to travel on decreases. In Alaska this is now just under 80 days a year. Further disruption for transport and industry on land seem likely.

Methane alert Siberia's peat bogs have been producing methane since they were formed at the end of the last ice age, but most of the gas is trapped in the permafrost. As the bogs thaw, they may release billions of tonnes of methane into the atmosphere.

Present sources of methane in the atmosphere:

about 55% is due to human activity (farming and rotting waste)

about 8% is from other natural sources

about 37% is released from wetlands

Methane as a greenhouse gas Methane makes up 13% of greenhouse gases. It stays in the atmosphere for only eight years or so, but traps 23 times more heat than carbon dioxide. Carbon dioxide is currently the biggest cause of global warming, but methane is very important too.

tundra, but also Earth's atmosphere.

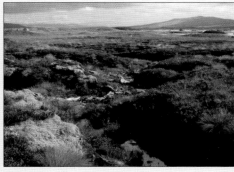

Shifting northwards As temperatures rise, the depth of the layer that thaws each year is increasing in many areas. The southern limit of permafrost will shrink and shift northwards several hundred kilometres during this century, reducing the tundra's extent.

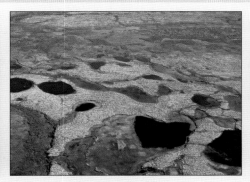

Pools in the permafrost In summer the layer of frozen soil keeps melting snow and ice from draining away. Over the surface, marshy pools and shallow lakes form. Widespread thawing will cause lakes to drain in some places and create new wetlands in other areas.

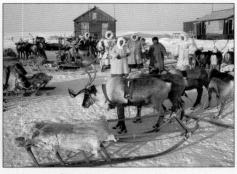

Life on frozen ground In Russia alone, 200,000 people live as nomads for part of the year, herding reindeer. Thawing permafrost means there are likely to be fewer reindeer and as a result the nomads will find it harder to survive too.

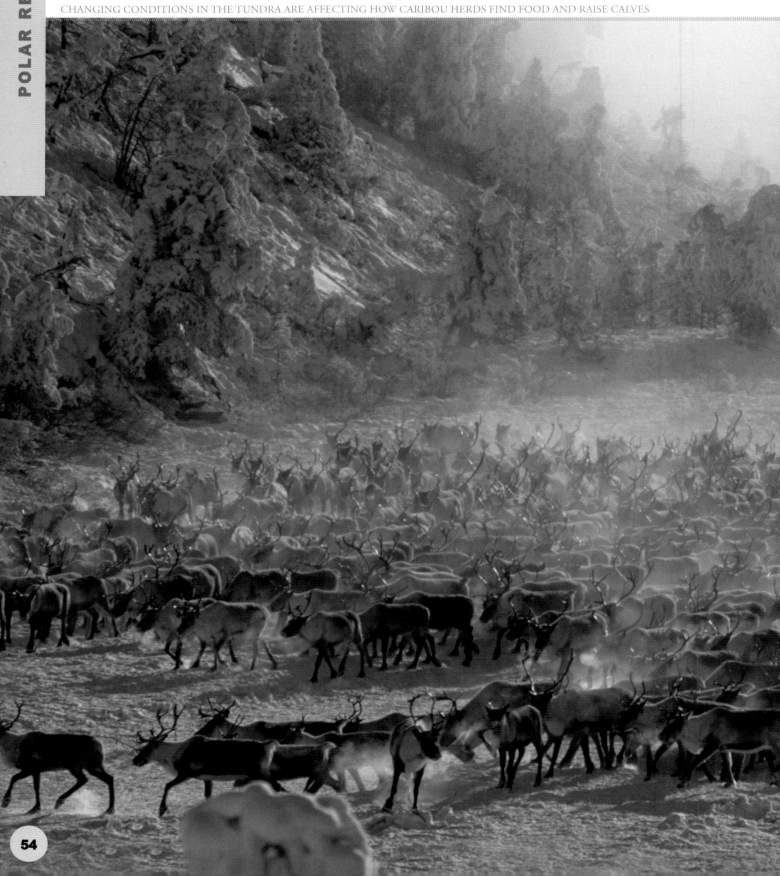

the caribou

CHANGING CONDITIONS IN THE TUNDRA ARE AFFECTING HOW CARIBOU HERDS FIND FOOD AND RAISE CALVES

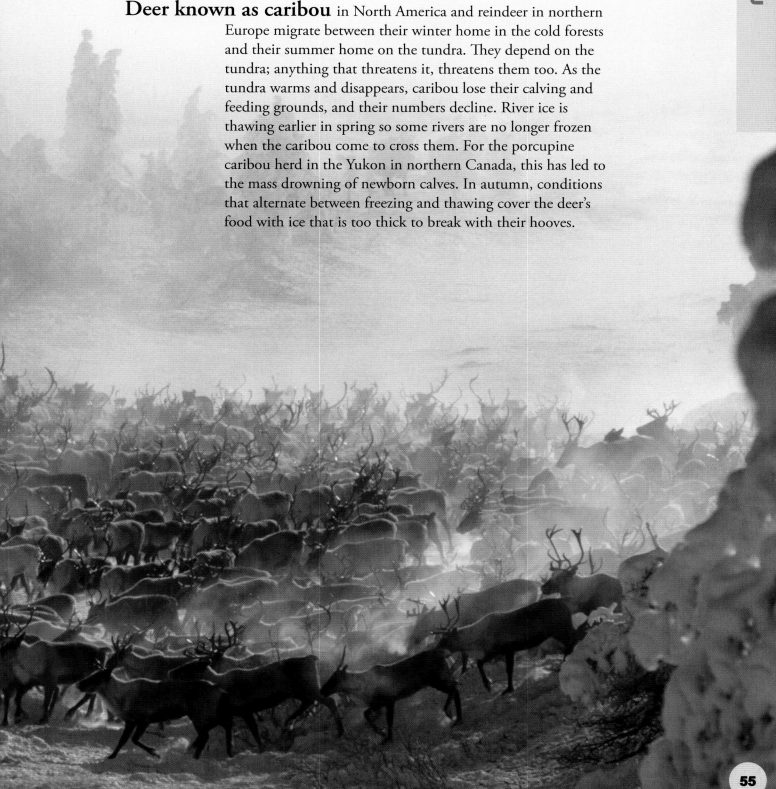

Caribou are found in northern North America, Greenland, and across northern Europe and northern Asia.

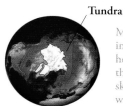

Tundra

Many Arctic peoples in Europe and Asia still herd caribou. They eat their meat and use their skins to make tents and warm clothes.

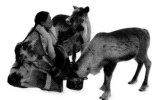

In some places, global warming is leading to heavier snow and rain. This freezes solid over the deer's main food – lichen.

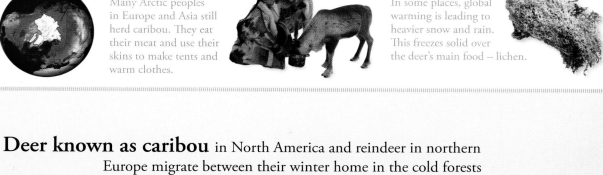

Deer known as caribou in North America and reindeer in northern Europe migrate between their winter home in the cold forests and their summer home on the tundra. They depend on the tundra; anything that threatens it, threatens them too. As the tundra warms and disappears, caribou lose their calving and feeding grounds, and their numbers decline. River ice is thawing earlier in spring so some rivers are no longer frozen when the caribou come to cross them. For the porcupine caribou herd in the Yukon in northern Canada, this has led to the mass drowning of newborn calves. In autumn, conditions that alternate between freezing and thawing cover the deer's food with ice that is too thick to break with their hooves.

antarctic ecosystem

Antarctica is Earth's last great wilderness: a land of rock and ice far from civilization. A cold ocean current, called the polar front, cuts off the Antarctic continent from the tropical waters and warmer lands above. Isolated and barren, this place is full of extremes. There are mountains as high as the Alps and even the smaller peaks are buried under several kilometres of ice. Three-quarters of the world's freshwater is locked up here in a massive ice sheet that's bigger than the United States of America.

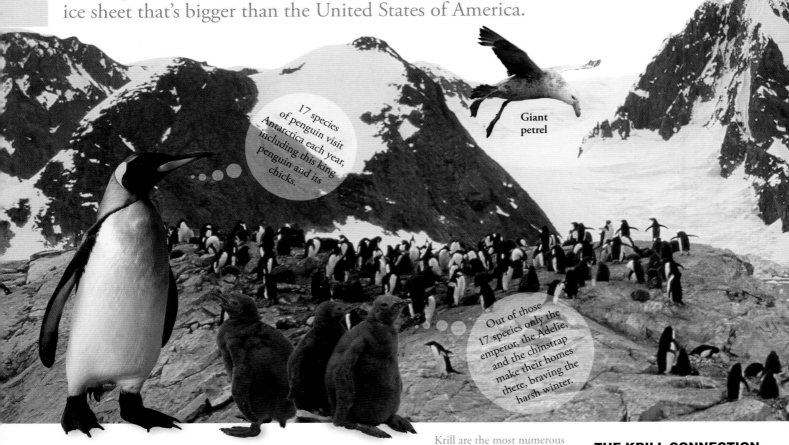

17 species of penguin visit Antarctica each year, including this king penguin and its chicks.

Giant petrel

Out of those 17 species only the emperor, the Adelie, and the chinstrap make their homes there, braving the harsh winter.

A harsh place to live Over 98 per cent of Antarctica is covered by ice, which makes life hard for mammals. The only animals that live here for the whole year are penguins and seals.

Krill are the most numerous animals on Earth.

THE KRILL CONNECTION
Perhaps the most important Antarctic species is krill. Krill are like shrimps. They form the bridge in the food chain between microscopic organisms and fish, birds, and mammals.

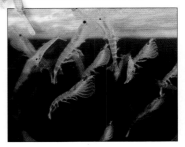

Land, sea, air Antarctica is essentially one big habitat: a huge rocky ice rink that doubles in size when the ocean freezes each winter. An Antarctic winter is like nothing else on Earth: little can survive in this cold, rainless, and windy desert. In summer, it bursts into life. On land, millions of penguins, seals, and seabirds arrive to breed, and underwater in the Antarctic ocean, sea life thrives.

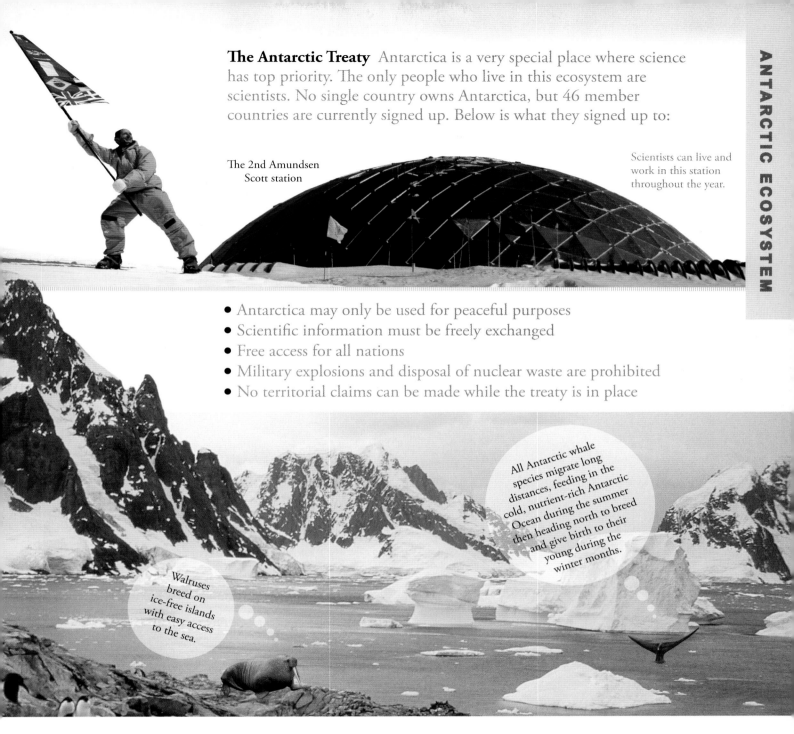

The Antarctic Treaty Antarctica is a very special place where science has top priority. The only people who live in this ecosystem are scientists. No single country owns Antarctica, but 46 member countries are currently signed up. Below is what they signed up to:

The 2nd Amundsen Scott station

Scientists can live and work in this station throughout the year.

- Antarctica may only be used for peaceful purposes
- Scientific information must be freely exchanged
- Free access for all nations
- Military explosions and disposal of nuclear waste are prohibited
- No territorial claims can be made while the treaty is in place

All Antarctic whale species migrate long distances, feeding in the cold, nutrient-rich Antarctic Ocean during the summer then heading north to breed and give birth to their young during the winter months.

Walruses breed on ice-free islands with easy access to the sea.

SEAL TEETH
Weddell seals use their teeth to keep open "trap doors" in the ice. Eventually, the ice grinds down their teeth so much that they cannot chew food, and they die.

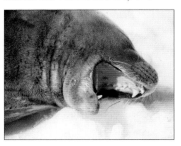

PINK SNOW
Algae in the ice bloom, turning ice caves pink. The pigments (colour chemicals) in the algae capture light to make energy via photosynthesis, while the snow provides moisture.

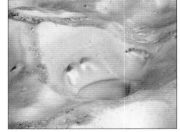

WHALE SPOTTING
Many whales visit Antarctica including the humpback whale, (below) and minke whale. They come to feast on the abundant krill.

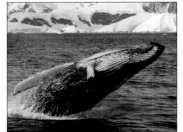

UNDER THE ICE
Beneath the ice, the warmer Antarctic ocean is packed with everything from microscopic bugs and plankton to squid, jellyfish, and starfish.

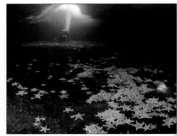

threatened antarctica

The South Pole is about 3,500 km (2,200 miles) from South America, the nearest continent (a vast distance slightly less than the width of the United States of America). Although this is an incredibly **remote** region – one of the only places where people have never settled – it is still threatened by human activities. Most of the threats to Antarctica, including *global warming* and *pollution*, are caused by things people are doing far away.

Ninety per cent of the world's ice is

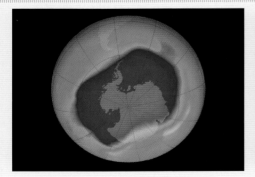

Ozone hole In 1985, scientists noticed a huge hole in the ozone layer over Antarctica. The ozone layer screens out ultraviolet radiation from the Sun. The chemicals, chlorofluorocarbons (CFCs), were to blame and so most countries began to phase them out. The hole is expected to disappear by about 2050.

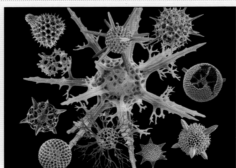

UV affects plankton Harmful ultraviolet rays can stop phytoplankton from growing properly. Phytoplanktons are the staple diet of krill, which in turn are eaten by the penguins, seals, and seabirds that breed in Antarctica. The hole in the ozone therefore threatens the Antarctic food web from the bottom up.

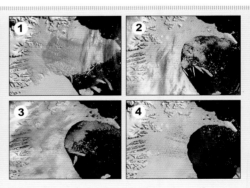

Melting ice Huge chunks of ice are falling into the sea due to global warming. This series of pictures shows the collapse of the Larsen B ice shelf. An area of ice 220 m (721 ft) thick and 3,250 sq km (1,255 sq miles) in size broke off. The ice, which had been in place for 12,000 years, took just 35 days to disappear.

A chemical mix Chemicals people pour into rivers or seas can be swept around the world by ocean currents, eventually washing up at the poles. Or they can be blown away with air pollution and fall onto Antarctica with snow. Scientists have found traces of harmful chemicals in Antarctic penguins, seals, whales, and seabirds. The chemicals include long-banned deadly pesticides such as DDTs.

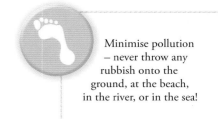

Minimise pollution – never throw any rubbish onto the ground, at the beach, in the river, or in the sea!

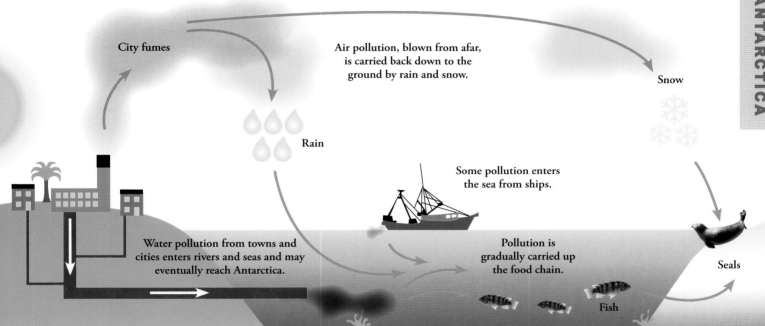

City fumes

Air pollution, blown from afar, is carried back down to the ground by rain and snow.

Snow

Rain

Some pollution enters the sea from ships.

Water pollution from towns and cities enters rivers and seas and may eventually reach Antarctica.

Pollution is gradually carried up the food chain.

Seals

Fish

locked in freezing Antarctica.

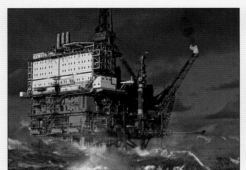

Oil mining Antarctica has been designated "a natural reserve dedicated to peace and to society" and nations have agreed not to explore for minerals or oil under the terms of the Antarctic Treaty. But as supplies of Earth's resources dwindle elsewhere, a time may come when it makes economic sense to develop Antarctica too.

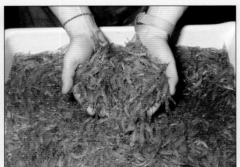

Rising krill catches Antarctic krill form dense concentrations in summer that can be several kilometres across and 20 m (65 ft) deep. These have attracted fishing fleets hoping to make krill a food for humans. Current catch levels are rising, but are not at a dangerous level yet.

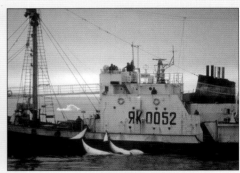

Whaling Whale hunting in the 19th century reduced the numbers of most species to the point where there were too few to hunt. Blue whales are at less than one per cent of their original numbers and are still not increasing despite years of protection. Now the whale fleets are setting off again...

emperor penguins

EMPEROR PENGUIN NUMBERS ARE GOING DOWN AS THEIR FOOD SUPPLY IS AFFECTED BY GLOBAL WARMING

Huddling in the cold and waddling on ice, diving through waves and tobogganing through snow, penguins are the icons of Antarctica. Of the 50 million or so penguins in Antarctica, only emperor penguins breed on the ice and snow. They are the ultimate polar survivors, breeding further south than any other animal. And they are perfectly adapted for the task. However, as Antarctica warms due to global warming, there will be less ice in the sea from one year to the next. This affects the food chain as reduced ice means reduced sea-ice algae (a major food for krill). This leads to fewer krill, which is the penguins' staple diet. Less food means fewer emperor penguins. Over the past 50 years, the population of Antarctic emperor penguins has declined by 50 per cent.

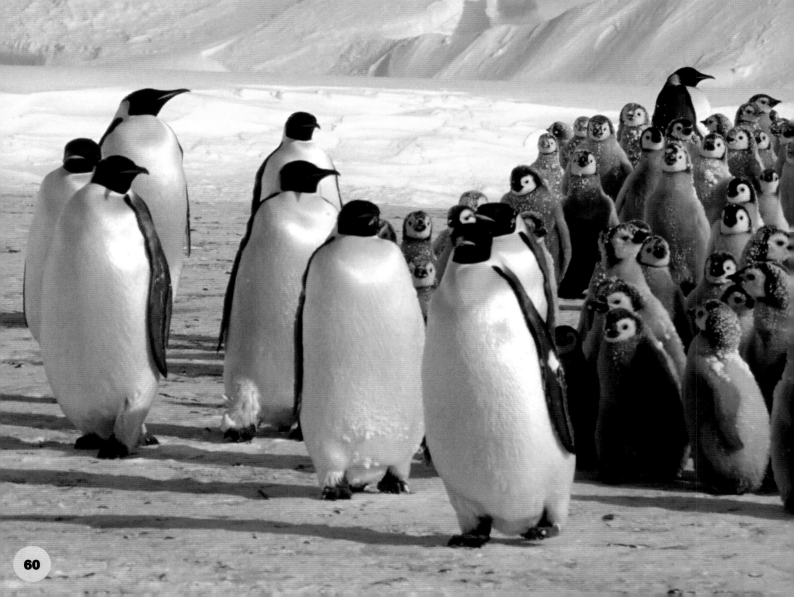

There are at least 40 different colonies of emperor penguins in the Antarctic. Some colonies comprise no more than 200 pairs, while the biggest ones can consist of more than 50,000 pairs.

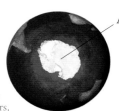

Antarctica

Much of a penguin's life is taken up with long feeding trips to the sea. They can't fly, so they have to waddle over rocks and skid down the ice instead. Their curved bodies make great toboggans, using their flippers to push along. In the water, they whizz along at up to 10 km/h (6 mph) – slightly faster than Olympic swimmers.

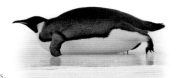

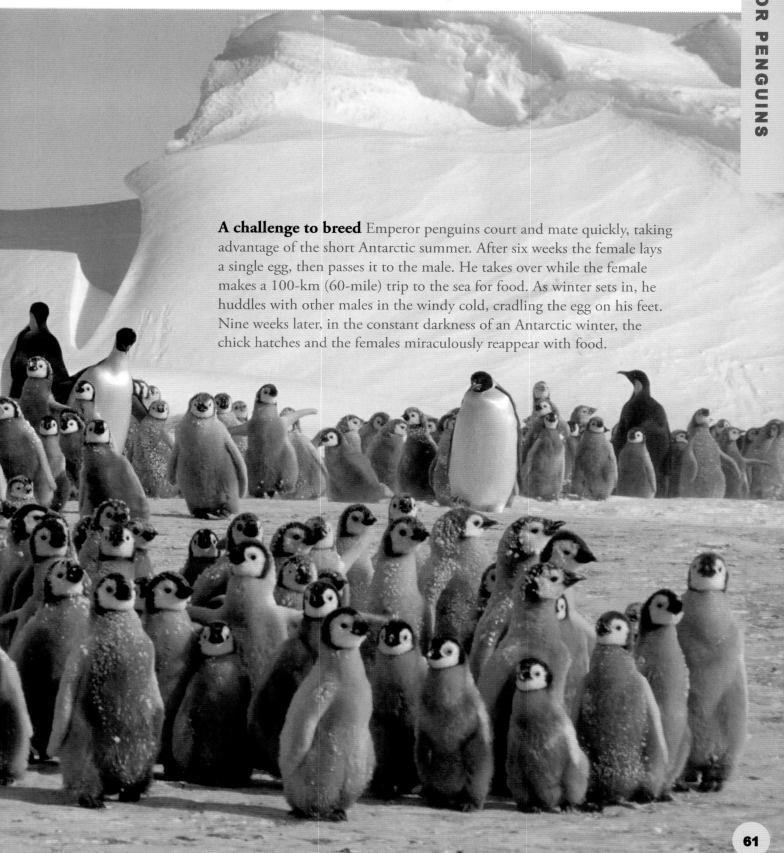

A challenge to breed Emperor penguins court and mate quickly, taking advantage of the short Antarctic summer. After six weeks the female lays a single egg, then passes it to the male. He takes over while the female makes a 100-km (60-mile) trip to the sea for food. As winter sets in, he huddles with other males in the windy cold, cradling the egg on his feet. Nine weeks later, in the constant darkness of an Antarctic winter, the chick hatches and the females miraculously reappear with food.

MAKING A DIFFERENCE

Use less energy and reduce your carbon footprint, thereby reducing the need for oil from polar regions. Avoid using the car. Turn off lights.

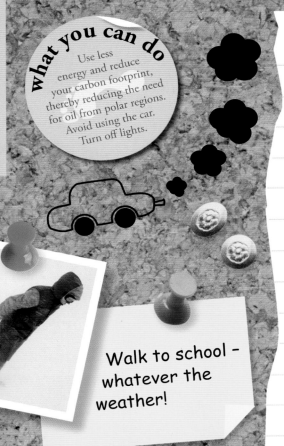

Walk to school – whatever the weather!

Rubbish in the waterways

The world's waterways are all connected by Earth's seas and oceans. A plastic bag in a river in England could end up in the Arctic. There it could be eaten by a sea bird or animal. What can you do?

what you can do

Next time someone asks what you want for your birthday – how about a polar bear? Look up adoption schemes on the internet. **www.charity-gifts.org/wwf-adopt-an-animal.php**

1. **Take part** in **beach** or **river clean ups**, or organise your own local clean-up. Try to get your school involved.

2. **Pick up** any litter and put it in the **BIN**.

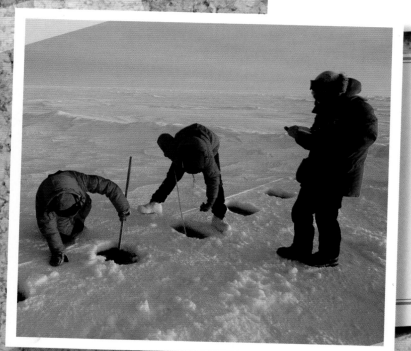

Arctic Research Assistant needed

Are you ready for a new challenge?

- **Most important** Must be passionate about the polar regions.
- **The job** Taking ice samples, temperature recordings, examining data, monitoring wildlife, and other outdoor work.
- **The environment** Extremely cold. Long, dark winters.
- **The successful applicant** You'll need a good sense of humour, to be able to work well as part of a team, and mix easily with people from different backgrounds, countries, and ages.
- **On the menu** Fishfingers

What can we do to make a difference to the poles? Even though they are far away, we can still do things to help.

KNOW THE DEBATE

developing the polar regions

- **Fishing around Antarctica** – the opportunities for fishing are immense (and stocks elsewhere are dwindling). Fishing could be increased from its present limits with plenty of fish to spare...
- **Tourism** – visitors help native people earn a living, and the more people that see the area, the more it will be in their memories as a place to protect.
- **A treasure trove of minerals** – mining could be done in a way that makes as little impact on the environment as possible. If people care about the Arctic and Antarctica, customers won't put up with companies that ruin it.
- **Drilling for oil** – as world resources of oil dry up, oil in the Arctic and Antarctica provide an answer. Again, the extraction process could be done with sensitivity to the environment.
- **In return for a licence** to mine resources, companies could pay for scientific research.

protecting the polar regions

- Squid, krill, and fish form the base of the food chain so fishing quotas must not be increased.
- **Mining companies have been destructive** to the environment in the past. They pollute and destroy habitat.
- Industrial waste has been dumped in the Arctic and **caused long-term pollution** and entered the food chain.
- **Tourism is destructive** and polluting. Rubbish dropped in freezing temperatures never biodegrades (breaks down).
- Scientists from over 25 countries have proved the **importance of Antarctica in learning about life on earth.**
- **Better to play safe,** than be sorry later.
- **The Antarctic Treaty proves nations can work together for the good of all mankind.** Let's leave it that way.

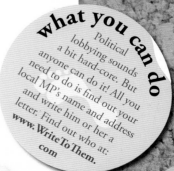

Dear Bob Black, MP

I am concerned about the polar regions. The ice is melting due to global warming. Animals, including polar bears and penguins, are losing their habitat. Fishing in the Arctic Ocean is endangering fish stocks, and mining for oil and minerals is also harmful.

We really need to act now to protect these special places.

Please make decisions that will bring an end to global warming and do all you can to inform people of the problems at the poles that could affect everyone.

Best wishes

Alex Potter

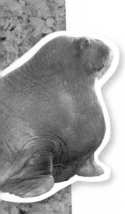

Get lobbying

Write a letter to the government to show that you care!

what you can do

Political lobbying sounds a bit hard-core. But anyone can do it! All you need to do is find out your local MP's name and address and write him or her a letter. Find out who at: www.WriteToThem.com

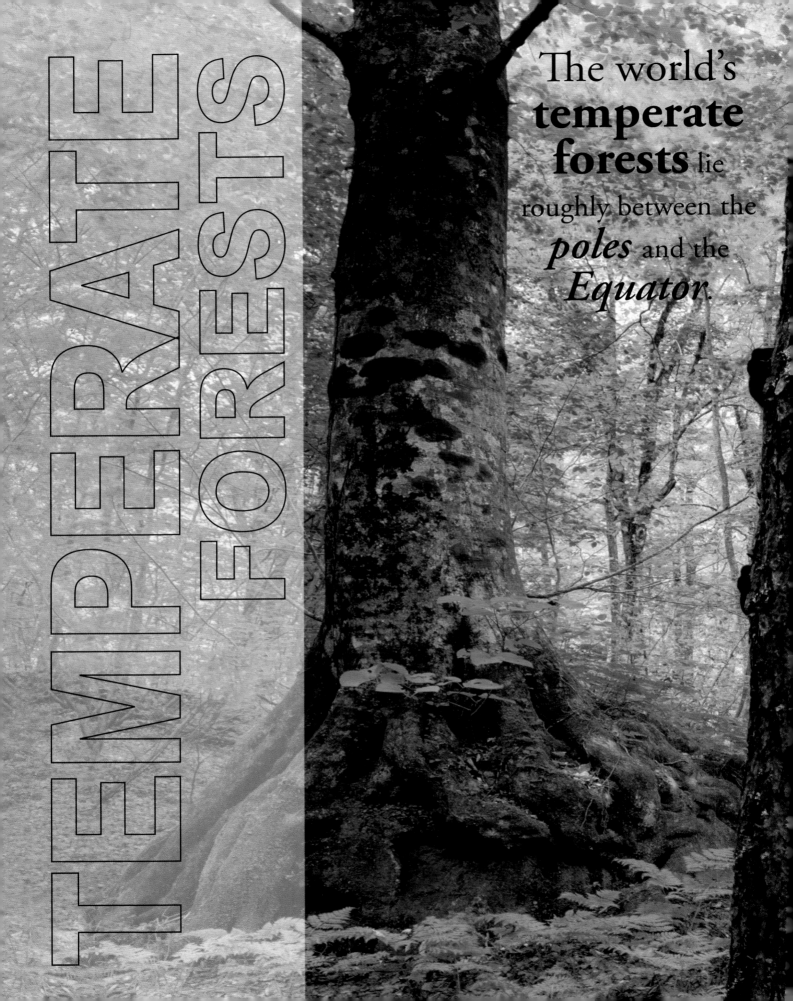

TEMPERATE FORESTS

The world's **temperate forests** lie roughly between the *poles* and the *Equator*.

The word temperate means "not extreme".
The temperate regions on Earth lie in the middle
latitudes, where there are distinct warm and cold
seasons that we call summer and winter.
Trees thrive in these areas, as long as there's
enough rainfall, and forests nurture a wondrous
variety of animals and plants.

TEMPERATE FORESTS

where on earth...?

Forests grow wherever in the world it's warm and wet enough for trees to thrive. Temperate forests grow in places where there is precipitation (rain and snow) throughout the year, but separate warm and cold seasons.

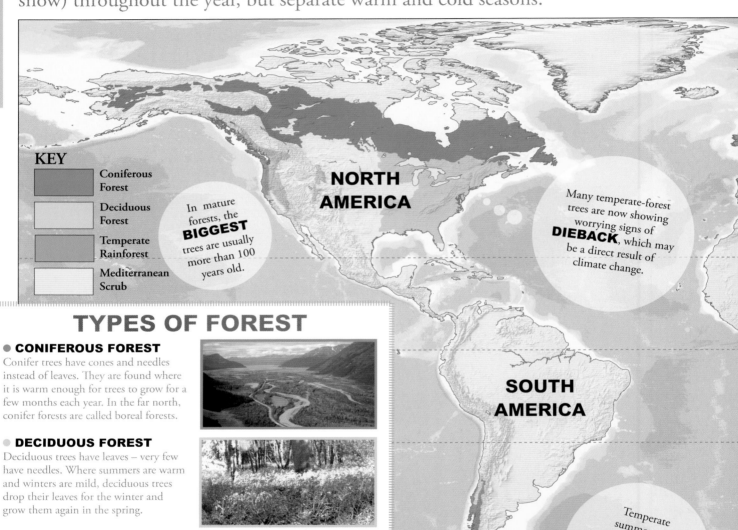

KEY

Coniferous Forest

Deciduous Forest

Temperate Rainforest

Mediterranean Scrub

NORTH AMERICA

In mature forests, the **BIGGEST** trees are usually more than 100 years old.

Many temperate-forest trees are now showing worrying signs of **DIEBACK**, which may be a direct result of climate change.

SOUTH AMERICA

Temperate summers are never as hot as the **TROPICS**, and winters are never as cold as the **POLES**.

TYPES OF FOREST

● **CONIFEROUS FOREST**
Conifer trees have cones and needles instead of leaves. They are found where it is warm enough for trees to grow for a few months each year. In the far north, conifer forests are called boreal forests.

● **DECIDUOUS FOREST**
Deciduous trees have leaves – very few have needles. Where summers are warm and winters are mild, deciduous trees drop their leaves for the winter and grow them again in the spring.

● **TEMPERATE RAINFOREST**
On the Pacific coast of North America, the climate is mild and wet. Here, there are tall, wide conifers covered in moss. These lush forests, and others like them, are called temperate rainforests.

● **MEDITERRANEAN SCRUB**
Shrubs and trees in this type of forest keep their leaves all year long. They are especially adapted to survive hot, dry summers, and to make the most of cool, moist winters.

Rooted to the spot Once a tree has taken root, it has to stand in the same place for the rest of its life. If the weather changes, or conditions become unsuitable, trees can't do anything about it, and they suffer stress.

SEASONS SHIFT
The seasonal change in temperature is a challenge for animals and plants. Their coping strategies, like hibernating in winter or flowering in spring, are timed to match the seasons, but the seasons are changing.

ON THE MOVE
As our climate warms up, ideal conditions for each species are moving towards the poles. Mobile creatures like birds can move easily, but temperate forests will have to move too, and they can't travel quickly.

CARBON STORES
Trees absorb and store carbon. Temperate rainforests store more carbon per hectare (acre) than any other land habitat. If they die, their carbon will add to the greenhouse gases.

ANCIENT WOODS
There have been conifers on the Earth for 300 million years – they once extended into the Arctic. Deciduous forests are a little more recent – they have been around for 65 million years.

LATE ARRIVAL
Compared to the other forests, Mediterranean scrub is relatively modern, arriving over the last 40 million years. Much of its wildlife is unique to each continent, because it evolved in isolation.

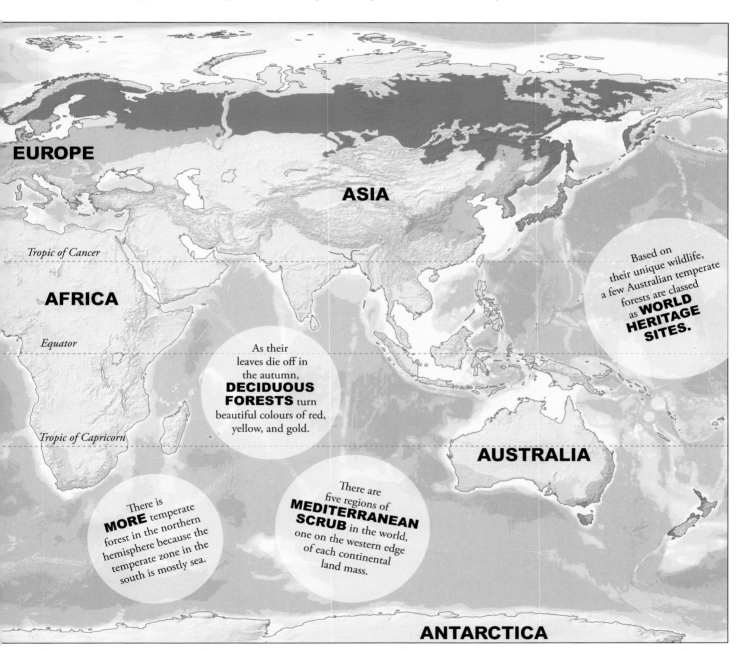

EUROPE

ASIA

Tropic of Cancer

AFRICA

Equator

Based on their unique wildlife, a few Australian temperate forests are classed as **WORLD HERITAGE SITES.**

As their leaves die off in the autumn, **DECIDUOUS FORESTS** turn beautiful colours of red, yellow, and gold.

Tropic of Capricorn

AUSTRALIA

There is **MORE** temperate forest in the northern hemisphere because the temperate zone in the south is mostly sea.

There are five regions of **MEDITERRANEAN SCRUB** in the world, one on the western edge of each continental land mass.

ANTARCTICA

When this happens year after year, trees are vulnerable to attack by disease and insects. Branches and shoots die (called "dieback") and sometimes the whole tree is killed. Often, this is triggered by summer drought, a sign of climate change.

One reason trees are so important is that other wildlife depends on them – mosses, ferns, and funguses, bugs, beetles, wasps, caterpillars, birds, snakes, and squirrels all live on, or in, the bark, leaves, and branches of trees.

boreal ecosystem

Boreal forest, also called the taiga, is named after Boreas, Greek God of the north wind. Made up of conifer trees, it's the world's largest biome on land, covering 17 per cent of Earth's vegetated land surface (more than 15 million sq km /5,800,000 sq miles), circling the planet in the northern hemisphere. The growing season, when there's enough warmth and sunlight for plants to grow, lasts just two or three months, and the winters are long and frozen. Average winter temperatures often fall to a bitter -30°C (-22°F).

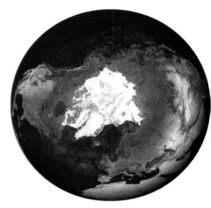

Patches of soil underneath the northern boreal forest are permanently frozen – this is called permafrost.

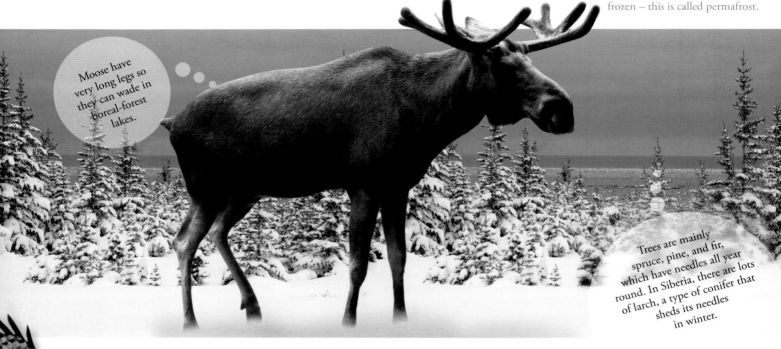

Moose have very long legs so they can wade in boreal-forest lakes.

Trees are mainly spruce, pine, and fir, which have needles all year round. In Siberia, there are lots of larch, a type of conifer that sheds its needles in winter.

Some species, like the moose, the Siberian tit, and the great grey owl, are found in all the world's boreal forests. Others live only on one or two continents – the snowshoe hare, for example, is found only in America, and the Siberian tiger is found only in Europe and Asia. The red squirrel, and many songbirds, have similar American and European versions.

BERRY BUSHES
The berries of small plants like bilberry and cowberry in Europe, and blueberry and bunchberry in North America, provide vital food for birds and mammals, including bears.

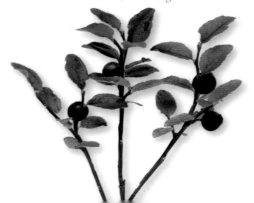

TIGER OF THE TAIGA
In the Russian far east, two rare cats prowl boreal forests. Siberian (Amur) tigers and Amur leopards both have long thick fur, long legs, and big feet to survive the months of snow.

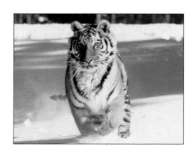

The need for needles

Because they have needles all year round, conifer trees waste none of the precious growing season producing new ones, so the trees can start growing new wood as soon as it's warm. Eventually, all needles do fall off and decay, creating a thick spongy carpet on the forest floor. Waxy and full of sticky resin, they rot slowly in the freezing temperatures. Acids are washed out of them into the soil. Mosses thrive on this shady, acidic ground, but few other plants survive.

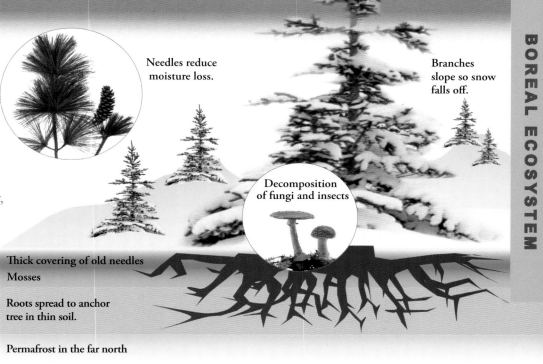

Needles reduce moisture loss.

Branches slope so snow falls off.

Decomposition of fungi and insects

Thick covering of old needles

Mosses

Roots spread to anchor tree in thin soil.

Permafrost in the far north

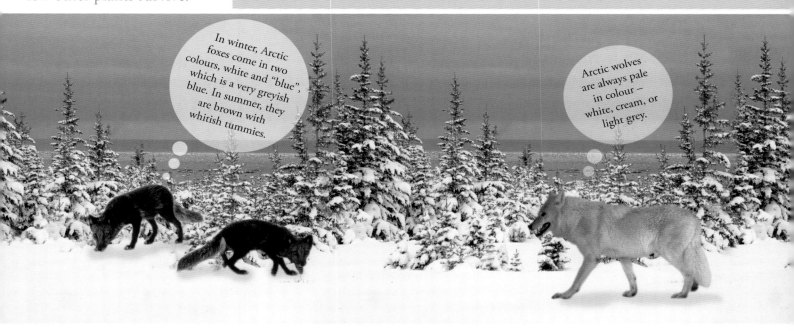

In winter, Arctic foxes come in two colours, white and "blue", which is a very greyish blue. In summer, they are brown with whitish tummies.

Arctic wolves are always pale in colour – white, cream, or light grey.

FOREST FIRES

Most boreal forest fires happen naturally. They are a vital part of the ecosystem since they help to release seeds, and provide ashes that nourish small plants.

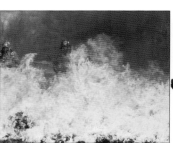

INSECT INVASIONS

Insects often invade the forest and strip the needles off older trees. Like fires, these insect attacks disturb the system, and are important for keeping a rich mix of tree species.

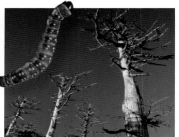

FOREST PEOPLE

At one time, native peoples lived in boreal forests. The Ojibway of North America built birch-bark wigwams as homes, dressed in furs, and even used moss as babies' nappies.

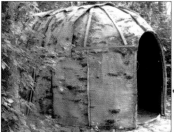

SAVING MOISTURE

Needles are narrow, tightly rolled leaves with a waxy coating. Because they don't lose much water by evaporation, needles stay in place through the very dry boreal winter when the water in the soil is frozen.

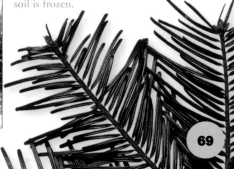

temperate rainforest

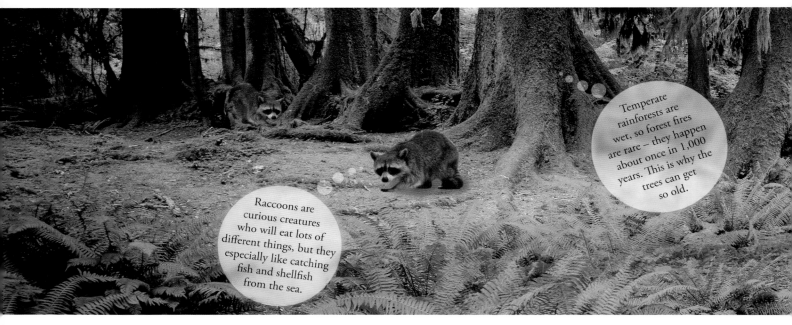

On the west coast of North America, between the sea and the Rocky Mountains, there's a very special kind of conifer forest called temperate rainforest. The weather is milder here than in boreal forest, and very wet, so the trees can keep growing for most of the year. They live for a long time and reach massive sizes, commonly 80 m (260 ft) high, with trunks two or three metres (6.5 ft–10 ft) across. In the dark, damp interior, the trees are draped with moss and supported by huge buttresses (trunks that spread out at the base like the legs of the Eiffel Tower).

Raccoons are curious creatures who will eat lots of different things, but they especially like catching fish and shellfish from the sea.

Temperate rainforests are wet, so forest fires are rare – they happen about once in 1,000 years. This is why the trees can get so old.

Red and green giants

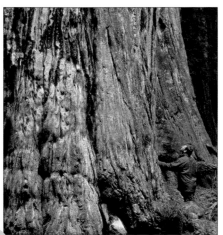

The southern part of North America's rainforest is home to the famous Californian redwood trees (left). Some are over 2,200 years old, and the tallest-ever specimen is 112 m (367 ft) high. Even these giants are not as big as their South American cousins, the alerce trees of Chile's Valdivian forest, which can reach 114 m (374 ft) – some are over 3,000 years old. Now, since many alerce trees have been cut down for timber, they are threatened with extinction.

DRIPPING FOGS

All year, fogs roll in from the sea and their moisture clings to the trees. Californian redwoods, which rely on these fogs for water, can only grow within 20 km (12.5 miles) of the coast.

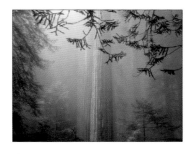

ecosystem

Between mountains and sea Mountains keep temperate rainforests wet. Moist air from the ocean is forced up to pass over them. As it rises, it cools, and the moisture falls as rain. On the far side of the mountains, in what's called the "rain shadow", the weather is much drier. Coastal temperate rainforests are found in Norway, southern Chile, New Zealand, Tasmania, and Japan.

Moisture turns to rain.

SUN

The air is dry because its moisture has already fallen as rain.

Moist air from the ocean

Temperate rainforest

Rain shadow

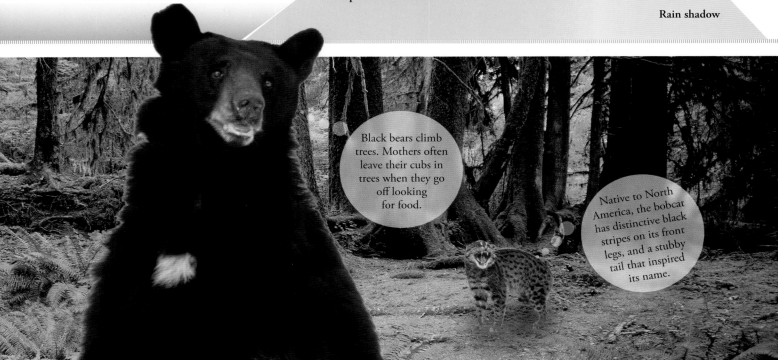

Black bears climb trees. Mothers often leave their cubs in trees when they go off looking for food.

Native to North America, the bobcat has distinctive black stripes on its front legs, and a stubby tail that inspired its name.

LIFE-SAVING SPECIES
Native Americans used the leaves and branches of the Pacific yew as medicine, and modern scientists use its bark in a cancer drug. It takes three mature trees to treat one patient.

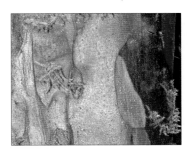

MYSTERY BIRD
Until 1974, no-one could find the home of the marbled murrelet, a seabird of North America's west coast, because it nests in inland forests. As these disappear, its numbers decline.

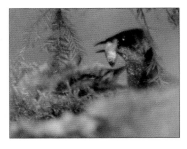

THUNDERBIRD
At one time, many Native American cultures lived in fear of the legendary thunderbird, a giant god-like bird that lived in the mountains to the east and ate killer whales from the sea. People believed it could throw lightning, and make thunder by clapping its wings. The feared bird was often represented on carved totem poles.

HIDE AND SEEK
Unlike tropical rainforests, temperate rainforests are still and quiet, and the animals stay hidden. Most, like this Roosevelt elk, are brown and mottled or stripy to blend into the forest shadows.

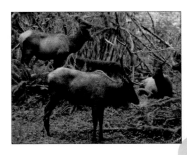

73

forest **and sea**

MANY OF THE EARTH'S FORESTS ARE NOURISHED FROM ITS OCEANS AND SEAS

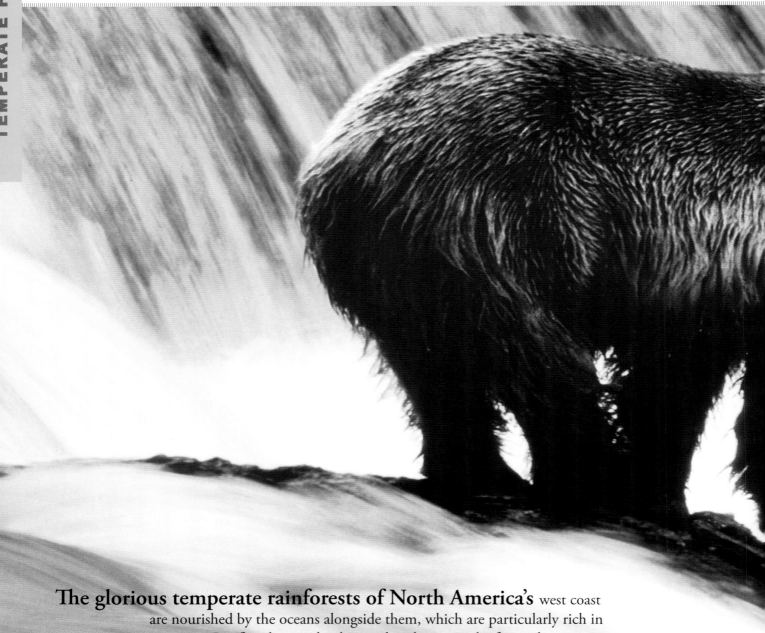

The glorious temperate rainforests of North America's west coast
are nourished by the oceans alongside them, which are particularly rich in
nutrients. Pacific salmon take these riches deep into the forests by swimming
up rivers and streams in large numbers to mate and lay their eggs, or "spawn".
These journeys are called salmon runs. Swimming up a single river, there can
be 20 million fish. There are so many salmon that they make easy prey for
grizzly bears. Normally solitary animals that only hunt at night, bears gather
around streams and rivers at spawning time and stand in fast-flowing rapids
to catch salmon as they leap. Getting past the bears is a dangerous game.
In Alaska, grizzlies consume 40 per cent of all sockeye salmon as they pass –
there is such a glut that bears often take a single bite out of one salmon
before discarding it and picking up another one.

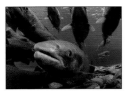

Adult salmon live at sea. In late summer, when they have matured, they return to the place where they were born. There they spawn, then die.

The rotting carcasses are eaten by scavenging birds, who then fly over the forest, distributing valuable fertilizer in the form of droppings.

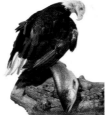

Salmon eggs

The next spring, the eggs hatch into young fish. These spend up to two years in fresh water before they head for the sea.

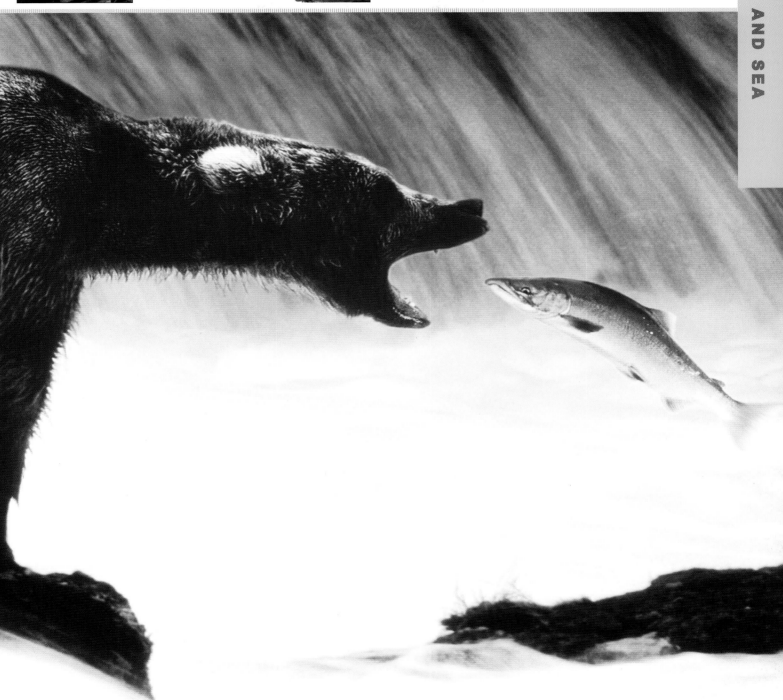

By eating salmon, bears transfer ocean nutrients such as nitrogen, potassium, and phosphorous, directly to the forest floor, feeding the trees. These are either in the form of bear droppings, or half-eaten fish carcasses dragged onto land. The dead fish are then devoured by maggots who carry the nutrients even further in their own droppings when they grow into flies.

deciduous **ecosystem**

Warm temperate forests are found where there are obvious cold and warm seasons, but where precipitation (rain and snow) falls evenly throughout the year. There are large areas of this type of forest in Europe, North America, and Asia, and small patches in the southern hemisphere. Trees are mainly deciduous, which means they lose their leaves in autumn, and stand naked through winter. Common examples of deciduous trees are maple, beech, oak, and chestnut.

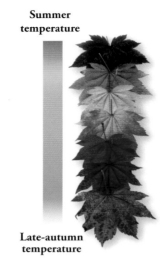

Summer temperature

Late-autumn temperature

The big drop

In the autumn, when temperatures fall and there is less light, the trees lose green chlorophyll from their leaves. The leaves turn brilliant shades of orange, red, and gold before they die and fall off.

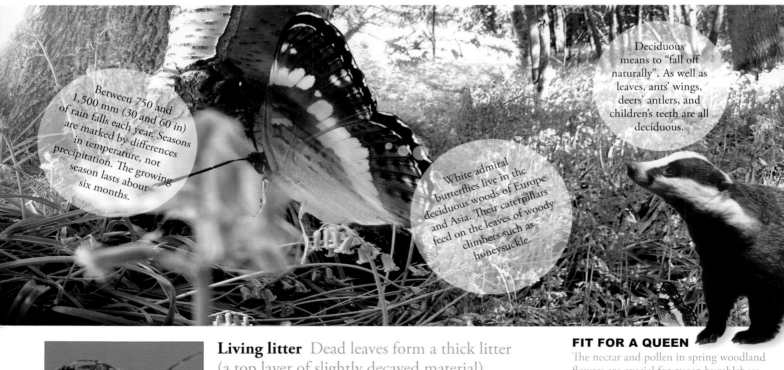

Between 750 and 1,500 mm (30 and 60 in) of rain falls each year. Seasons are marked by differences in temperature, not precipitation. The growing season lasts about six months.

White admiral butterflies live in the deciduous woods of Europe and Asia. Their caterpillars feed on the leaves of woody climbers, such as honeysuckle.

Deciduous means to "fall off naturally". As well as leaves, ants' wings, deers' antlers, and children's teeth are all deciduous.

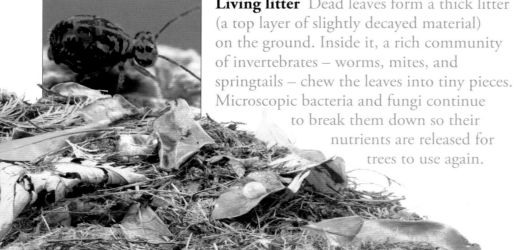

Living litter Dead leaves form a thick litter (a top layer of slightly decayed material) on the ground. Inside it, a rich community of invertebrates – worms, mites, and springtails – chew the leaves into tiny pieces. Microscopic bacteria and fungi continue to break them down so their nutrients are released for trees to use again.

FIT FOR A QUEEN

The nectar and pollen in spring woodland flowers are crucial for queen bumblebees, which are the only bees to survive the winter. All the others – males and female workers – die off in autumn, and queens found new colonies alone.

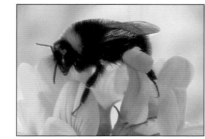

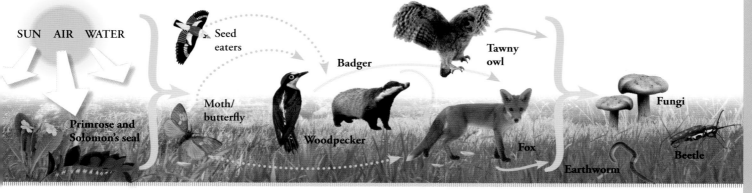

Deciduous forest food chain
Small birds, insects, and small mammals live off plants; larger birds and mammals eat insects and smaller birds and mammals; and top predators eat lots of other creatures.

SUN   AIR   WATER

Seed eaters

Moth/ butterfly

Badger

Tawny owl

Primrose and Solomon's seal

Woodpecker

Fox

Fungi

Earthworm

Beetle

PRODUCERS
At the bottom of the deciduous food chain are a variety of trees, flowers, and large, tufty woodland grasses.

PRIMARY CONSUMERS
Moth and butterfly caterpillars eat tree leaves, while birds and squirrels eat seeds and nuts.

SECONDARY CONSUMERS
Woodpeckers eat insects and caterpillars, and badgers eat earthworms, insects and mice.

PREDATORS
Tawny owls, foxes, and other top predators live on small mammals and birds.

DECOMPOSERS
Funguses, earthworms, and bacteria break down fallen leaves. Wood-eaters like bracket fungi and beetles rot branches and dead trees.

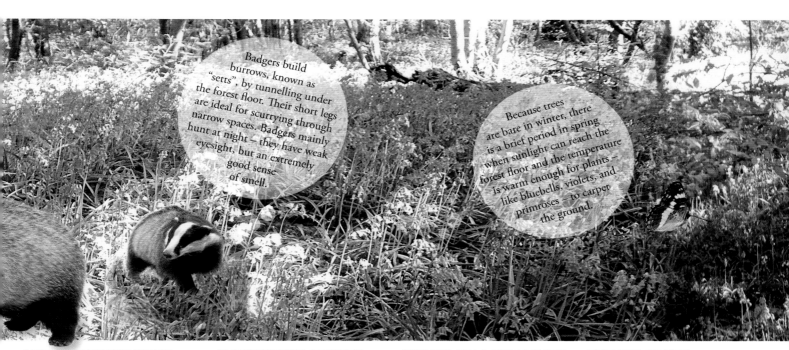

Badgers build burrows, known as "setts", by tunnelling under the forest floor. Their short legs are ideal for scurrying through narrow spaces. Badgers mainly hunt at night – they have weak eyesight, but an extremely good sense of smell.

Because trees are bare in winter, there is a brief period in spring when sunlight can reach the forest floor and the temperature is warm enough for plants – like bluebells, violets, and primroses – to carpet the ground.

UNDERGROUND WEBS
The litter is laced with networks of microscopic fibres like underground webs. These are the bodies of woodland fungi – each one is called a mycelium. Fungi, which digest living or dead plant matter, are vital for breaking down leaf litter. When two mycelia meet underground, they grow fruiting bodies, which we call mushrooms. These produce thousands of tiny spores that grow into the next generation of fungi.

HARVESTING FENCES
Beneath the tallest branches are small trees like dogwood and hazel. In Europe, these were once cut down every few years ("coppiced") to make tool handles or fence posts.

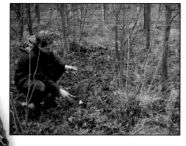

WHERE DID I PUT THAT?
In autumn, squirrels, chipmunks, and jays gather large seeds like acorns, chestnuts, and hazlenuts, and store them in the ground. If seeds are never collected, they grow into new trees.

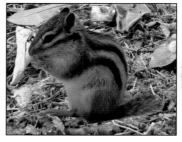

THE BIG SLEEP
Like this hedgehog, many mammals hibernate (go into a deep sleep) to survive the winter. Their temperature drops, their breathing slows, and they are hard to wake.

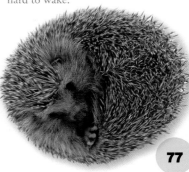

fallen forests

Deciduous forests have been more **affected** by human activity than *any other biome*, since they grow in the areas of fertile soil and relatively gentle climate that are most popular for humans to live in. Huge areas, especially in **China** and **Europe**, were *cut down* long ago to make way for cultivation. Most existing deciduous forest is *regrown* (so it's called "secondary forest"), and only tiny *fragments* of original **forest** remain.

Creatures in a broken-up forest can't

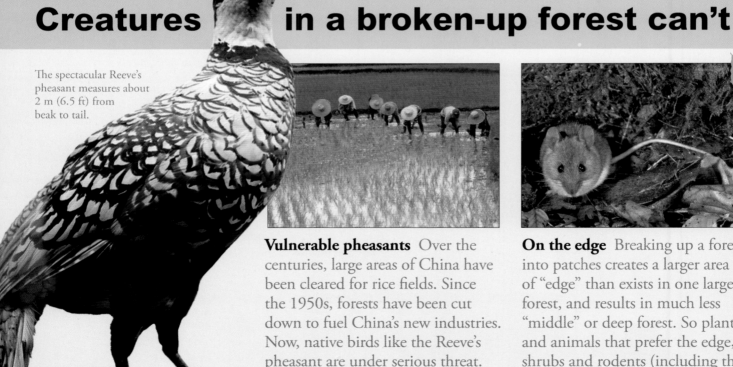

The spectacular Reeve's pheasant measures about 2 m (6.5 ft) from beak to tail.

Vulnerable pheasants Over the centuries, large areas of China have been cleared for rice fields. Since the 1950s, forests have been cut down to fuel China's new industries. Now, native birds like the Reeve's pheasant are under serious threat.

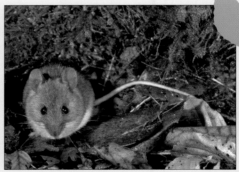

On the edge Breaking up a forest into patches creates a larger area of "edge" than exists in one large forest, and results in much less "middle" or deep forest. So plants and animals that prefer the edge, like shrubs and rodents (including the yellow-necked mouse, above) thrive, and those that like deep forest suffer.

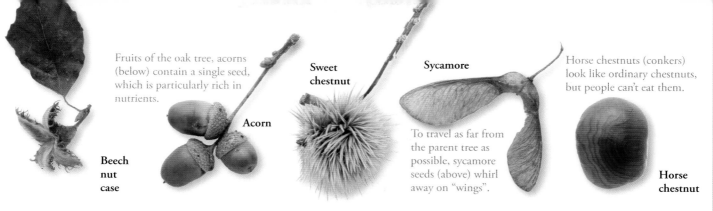

Fruits of the oak tree, acorns (below) contain a single seed, which is particularly rich in nutrients.

Sweet chestnut

Acorn

Sycamore

To travel as far from the parent tree as possible, sycamore seeds (above) whirl away on "wings".

Horse chestnuts (conkers) look like ordinary chestnuts, but people can't eat them.

Beech nut case

Horse chestnut

Seed bounty Every few years, deciduous trees produce far more seeds than usual. These are called mast years. During mast years, there are too many seeds for animals like mice and birds to eat, so lots of seeds survive and grow into new trees. But because this seed glut doesn't happen every year, the population of seed-eating birds and mice doesn't increase. Scientists don't really know what triggers mast years, but in some plants they are related to very high temperatures the year before. As temperatures rise because of climate change, mast years may happen more often. If they do, seed eaters could increase in number and eat more seeds, leaving very few to grow into new trees.

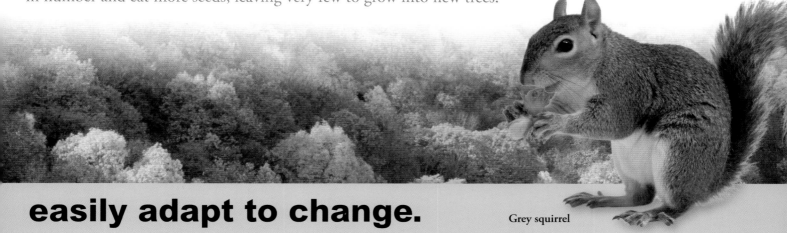

easily adapt to change.

Grey squirrel

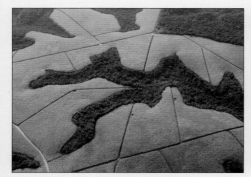

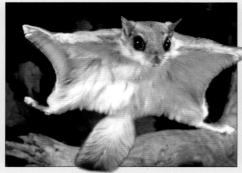

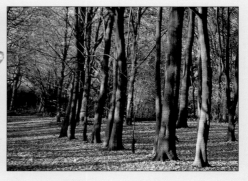

Leafy corridors Small patches of forest are like islands in a sea of open land, and this makes it hard for forest species to change their location in response to climate change. One solution is to link the patches with narrow strips of specially planted forest that animals can move through.

On the move To keep pace with climate change, woodland plants and animals will have to migrate towards the poles. Experts think the right climate for temperate forests will move about 1,000 m (3,280 ft) a year. But plants and animals, such as the southern flying squirrel, can't keep up.

Dry and drier With climate change, summer heat waves and droughts may increase, making trees dry and parched. The European beech tree, which has shallow roots, will struggle to survive in dry summers, and may disappear altogether from the southern edge of its range.

coming together

THE FASCINATING SEASONAL LINK BETWEEN THE GREAT TIT, THE OAK TREE, AND THE WINTER-MOTH CATERPILLAR

When great-tit chicks hatch in spring, their parents need a good supply of small caterpillars to feed them. In European woodlands, they rely on the winter moth, whose caterpillars eat oak leaves. Once the caterpillars start eating, there is a huge abundance of them, but this period lasts only a few weeks, and it happens more quickly if the weather is warmer. Songbirds such as great tits need to time their egg laying so they have hungry mouths to feed just when there are lots of caterpillars. With climate change, spring temperatures have been increasing for the past 25 years in Northern Europe, and oak buds are opening about 10 days earlier. But it's not easy for the moth and the great tit to change their timing to match. In some places, young great tits are missing out on the feast because their mother does not lay her eggs early enough.

Feed the birds in your garden to help them survive while they are adjusting to climate change.

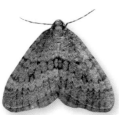 Adult winter moths mate and lay eggs in winter, and the eggs should hatch just as the new oak leaves start to grow.

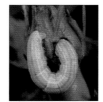 If the caterpillars hatch too early, they will starve. If they hatch too late, the oak leaves will be too old, too tough, and too full of bitter tannin to eat.

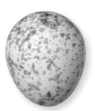 As spring gets earlier, great tits are at risk because they are not laying their eggs in time to catch the earlier caterpillar glut.

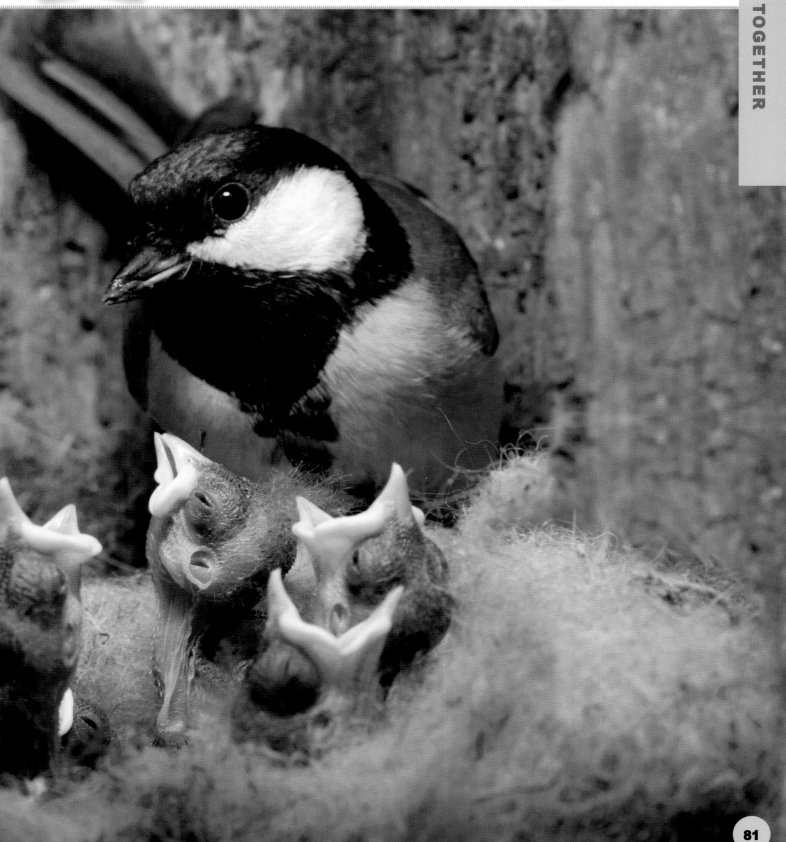

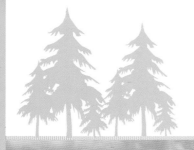

logging

THE GOOD, THE BAD, AND THE CRIMINAL

People need wood — in theory, wood is a sustainable resource that we *should* use for buildings and fuel. In well-managed forests, a tree is planted for every tree that's cut down so the total amount of forest doesn't change. But because there are more and more people on the Earth all the time, more and more wood is being used. (During the last 40 years, global timber use has more than doubled, and paper use in particular has more than *trebled*.) In tropical countries, the total amount of forest cover on the land has dropped from 53 per cent in 1985 to 46 per cent in 2005. Much of the forest that's left is being damaged by logging activities, or replaced by plantations of tree crops. Over the same period, forest cover in the temperate regions of Asia, Europe, and North America has risen from 22 per cent to 27 per cent because more forest is being planted than cleared in these areas. About three per cent of the world's forests have been planted just to produce wood, but these unnatural forests don't provide homes for local wildlife the way natural forests do.

Reduce paper consumption by cleaning up kitchen spills with a cloth instead of paper towel.

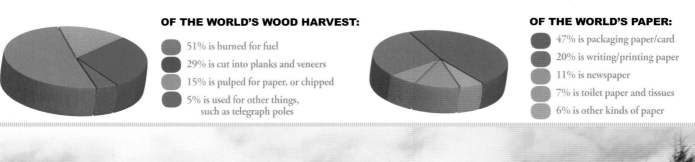

OF THE WORLD'S WOOD HARVEST:

- 51% is burned for fuel
- 29% is cut into planks and veneers
- 15% is pulped for paper, or chipped
- 5% is used for other things, such as telegraph poles

OF THE WORLD'S PAPER:

- 47% is packaging paper/card
- 20% is writing/printing paper
- 11% is newspaper
- 7% is toilet paper and tissues
- 6% is other kinds of paper

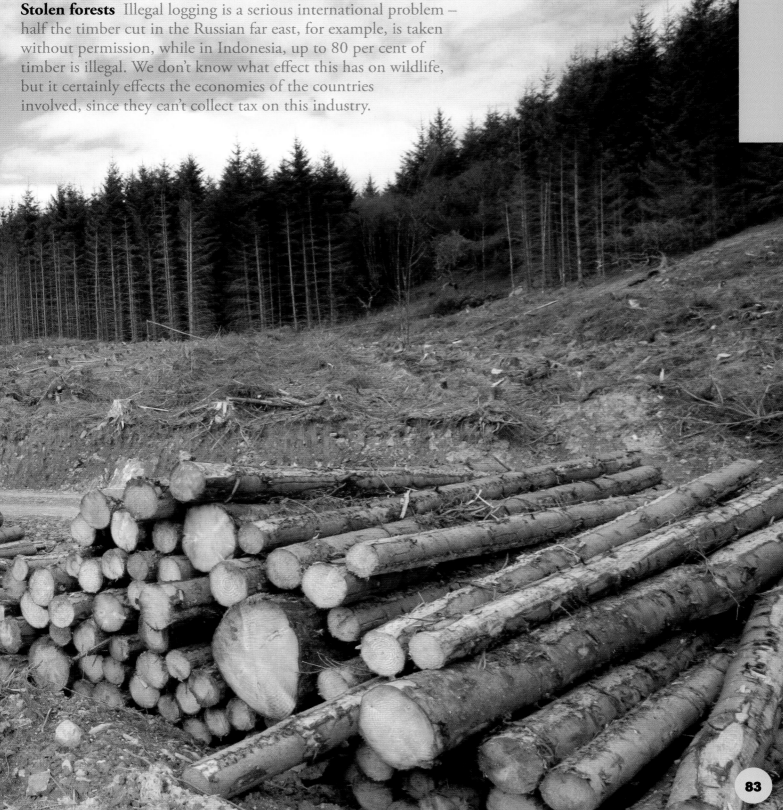

Stolen forests Illegal logging is a serious international problem – half the timber cut in the Russian far east, for example, is taken without permission, while in Indonesia, up to 80 per cent of timber is illegal. We don't know what effect this has on wildlife, but it certainly effects the economies of the countries involved, since they can't collect tax on this industry.

mediterranean

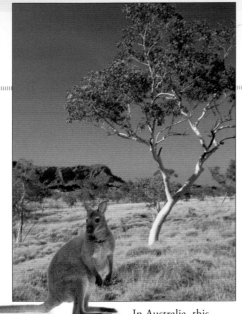

In Australia, this scrubland is called the Mallee. Here, there are lots of eucalyptus plants and a few kangaroos.

On the western edge of each continental land mass, there are places where winters are wet, but summers are hot and dry. Here, where the average temperature is 25°C (77°F), and it often reaches 35°C (95°F), there is a special biome. There are five of these, but the biggest is near the Mediterranean Sea, which gives the biome its name. Because so many people live there, lots of woodland is already lost – trees have been cut or burned, and the land is grazed by livestock. What's left is mostly scrub, with evergreen shrubs instead of trees.

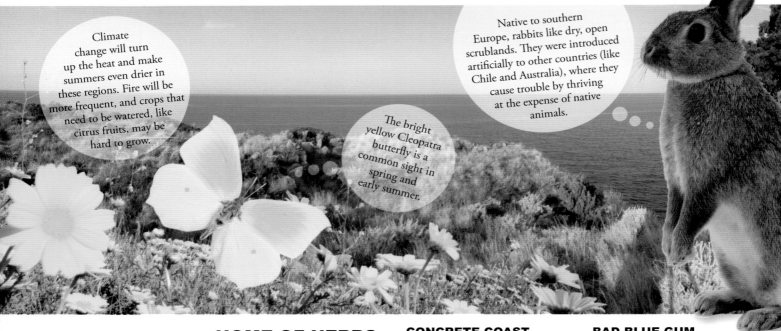

Climate change will turn up the heat and make summers even drier in these regions. Fire will be more frequent, and crops that need to be watered, like citrus fruits, may be hard to grow.

The bright yellow Cleopatra butterfly is a common sight in spring and early summer.

Native to southern Europe, rabbits like dry, open scrublands. They were introduced artificially to other countries (like Chile and Australia), where they cause trouble by thriving at the expense of native animals.

HOME OF HERBS

Lavender

Herbs like thyme, lavender, and rosemary make their home in the Mediterranean scrub ecosystem. Their small, waxy leaves conserve water, and their scented oils protect the leaves from fungi and grazing animals.

CONCRETE COAST

Each summer, 220 million tourists holiday in the Med. As well as damaging sea life, these people use up precious fresh water – swimming pools and golf courses alone need millions of litres every day.

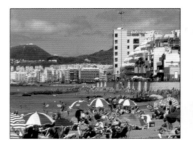

BAD BLUE GUM

Australian blue gum trees have been planted in the Mediterranean for wood and paper. The plantations don't support much wildlife, and the trees suck up water from deep underground and leave the soil dry.

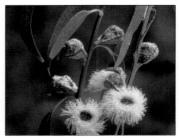

scrub ecosystem

Agile beasts Wild goats, sheep, and other climbers who live here look for food over large areas. Predators like lynx, hawks, and eagles feed on small mammals. There are many reptiles and insects in the scrub.

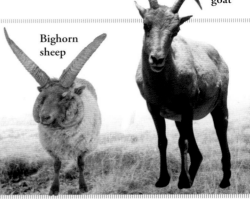
Wild goat

Bighorn sheep

Protea flower

Hummingbird

Spanish imperial eagle

Gryfon vulture

PROTEA
With heads up to 30 cm (12 in) across, proteas thrive in the poor scrub soil.

HUMMINGBIRD
Native to the Americas, tiny hummingbirds feed on flowers and insects.

EAGLE
An endangered species, the Spanish imperial eagle eats small birds and mammals.

VULTURE
A large, fierce bird of prey, the gryfon vulture (also griffin, griffon, or gryphon) mates for life.

BIGHORN SHEEP
Bighorn sheep graze on grasses and shrubs, and absorb minerals by licking salty stones.

WILD GOAT
Another creature that feeds on grass, the wild goat has small hooves with special non-slip ridges.

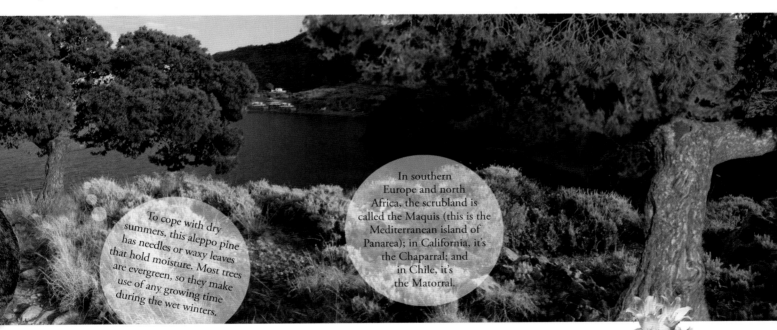

To cope with dry summers, this aleppo pine has needles or waxy leaves that hold moisture. Most trees are evergreen, so they make use of any growing time during the wet winters.

In southern Europe and north Africa, the scrubland is called the Maquis (this is the Mediterranean island of Panarea); in California, it's the Chaparral; and in Chile, it's the Matorral.

ROMAN RICHES
The Mediterranean region was the seat of the Roman Empire, which ruled Europe for 500 years from the first century BCE. Its riches were partly built on the oil from olive trees native to this area.

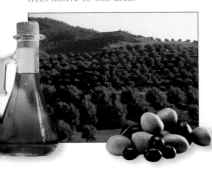

CLEVER CORK
The traditional management of cork-oak forest is the best example of low-impact, sustainable forestry in the world, since trees are never cut down. The cork bark is stripped off every ten years, but it always grows back.

Cork bark, bottle-stops, tile

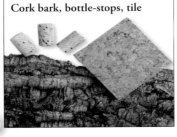

LOVE TO BURN
Fire, fanned by strong, dry winds, often burns vegetation in summer. Some trees, like eucalyptus and scrub oak, quickly re-grow from underground roots. Others, like pines or Australian Banksia shrubs, need the heat from fire to release their seeds from cones or woody fruits. Flowers like the fire lilies of southern Africa (right) wait underground for the heat or ash from fires to trigger their growth. The year after a fire, orchids flower profusely in the blackened earth.

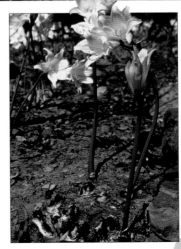

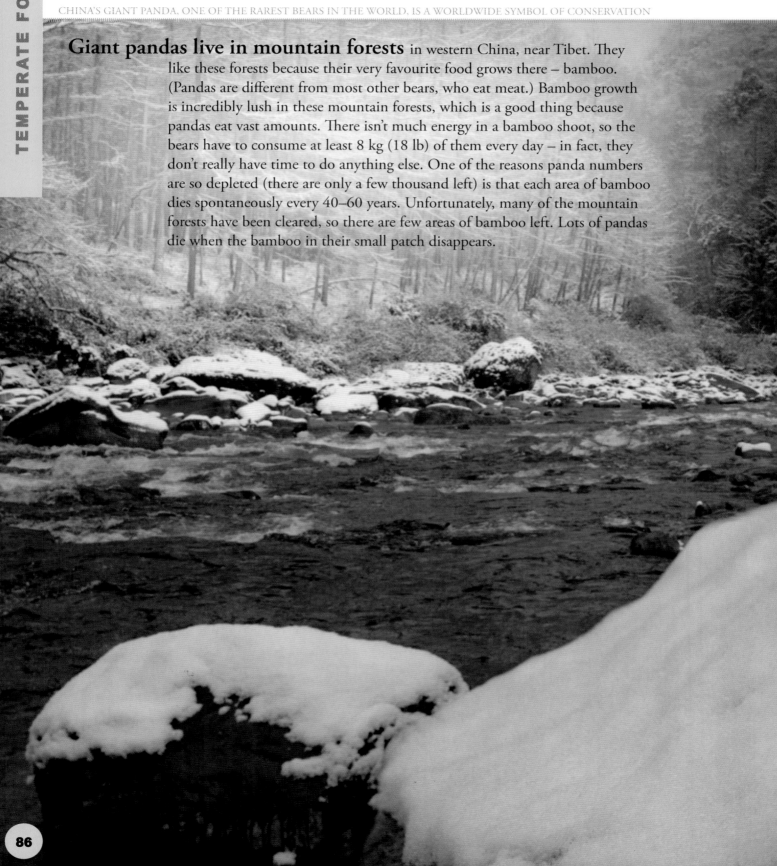

the giant panda

CHINA'S GIANT PANDA, ONE OF THE RAREST BEARS IN THE WORLD, IS A WORLDWIDE SYMBOL OF CONSERVATION

Giant pandas live in mountain forests in western China, near Tibet. They like these forests because their very favourite food grows there – bamboo. (Pandas are different from most other bears, who eat meat.) Bamboo growth is incredibly lush in these mountain forests, which is a good thing because pandas eat vast amounts. There isn't much energy in a bamboo shoot, so the bears have to consume at least 8 kg (18 lb) of them every day – in fact, they don't really have time to do anything else. One of the reasons panda numbers are so depleted (there are only a few thousand left) is that each area of bamboo dies spontaneously every 40–60 years. Unfortunately, many of the mountain forests have been cleared, so there are few areas of bamboo left. Lots of pandas die when the bamboo in their small patch disappears.

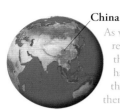

China

As well as keeping pandas in special reserves, scientists are monitoring them in the wild, mapping their habitats, and trying to understand their mating habits in order to help them breed more easily.

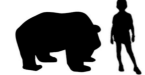

Although pandas are quite large bears, their babies are incredibly tiny. They're about the length of a pencil when they're born, and pink all over with a small amount of white fur.

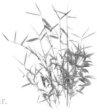

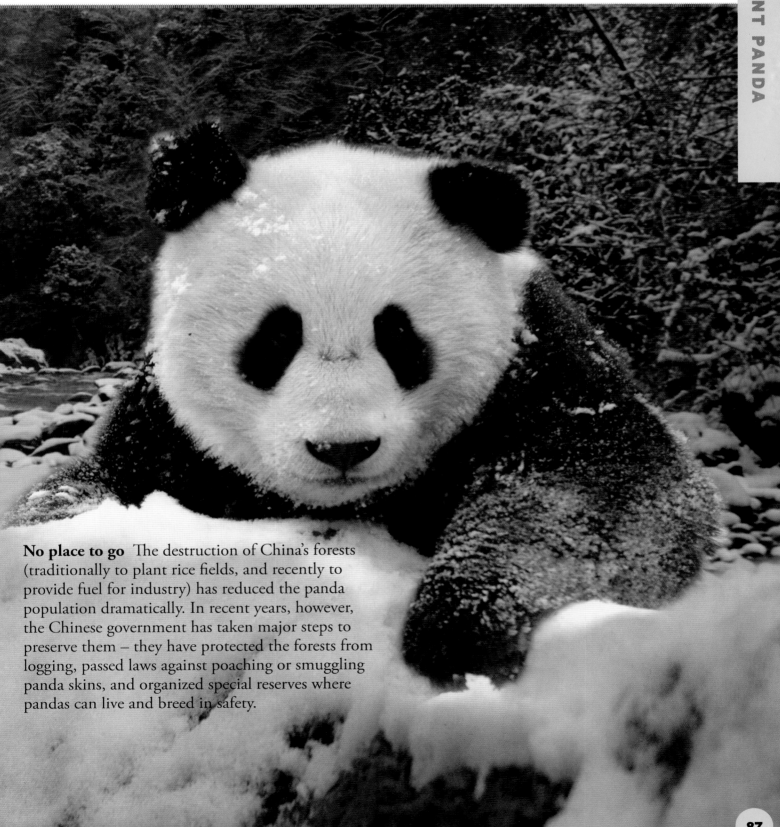

No place to go The destruction of China's forests (traditionally to plant rice fields, and recently to provide fuel for industry) has reduced the panda population dramatically. In recent years, however, the Chinese government has taken major steps to preserve them – they have protected the forests from logging, passed laws against poaching or smuggling panda skins, and organized special reserves where pandas can live and breed in safety.

MAKING A DIFFERENCE

Temperate forests are awesome places.

They can be terrifying and creepy, like the Forbidden Forest near Harry Potter's school or the woods where Hansel and Gretel were lost. Or they can be safe sanctuaries, like Robin Hood's Sherwood Forest or Lothlorien, where the Galadrim elves live in *Lord of the Rings*. However they are seen, temperate forests are precious. When we cut down trees, we should do it wisely so the forests can thrive along with all the creatures that use them.

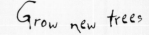

Grow new trees

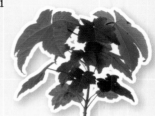

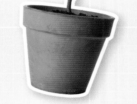

Don't throw it away

When you've finished with paper, recycle it. Paper can be recycled about six times before its fibres are too broken to be strong enough. Then it can be mixed with new wood pulp to strengthen it. Buy recycled paper products whenever you can.

what you can do

Always tuck a clean cotton handkerchief into your pocket or purse – tissues waste a huge amount of paper.

© Look out for the Forest Stewardship Council logo on books, paper, furniture, shelving, and timber.
FSC
There are over 90,000,000 hectares (222,400,000 acres) of FSC-certified forests around the world, and several thousand different products are made from their wood.

www.fsc.org

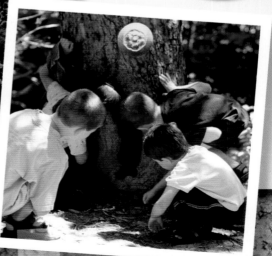

Children who care about trees will look after them when they grow up.

"He that plants trees loves others beside himself."

Thomas Fuller, English writer, 1732

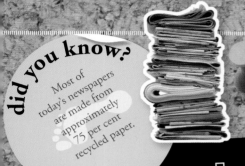

did you know? Most of today's newspapers are made from approximately 75 per cent recycled paper.

KNOW THE DEBATE

what's being done

- **The Forest Stewardship Council (FSC)** was set up to guarantee that every forest its wood comes from, and the people who live in or near each forest, are well looked after.
- **Lots of different countries** are passing laws to protect their precious forests from logging, clearing, mining, and similar exploitation.
- **National networks** are gathering people's information and observations about nature so they can monitor the effects of climate change. This will only work if lots of people record things like when a particular butterfly appeared in spring, when the first swallow arrived, and how often the grass needs cutting.

what we can do

- **Plant trees** and look after them for a long time to help control climate change. Trees absorb carbon dioxide and store the harmful carbon in their wood.
- **Look for a charity** that will help you to sponsor a tree in a protected forest – or give one as a present!
- **Support the natural cork industry.** Encourage wine-producers to seal bottles with cork stoppers rather than metal or plastic caps.
- **Spend time in your nearest wood.** Walk in it, smell it, and find its secrets. Watch the seasons change, and above all, enjoy it.

If you go into a forest for a walk or a picnic, don't drop litter or leave a fire smouldering – forest fires destroy trees and cause pollution.

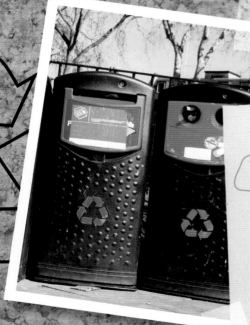

Use less paper

Never throw away a piece of paper that has not been covered on both sides. Open envelopes carefully, so you can use them more than once. Find information on the Internet instead of buying magazines, and look for paper made from other fibres, like hemp or straw. Re-use greeting cards by cutting off the front to make post cards or gift tags. And, of course, **USE RECYCLING BINS!**

what you can do

Buy or build a bird box for your garden to provide protection and shelter for local species.

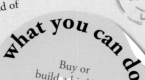

89

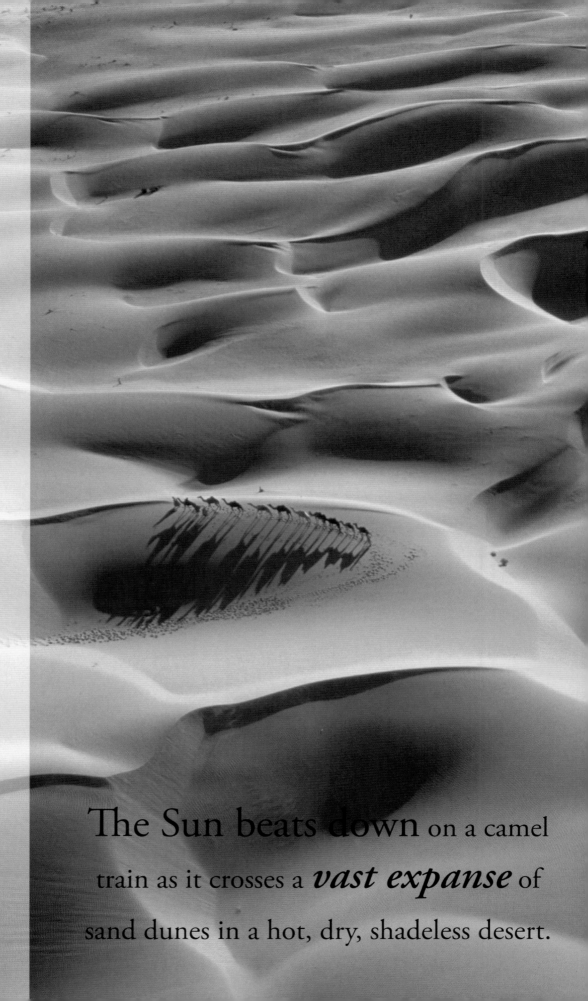
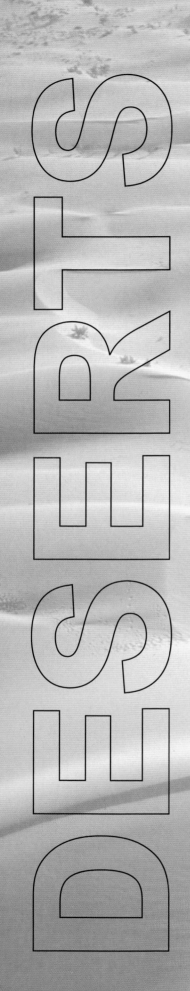

DESERTS

The Sun beats down on a camel train as it crosses a *vast expanse* of sand dunes in a hot, dry, shadeless desert.

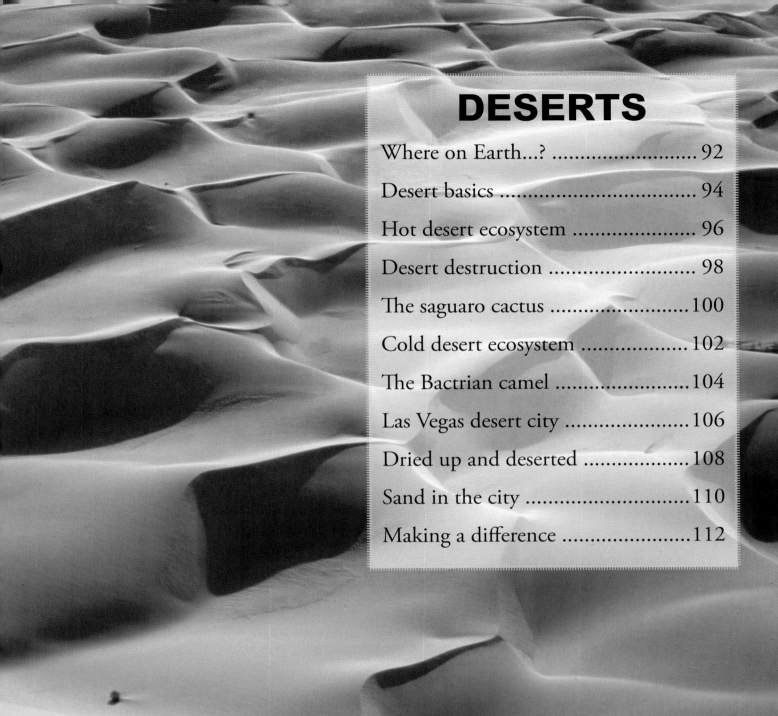

DESERTS

But is the desert as empty as it appears? Insects scuttle around on the sand, plant seeds lie dormant below the surface, and many animals from rodents to reptiles seek shelter in underground burrows, waiting to come out in the cool night air to hunt for food.

where on earth...?

Deserts are arid areas of land that receive less than 25 cm (10 in) of rain a year. Deserts currently cover about one-fifth of the Earth's land surface. They can be found in all sorts of locations, from mountains to coasts – and even Antarctica.

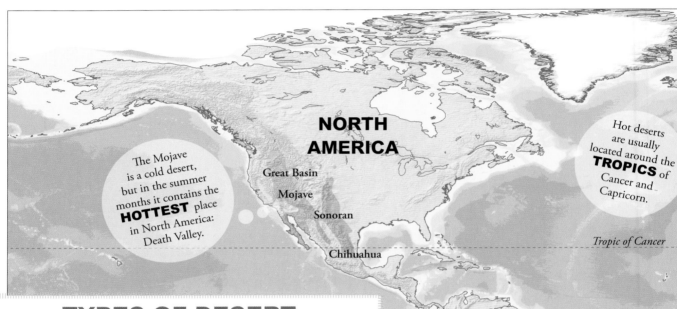

NORTH AMERICA

Great Basin

Mojave

Sonoran

Chihuahua

The Mojave is a cold desert, but in the summer months it contains the **HOTTEST** place in North America: Death Valley.

Hot deserts are usually located around the **TROPICS** of Cancer and Capricorn.

Tropic of Cancer

Equator

SOUTH AMERICA

Atacama

Tropic of Capricorn

Patagonia

There are places in the Atacama where rainfall has never been recorded, making it the world's **DRIEST DESERT.**

TYPES OF DESERT

● **HOT** Most hot deserts, such as the Sahara, are subtropical: they occur near the Tropics of Cancer and Capricorn. They are extremely hot during the day all year round, but there is a big difference in the temperature at night, when it may plummet to below freezing.

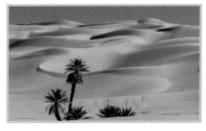

● **COLD** Cold deserts are often far from the sea, and can occur at high altitudes or in the rain shadows of mountains. The big difference in cold desert temperatures is between summer and winter. In the winter daytime, it's cold enough for snow, but summer days are hot.

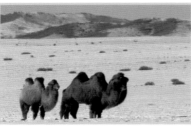

● **COASTAL** Where deserts have coastlines, their climate may be affected by cold offshore ocean currents. Cold currents lower the air temperature, and also make the air even more dry. Not every desert on the coast is affected because not every coast has a cold current.

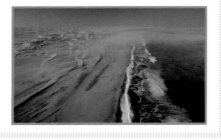

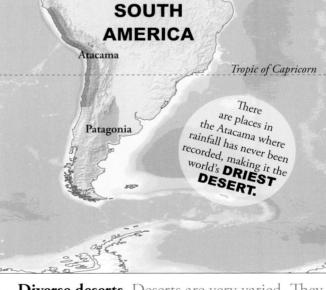

Diverse deserts Deserts are very varied. They may be large or small, and can be found all over the world, in tropical and temperate areas and at high and low altitudes. But they do have things in common: strong sunshine,

WHAT CAUSES DESERTS?

As air moves around the Earth, it collects water through evaporation and loses it again through precipitation (rain, snow, hail, and sleet). Dry air contains little water vapour, so the land it passes over receives little rain.

TYPES OF DESERT

Deserts can be classified in various ways, such as by temperature (hot or cold), or physical characteristics (sandy or rocky). In this book deserts are described as hot or cold. Both types may be affected by ocean currents, turning parts of them into coastal deserts.

DESERT MARGINS

A desert is a place with little rain, but towards the edge of a desert, more rain falls. This means more plants can grow, and the land turns from a desert into grassland. Most desert people live in these semi-arid areas between a desert and a grassland.

PROTECTING THE DESERT

You might think that climate change can't affect deserts, which are already hot and dry – but it may make them hotter and drier. Water would become even scarcer and so plants would die off, leaving no food for animals.

DESERTIFICATION

An even bigger problem than climate change is that of desertification – the spread of desert conditions into other biomes. Nearly three-quarters of the world's drylands (grassland and dry forest) are at risk of drying up and turning into desert.

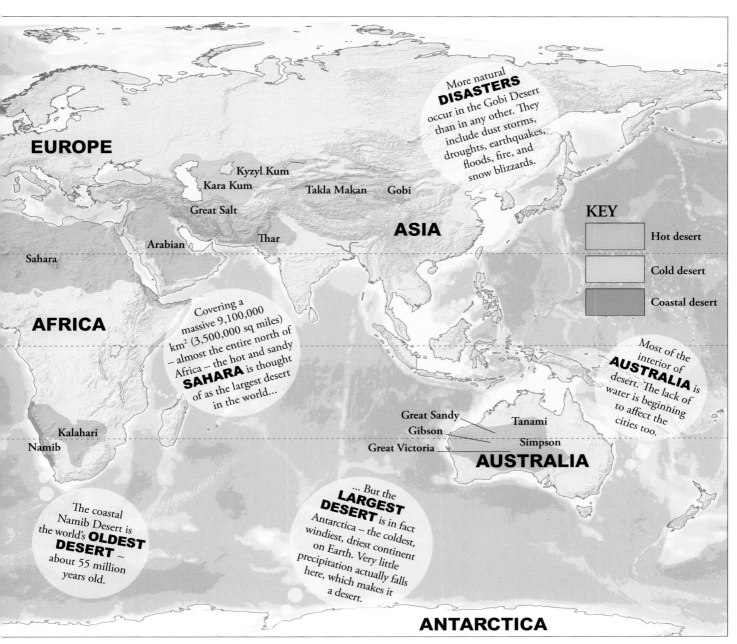

EUROPE

Kyzyl Kum
Kara Kum
Great Salt
Arabian
Thar
Takla Makan
Gobi

ASIA

Sahara

AFRICA

More natural **DISASTERS** occur in the Gobi Desert than in any other. They include dust storms, droughts, earthquakes, floods, fire, and snow blizzards.

KEY
Hot desert
Cold desert
Coastal desert

Covering a massive 9,100,000 km² (3,500,000 sq miles) – almost the entire north of Africa – the hot and sandy **SAHARA** is thought of as the largest desert in the world...

Most of the interior of **AUSTRALIA** is desert. The lack of water is beginning to affect the cities too.

Kalahari
Namib

Great Sandy
Gibson
Great Victoria
Tanami
Simpson

AUSTRALIA

The coastal Namib Desert is the world's **OLDEST DESERT** – about 55 million years old.

... But the **LARGEST DESERT** is in fact Antarctica – the coldest, windiest, driest continent on Earth. Very little precipitation actually falls here, which makes it a desert.

ANTARCTICA

harsh winds – and, of course, dryness. There are occasional, sudden downpours, but most of the time rainfall is so low that not many plants can grow, which means there is little food for animals. Plants also provide ground cover. Without them, soil can blow away, leaving just sand and rock. This bare ground reflects heat from the Sun, warming the air. Warm air holds in more water than cold air, so now there's even less chance of rain falling in the desert.

desert basics

TROPICAL RAINFORESTS get more than **180 cm** (70 in) of rain per year, which is why they have such lush vegetation.

TEMPERATE FORESTS get **50–200 cm** (20–80 in) of rain per year.

GRASSLANDS get **25–75 cm** (10–30 in) of rain per year. It is enough to support grass, but not many trees.

DESERTS usually get less than **25 cm** (10 in) of rain per year, which is not enough for most plants to grow.

There are four things that all *deserts* have in common: **lack of rainfall**, strong **sunshine**, and **wind**, which all together make a **sparse landscape**. All animals and plants that live in deserts have *adapted* to survive the harsh environment.

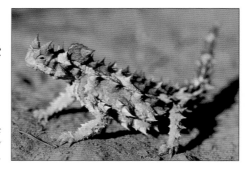

A thorny devil makes the most of the little water found in Australian deserts by drinking dew that collects in its spines.

How much rain? Rainfall is one of the factors that makes an area a particular biome. A desert is a desert because it gets very little rain, so not many plants can grow there. Where more rain falls, more plants grow, making grassland. Where lots of rain falls, enough trees can grow to create forests.

Wind shapes the landscape, causing

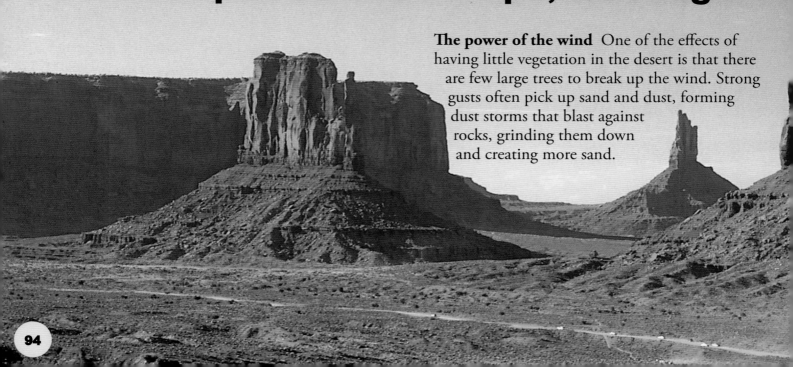

The power of the wind One of the effects of having little vegetation in the desert is that there are few large trees to break up the wind. Strong gusts often pick up sand and dust, forming dust storms that blast against rocks, grinding them down and creating more sand.

Strong sunshine

Stand in the middle of a desert, look up at the sky, and it's easy to see why deserts are hot: there are no clouds to block out the sunshine. It's the same reason why deserts are cold at night – there are no clouds to keep in the heat.

JUST ADD WATER!

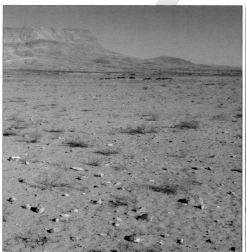

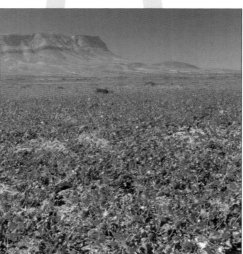

Springing into action

Most of the time, there are few plants to be seen in the desert because of the lack of rain. But when it falls, there can be a brief, beautiful blooming. Seeds lie dormant under the sand, waiting perhaps years for the unpredictable rain. Then they quickly germinate, bloom, and create new seeds for the next generation of plants – all within a few weeks.

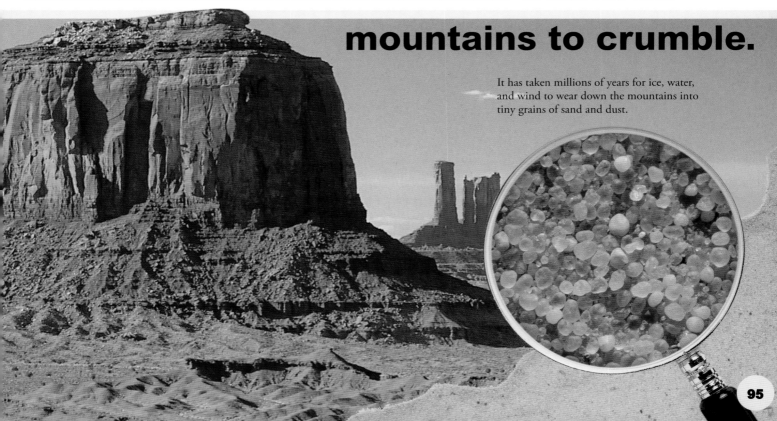

mountains to crumble.

It has taken millions of years for ice, water, and wind to wear down the mountains into tiny grains of sand and dust.

hot desert ecosystem

The Sahara Desert, in Africa, is the world's largest hot desert. Seemingly empty but for sand and rocks, the land actually supports a variety of wildlife – but it's a battle to survive in such an extreme environment. There are few plants to give shade, and winds can be strong. The clear blue sky has no clouds for rain or to protect against the Sun, so daytime temperatures are very high. The lack of cloud cover also lets the heat escape at night, so the hot desert turns very cold when the Sun goes down.

Average Saharan temperatures
Daytime: 58°C (136°F)
Night time: -10°C (14°F)

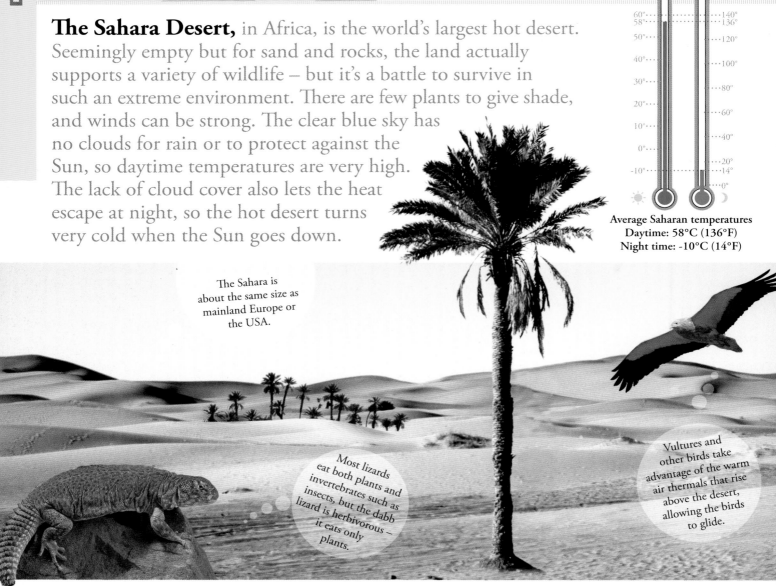

The Sahara is about the same size as mainland Europe or the USA.

Most lizards eat both plants and invertebrates such as insects, but the dabb lizard is herbivorous – it eats only plants.

Vultures and other birds take advantage of the warm air thermals that rise above the desert, allowing the birds to glide.

Survival skills It's hard to find food and water in the desert. The resources are scarce, and the extreme heat and lack of shade makes searching difficult. Desert animals are adapted to this type of existence; for example, some get all their water from their food. They also have ways of keeping cool, such as spending the day in cool burrows, coming out at night to hunt.

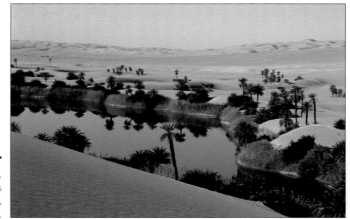

WATER IN THE DESERT
The lushest scenery in the desert is at an oasis. These pools form where underground water comes to the surface. Oases are a shady haven for animals, which come to fill up on leafy food as well as water.

Desert food chain Life in the desert relies on vegetation. Even carnivorous animals that do not eat plants, eat animals that do. But there are not many plants in the desert to support the chain, so the animals here are generally smaller and fewer in number than in other ecosystems.

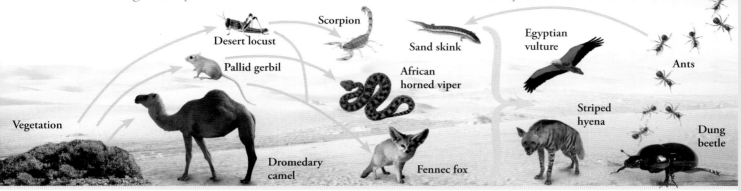

Desert locust

Scorpion

Pallid gerbil

Sand skink

Egyptian vulture

Ants

Vegetation

African horned viper

Striped hyena

Dung beetle

Dromedary camel

Fennec fox

PRODUCERS
Plants need three things to grow: sunshine, nutrients from the ground, and water. Sunshine and nutrients are plentiful, but water is often in short supply.

PRIMARY CONSUMERS
While the majority of plant eaters are invertebrates such as insects, there are some small and large mammals that are herbivorous too.

SECONDARY CONSUMERS
Being quite small animals, desert carnivores aim for small prey. They would not kill a full-grown camel, although a baby may be targeted. The predators may eat other meat eaters as well as herbivores.

SCAVENGERS & DECOMPOSERS
Scavengers such as vultures and hyenas aid decomposition by breaking up and eating dead animals. Ants take bits of carcass underground, where "leftovers" act as fertilizer. Dung beetles do the same thing with faeces, to the same effect. Any other waste is broken down by bacteria.

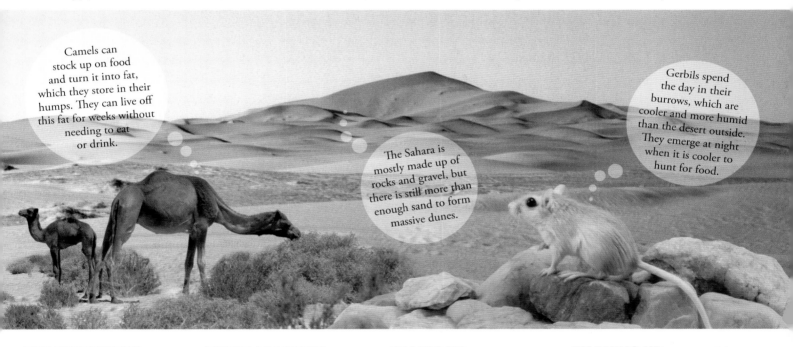

Camels can stock up on food and turn it into fat, which they store in their humps. They can live off this fat for weeks without needing to eat or drink.

Gerbils spend the day in their burrows, which are cooler and more humid than the desert outside. They emerge at night when it is cooler to hunt for food.

The Sahara is mostly made up of rocks and gravel, but there is still more than enough sand to form massive dunes.

THE BURROWERS
The jerboa is an expert recycler. Sealing itself in an underground den away from the heat, it is able to recapture the moisture from its breath, so it rarely needs to drink.

TWICE AS USEFUL
Hunting in the dark, the Fennec fox uses its large ears like satellite dishes to pinpoint the position of its prey. The ears' large surface area also loses heat, helping to keep the fox cool.

FILLING UP
Camels can go without water for up to two weeks. When thirsty, they can drink up to 120 litres (26 gallons) – a volume that would be fatal to most animals.

WARMING UP
The desert heat has its advantages. Reptiles are cold-blooded: they warm up and cool down depending on the environment. They need the sunshine to warm up and get active.

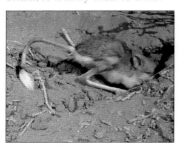
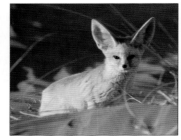
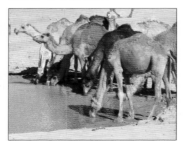
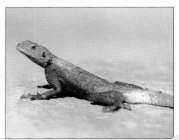

desert destruction

Deserts have always been subject to *natural* change, growing or shrinking with changes in rainfall. Millions of years ago, North Africa was covered by a sea; today it is home to the world's biggest hot desert. The main threat to deserts is not nature, but people. **Human activity** is having an enormous effect on desert wildlife, as well as the landscape. Plants and animals that have evolved to survive in the desert cannot cope with the rapid changes brought about by people, and so they die out.

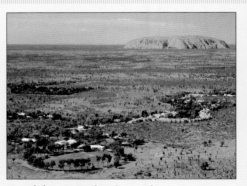

This fossil of a sea creature was found in the Sahara Desert, proving that the now arid area was once under water.

Arid areas are thought of as untouched,

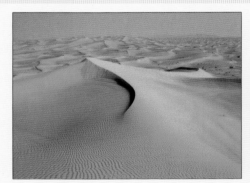

Climate change Already hot and dry, deserts are under threat of becoming hotter and drier due to climate change. Without water, no plants can grow. Without plants, the whole food chain collapses. Once the plants and animals disappear, there is little hope of the desert recovering.

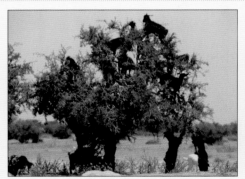

Overgrazing The introduction of non-native species into deserts has been devastating. Brought in by farmers who need the meat, milk, wool, and leather, domestic animals such as goats compete with wild animals for food. They also strip the plants bare, which can kill the plant, leaving the ground open to wind erosion.

Building Whether it's a tourist resort or a town, building settlements in the desert puts a strain on resources. Nomads move from place to place, so when water and pasture for animals run low, they move on and the stocks can recover. But when people stay in one place, there is no chance for the land to replenish itself.

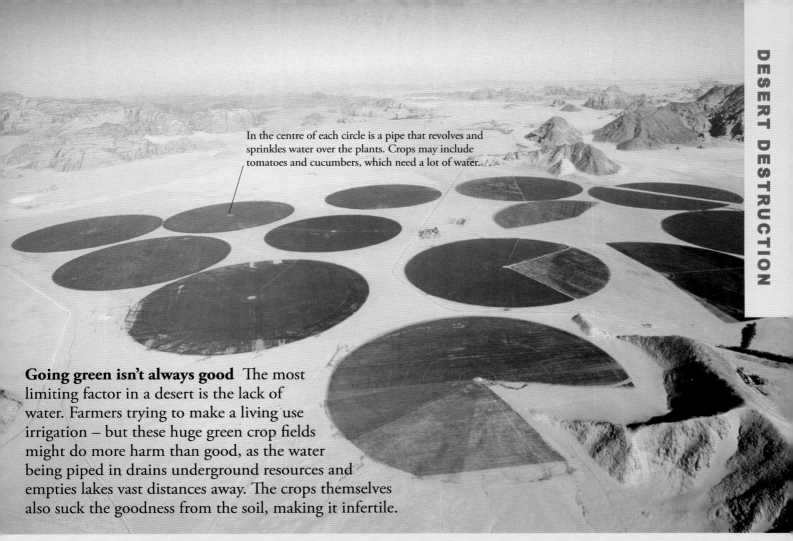

In the centre of each circle is a pipe that revolves and sprinkles water over the plants. Crops may include tomatoes and cucumbers, which need a lot of water.

Going green isn't always good The most limiting factor in a desert is the lack of water. Farmers trying to make a living use irrigation – but these huge green crop fields might do more harm than good, as the water being piped in drains underground resources and empties lakes vast distances away. The crops themselves also suck the goodness from the soil, making it infertile.

but people are changing the landscape.

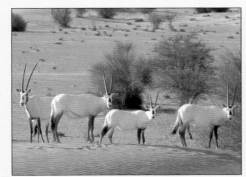

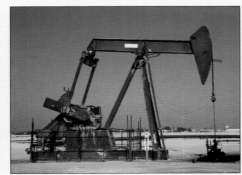

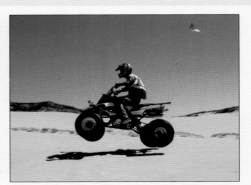

Overhunting The main threat to the balance of wildlife in the desert is overhunting, which is done for meat, fur, or even sport. The oryx is under threat of extinction, but, like every species, they have a place in the ecosystem. The food chain and the environment will suffer if any part of it is missing.

Mining Below the surface of most deserts lie rich deposits of minerals, from oil to diamonds and gold. In the past, it was hard to access the minerals in deserts, but modern technology has overcome this. However, in doing so, the land is being ripped up, killing off the plants that provide food for animals.

Dune riding Hurtling over dunes in a quad bike or jeep looks like fun, but it actually destroys the dunes. It can cause the sand to slip, and also kills animals that hide below the sand's surface.

Be an ecotourist! If you visit a desert, stay in a resort that looks after the environment – and avoid dune buggies.

the saguaro cactus

PROTECTING A NATIONAL TREASURE OF NORTH AMERICA – AND THE ANIMALS THAT DEPEND ON IT FOR FOOD AND SHELTER

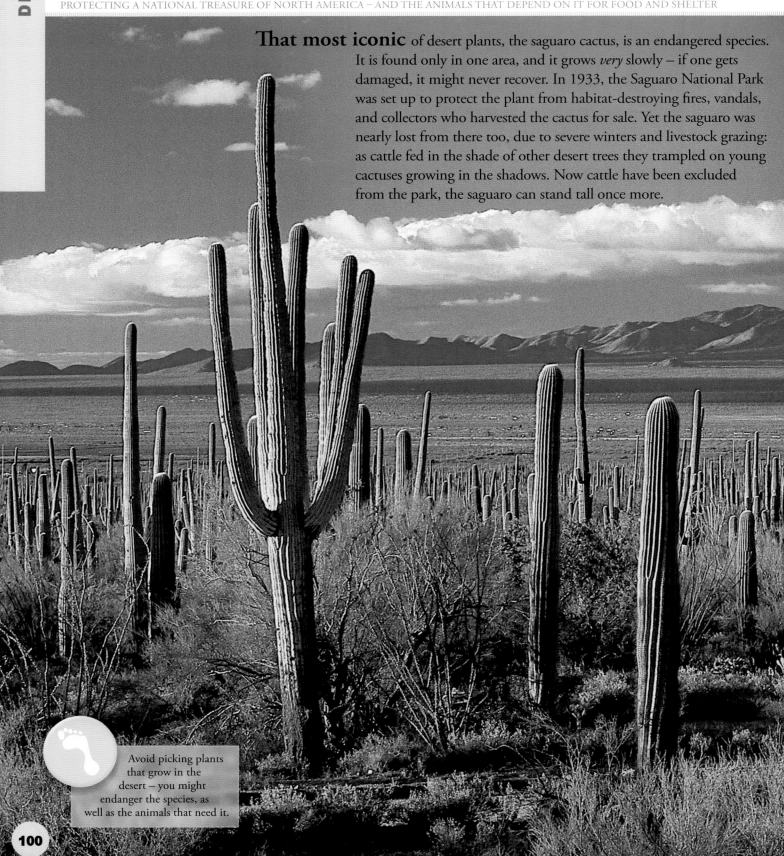

That most iconic of desert plants, the saguaro cactus, is an endangered species. It is found only in one area, and it grows *very* slowly – if one gets damaged, it might never recover. In 1933, the Saguaro National Park was set up to protect the plant from habitat-destroying fires, vandals, and collectors who harvested the cactus for sale. Yet the saguaro was nearly lost from there too, due to severe winters and livestock grazing: as cattle fed in the shade of other desert trees they trampled on young cactuses growing in the shadows. Now cattle have been excluded from the park, the saguaro can stand tall once more.

Avoid picking plants that grow in the desert – you might endanger the species, as well as the animals that need it.

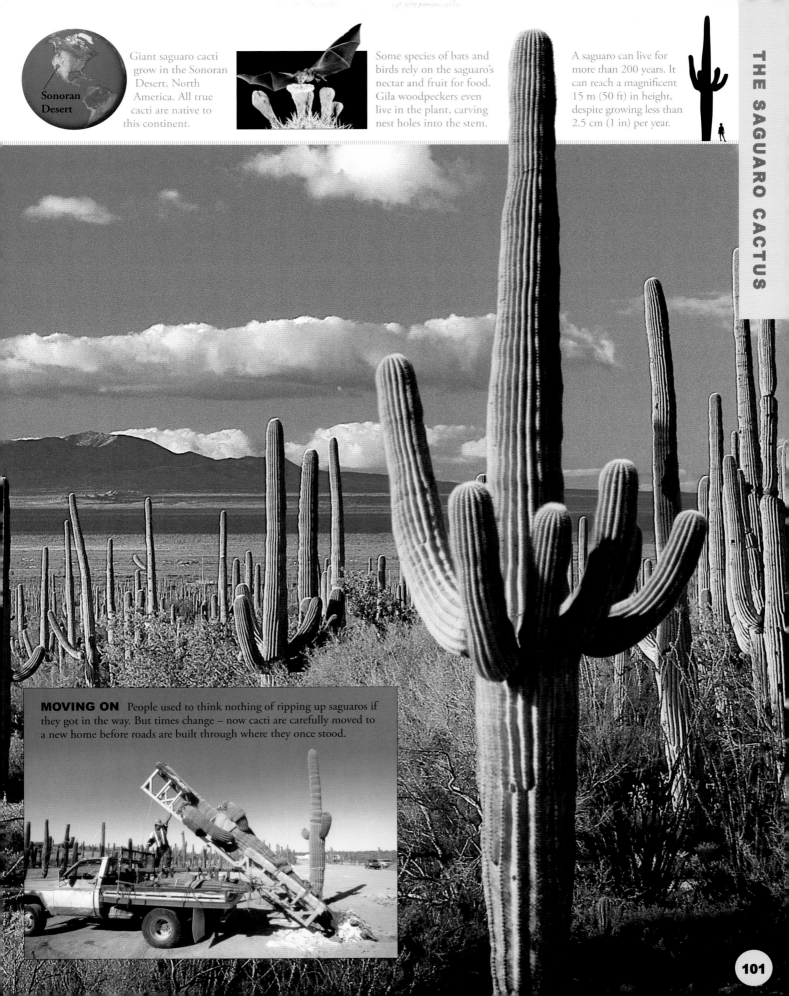

Sonoran Desert

Giant saguaro cacti grow in the Sonoran Desert, North America. All true cacti are native to this continent.

Some species of bats and birds rely on the saguaro's nectar and fruit for food. Gila woodpeckers even live in the plant, carving nest holes into the stem.

A saguaro can live for more than 200 years. It can reach a magnificent 15 m (50 ft) in height, despite growing less than 2.5 cm (1 in) per year.

MOVING ON People used to think nothing of ripping up saguaros if they got in the way. But times change – now cacti are carefully moved to a new home before roads are built through where they once stood.

cold desert ecosystem

Cold deserts share many features with hot deserts, such as strong winds and a sparse landscape. But they have one major difference: they freeze in the winter. Many cold deserts are actually drier than hot ones, because most of the precipitation falls as snow rather than rain, which animals cannot drink. It also covers the vegetation, making food hard to find. The best time of year is spring, when melting snow provides a little water for plants and animals. Come the summer, the hot Sun dries the land once more.

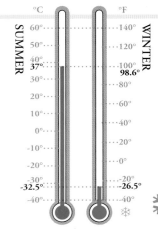

Average Gobi temperatures
Summer: 37°C (98.6°F)
Winter: -32.5°C (-26.5°F)

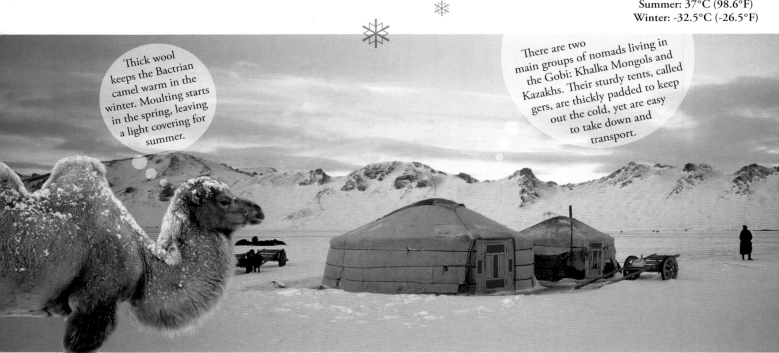

Thick wool keeps the Bactrian camel warm in the winter. Moulting starts in the spring, leaving a light covering for summer.

There are two main groups of nomads living in the Gobi: Khalka Mongols and Kazakhs. Their sturdy tents, called gers, are thickly padded to keep out the cold, yet are easy to take down and transport.

Life in the Gobi Desert In a cold desert, low winter temperatures are more of a problem than heat for plants and animals, and it is made even colder by windchill. It can be difficult for animals to find enough to eat, so to avoid this shortage some animals store fat, while others hibernate.

Traditional desert life

The Khalka Mongols that live in the Gobi are pastoralists – they keep livestock, living off the meat, milk, and wool that the animals provide. They live in tune with the desert, moving to new pasture up to 10 times a year, which gives the vegetation time to recover.

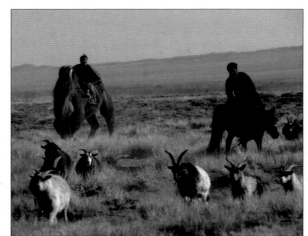

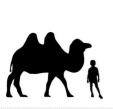

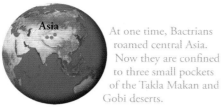

Asia

At one time, Bactrians roamed central Asia. Now they are confined to three small pockets of the Takla Makan and Gobi deserts.

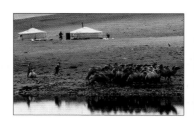

Wild Bactrians will not come to this oasis: domestic animals (including camels) and people scare them. The livestock also eats most of the plants in the desert, leaving none for the Bactrian.

Las Vegas desert city

IS THE DESERT A GOOD PLACE TO BUILD NEW HOMES FOR A GROWING POPULATION? OR HAS LAS VEGAS GONE TOO FAR?

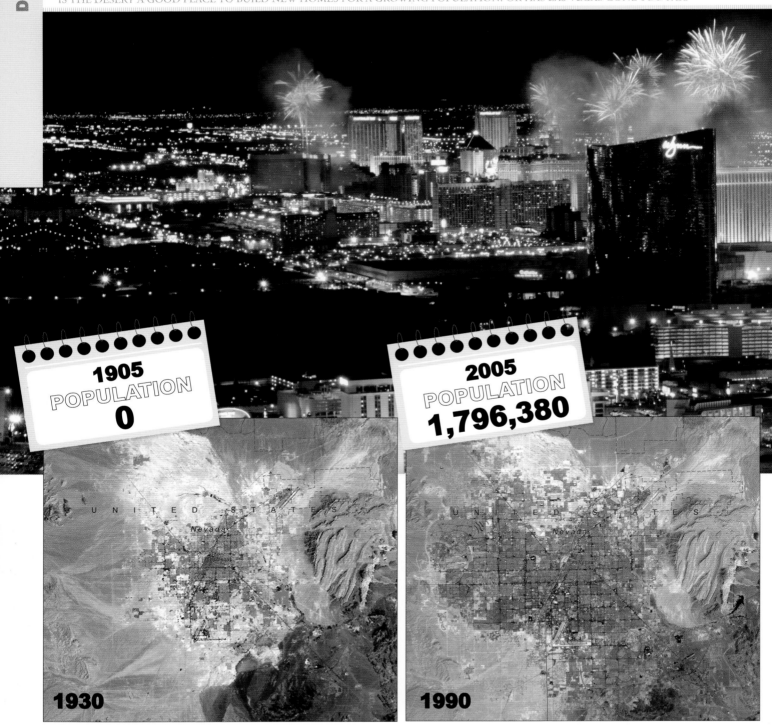

1905
POPULATION
0

2005
POPULATION
1,796,380

1930

1990

FROM SMALL BEGINNINGS...

People first went to Las Vegas for its freshwater spring – an oasis in the desert. The town grew to become a railroad stop, and by 1930, 5,000 people were living there. To meet the water needs of the population, the Hoover dam was completed in 1935, creating Lake Mead as a reservoir.

... TO SPRAWLING CITIES

Since the end of the Second World War, when there was a boom in tourism and gambling, the city has not stopped growing. In 1990 nearly a million people were living in Clark County, a number that has almost doubled again today. There is simply not enough water in Lake Mead for them all.

The need for fresh water in Las Vegas, the USA's fastest

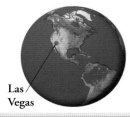

Las Vegas lies in the Mojave Desert. The city, in Nevada, USA, is part of a larger urban area called Clark County.

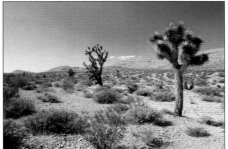

Building site? A desert might seem an ideal empty site for a city, but animals and plants are put under threat as their sources of shelter, food, and water are lost. Transport links to and from the city also carve up the desert, destroying even more land.

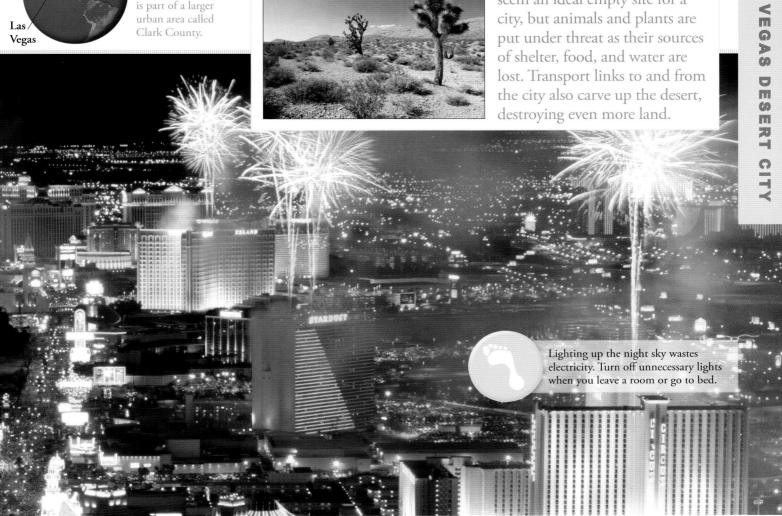

Lighting up the night sky wastes electricity. Turn off unnecessary lights when you leave a room or go to bed.

More than a DROP in the desert...

As well as its 1.8 million residents, Las Vegas attracts 30 million tourists a year. With pools, fountains, water-based shows, and personal use, it works out that each person in the city uses 40 per cent more water than the US national average. But water supplies, which are already limited in a desert, are predicted to run too low to meet demands by 2025. With hotels relying on their attractions to bring in money, this won't be an easy problem to solve.

(litres per person per day)

Las Vegas
1165
(307 gallons)

USA average
720
(190 gallons)

Los Angeles
530
(140 gallons)

TRANSPORT TENSION

Water isn't the only issue to consider when building in the desert. They have few natural resources, so Las Vegas is not able to produce much. Almost everything needed in the city, from food to clothing, is brought in by road or air, which causes pollution.

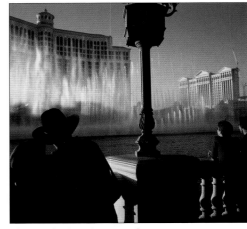

If water displays disappear from Las Vegas, will the tourists still come?

dried up and deserted

Desertification is what happens when once-fertile land becomes *useless* and turns to desert – and it's mainly due to *human activity.* Misusing the land causes vegetation to die out, which leads to soil erosion. Seventy per cent of drylands, such as grasslands and forests, are at risk of becoming desert – that's one-third of all the land on Earth, affecting 1 billion people and countless animals and plants.

Ostriches are native to South African grasslands, areas that are turning to desert. Many animals living there will die out if they have nowhere to go for food and shelter.

Wherever you live in the world, it's important not to waste water. You could turn off the tap while you brush your teeth.

Some causes of desertification...

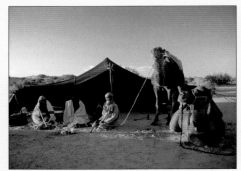

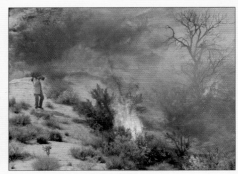

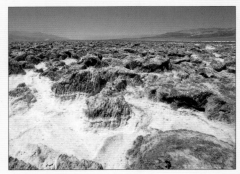

Overpopulation Many nomads have settled in desert margins where there is more vegetation, but there are too many people for the land to support. The soil becomes exhausted by farming, and livestock overgraze the plants. Left bare and exposed, the wind carries away the topsoil, leaving sand and rocks – and creating desert.

Fire People in urbanized desert margins set fires on purpose as a way of controlling natural fires. They clear the land of vegetation that might burn uncontrollably, creating fire breaks to protect their property. But this kills off slow-growing native plants, and also destroys sources of food and shelter for animals.

Salinization Irrigation provides water for plants, but it can also turn the land infertile. Minerals left behind when water evaporates leave a salty crust on the ground, which stops plants growing. Salinization also occurs where there are no plants – when soil gets blown away, minerals in the ground can come to the surface.

1963 **1973** **2001**

Lake Chad is in the Sahel, an area south of the Sahara that is quickly turning to desert. The lake contains just 5 per cent of the water it held 40 years ago.

Less in, more out

Lake Chad is a vital source of water in central Africa. People use the water for their animals and crops – it is even piped into the Sahara for irrigation. But there is only a limited amount of water, and it's running out. There is less rainfall in the area now, and the river that feeds the lake has been diverted for use elsewhere. The lake cannot replenish and it is shrinking fast.

... and some of the ways to prevent it.

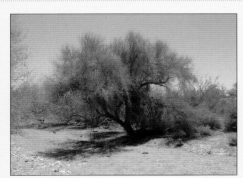

Protect native trees Tall plants help to keep land stable by acting as windbreaks, slowing down the wind to help prevent soil erosion. Native trees survive on less water than non-native, putting less strain on the habitat. Their roots are also important: they are very long or widespread to reach water, and this helps to bind and stabilize the soil.

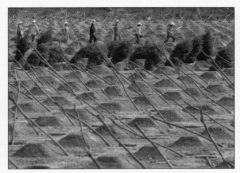

Sand fences Where trees have been removed, it is possible to plant new vegetation and create a sand fence to stop the desert creeping into, and taking over, neighbouring land. In China, a massive project called "The Green Wall" has been started to try to stop the spread of the Gobi Desert into exhausted farmland.

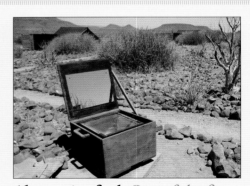

Alternative fuel One of the first sand fences in Africa proved to be a success – until people chopped down the trees for cooking fuel. Many desert dwellers live in poverty and use whatever resources they can find. By supplying alternatives such as solar-powered ovens, both the people and the land benefit.

sand in the city

STRONG WINDS OVER THE GOBI DESERT BRING MISERY (AND LOTS OF DUST) TO BEIJING, CHINA

The people of Beijing are getting used to a major problem that hits their city many times a year: dust. Blown in from the Gobi Desert, the fine yellow particles fill the air, causing reduced visibility and breathing difficulties. Airports are closed, cars are damaged, and people cannot work because dust even gets inside machines and computers that are kept indoors. Such storms are a natural occurrence in deserts, but as desertification swallows up farmland on the margins of the Gobi, the storms are brought closer to the cities, appearing more frequently and travelling further. Apart from forecasting when the storms are about to hit, there is little that anyone can do except try to prevent them from getting worse. And the only way to do this is to stop desertification.

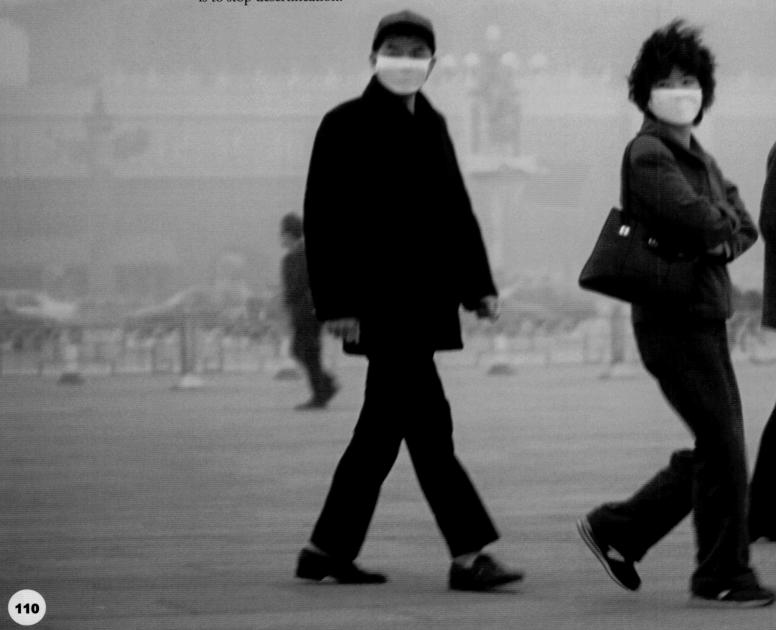

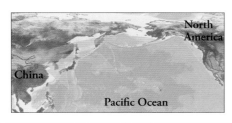

China

North America

Pacific Ocean

Dust storms can travel enormous distances. In a desert, both sand and dust get blown about, but sand is heavy and does not get lifted far – around 50 cm (2 ft) above the ground. Dust, however, can travel for thousands of kilometres. Gobi dust can reach the west coast of America, turning sunsets red and making cars dusty. It also drops into the Pacific Ocean between the continents, clogging up coral reefs. The Sahara Desert, in Africa, is to blame for dust in Europe and eastern America. Yet it does have one benefit: the fertile dust drops into and "feeds" the Amazon Rainforest.

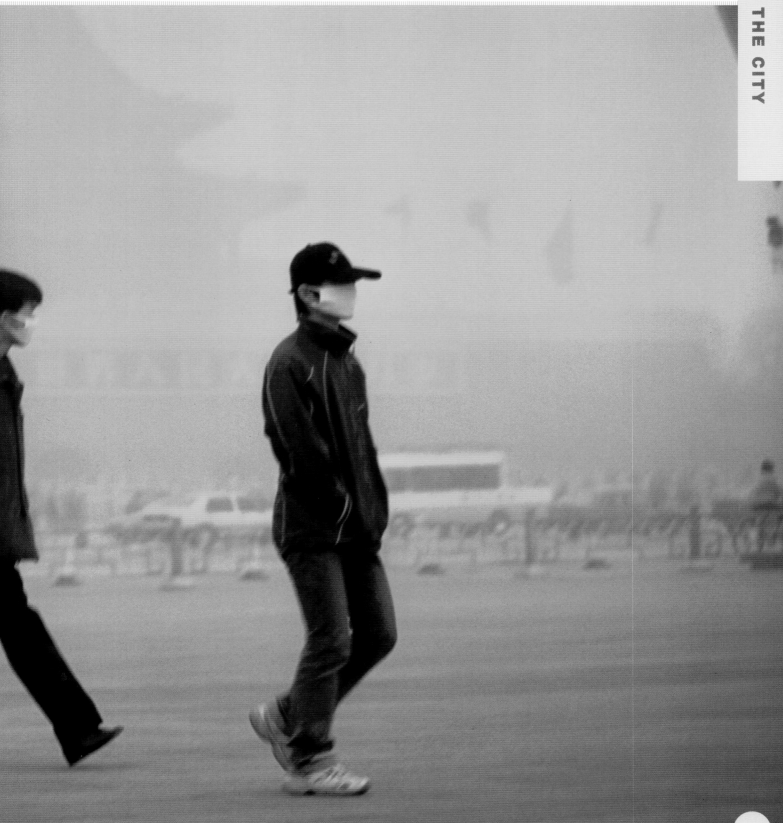

MAKING A DIFFERENCE

WHAT's it got to do with ME?

So you live in a town far away from a desert. Think desertification has nothing to do with you? **Think again!**

Don't waste water Water shortages occur in many parts of the world, but it's easy to get into the habit of saving water... ★ turn off taps ★ take a shower rather than a bath ★ water the garden with washing-up water or cold tea ★ use a bucket of water rather than a hose to wash a car

Get planting Stop soil erosion in arid areas by replacing trees. ★ Tree Aid is a charity that plants trees in Africa and supports poor communities that use the wood for fuel www.treeaid.org.uk

Got a garden?

Grow plants that are suitable for your climate.

what you can do

Are you visiting a desert area? (Don't forget this includes Las Vegas and Australia!) Be an ecotourist and limit the water you use. Do you need clean towels every day?

the search for water in dry land

Many desert dwellers live in poverty and have limited resources. For them, getting water isn't as simple as turning on a tap. But there are ways of making access to water easier.

Johads In the Thar Desert, small dams called johads are built across streams. When rain falls, the water collects behind the dam, creating a reservoir for people to use. The water also seeps into the ground, providing enough moisture for plants to grow.

Fog catchers In the Atacama Desert, water comes not from rain but from fog. Huge nets "catch" the fog, which condenses into water. Chlorine is added, the water is boiled, and people have enough safe water to drink, wash in, and cook with.

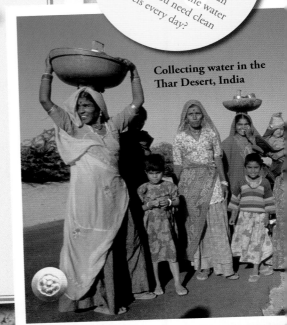

Collecting water in the Thar Desert, India

The best way to combat desertification is to prevent it happening in the first place – wherever you live in the world.

what you can do
Plan an event to mark World Day to Combat Desertification, held every year on 17 June. As well as raising awareness, you could raise funds for charity.

IYDD
International Year of Deserts and Desertification

● The year 2006 was declared International Year of Deserts and Desertification (IYDD) by the **United Nations** as part of their **Convention to Combat Desertification (UNCCD).**

● **Sub-Saharan Africa** and **South Asia** were identified as being most at threat from desertification. Other at-risk regions include Latin America and central and eastern Europe.

● One billion people in over 100 countries are affected by desertification. Many are **poor** and are **politically weak**.

● As a result of the IYDD, **national action programmes** encourage governments to work with local people to preserve the land, while still being able to earn a living.

● Countries not immediately affected by desertification offer technical and financial help through **partnership agreements**.

practical ACTION

● Desertification is not just about land, but people too. Those who live in desert margins have a vital job in protecting the land. But they still need to make a living for themselves, and often this causes a conflict of interest.

● It's important to **educate local people** in how to use desert resources. The UN has produced **kits** for children in primary schools to learn about causes and effects of desertification. Newspapers, radio, and TV all help to spread information too.

● What **hidden assets** are there in the area? Instead of raising non-native animals for food, which compete with native species, people in Africa could eat ostrich meat, or kangaroos in Australia.

● With enough know-how and money, **technology** can solve many problems: instead of using trees for fuel, **wind turbines** provide energy and **solar ovens** replace wood-burners. Solar-powered **desalination systems** make drinking water available.

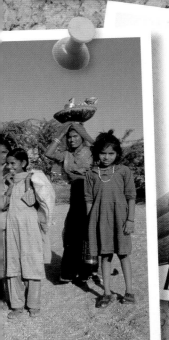

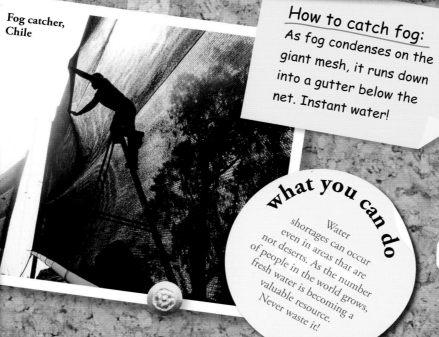

Fog catcher, Chile

How to catch fog:
As fog condenses on the giant mesh, it runs down into a gutter below the net. Instant water!

what you can do
Water shortages can occur even in areas that are not deserts. As the number of people in the world grows, fresh water is becoming a valuable resource. Never waste it!

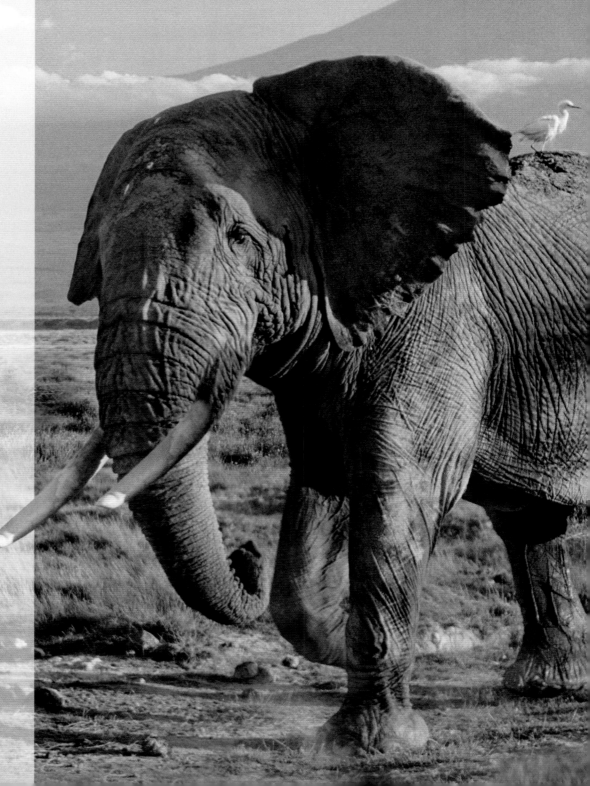

GRASSSLANDS

The grassland biome is a gentle landscape, but it contains a variety of *complex* and *diverse* habitats.

It may not look as impressive as a mountain range or rainforest, but the largest and fastest land animals live here, supported by the most common of plants: grass. This is the habitat in which humans evolved – and in which we have had a most profound influence.

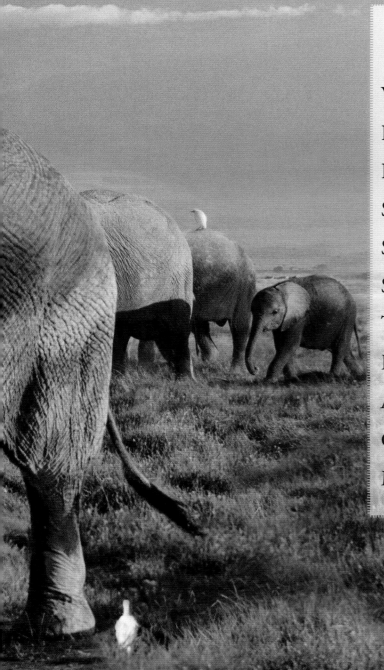

GRASSLANDS

where on earth...?

Grasslands are among the world's most productive biomes. The climate in these ecosystems falls between those of deserts and forests: they are usually hot – at least in summer – and have more rainfall than a desert, but not enough to support many trees.

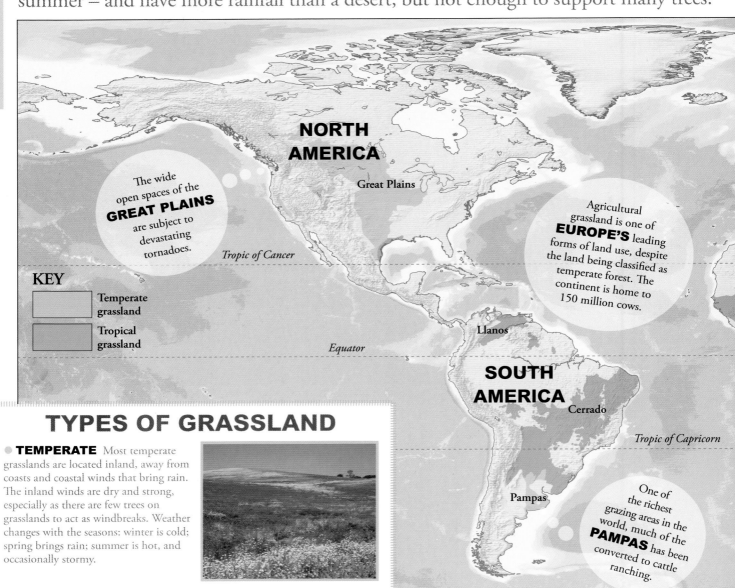

NORTH AMERICA

Great Plains

The wide open spaces of the **GREAT PLAINS** are subject to devastating tornadoes.

Tropic of Cancer

Agricultural grassland is one of **EUROPE'S** leading forms of land use, despite the land being classified as temperate forest. The continent is home to 150 million cows.

KEY

Temperate grassland

Tropical grassland

Llanos

Equator

SOUTH AMERICA

Cerrado

Tropic of Capricorn

Pampas

One of the richest grazing areas in the world, much of the **PAMPAS** has been converted to cattle ranching.

TYPES OF GRASSLAND

● **TEMPERATE** Most temperate grasslands are located inland, away from coasts and coastal winds that bring rain. The inland winds are dry and strong, especially as there are few trees on grasslands to act as windbreaks. Weather changes with the seasons: winter is cold; spring brings rain; summer is hot, and occasionally stormy.

● **TROPICAL** Also called savanna, tropical grassland areas have two seasons – wet and dry – rather than four. It is warm all year round, but rain tends to fall only during the wet season. With the help of the heavy downpours, or monsoons, some savanna grasses can grow to several metres tall.

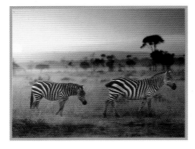

With grasslands appearing all over the world, it's hardly surprising that there is a great diversity of animals living in these ecosystems. There is as much activity below ground as above it. Grasslands are open spaces where

116

GIVE AND TAKE
Grassland covers half the Earth's land surface. Much of the natural grassland has been lost to agriculture, but the total amount of grassland across the world remains the same as large areas of forest are felled to create pasture (grassland used for grazing).

GRASS OR SHRUB?
Grasslands are not just made up of grass: plenty of non-woody, flowering plants with broad leaves – such as daisies – grow there too. Some trees and shrubs grow on grasslands, but when there are more woody plants than grass, the land is known as shrubland.

HARD GARDENING
Many extreme natural events occur on grasslands, from monsoons, wildfires, and tornadoes to droughts and freezing temperatures. Yet far from causing problems, these events help to maintain grassland, for example by weeding out plants that compete with the grass.

WIND POWER
In the summer, strong gusts of wind spread fires across open grassland. While fire can help grass – for example, the ash acts as fertilizer – blazes can have devastating effects. Wildlife and people can lose their homes, local sources of food, and even their lives.

WHAT ABOUT EUROPE?
This continent may be known for its rural scenery of gently rolling grassy fields and "patchwork" farms, but technically Europe is classified as temperate forest – despite much of it being cleared to create meadows or urban areas.

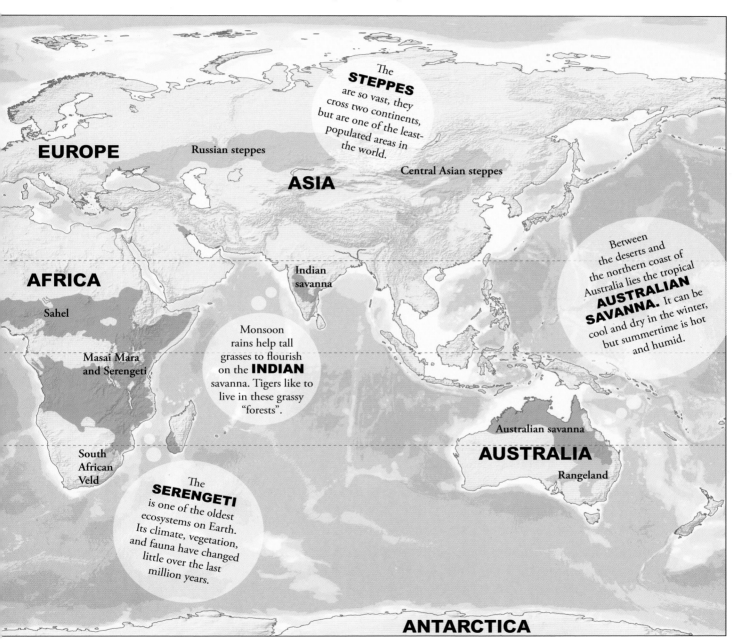

The **STEPPES** are so vast, they cross two continents, but are one of the least-populated areas in the world.

Russian steppes

Central Asian steppes

ASIA

EUROPE

AFRICA

Sahel

Masai Mara and Serengeti

Indian savanna

Between the deserts and the northern coast of Australia lies the tropical **AUSTRALIAN SAVANNA.** It can be cool and dry in the winter, but summertime is hot and humid.

Monsoon rains help tall grasses to flourish on the **INDIAN** savanna. Tigers like to live in these grassy "forests".

South African Veld

Australian savanna

AUSTRALIA

Rangeland

The **SERENGETI** is one of the oldest ecosystems on Earth. Its climate, vegetation, and fauna have changed little over the last million years.

ANTARCTICA

there are few places to hide from predators, so animals such as prairie dogs and voles dig burrows to shelter underground. Many non-burrowing herbivores, such as antelope, rely on speed to out-run carnivores. The grasses that form the basis of the herbivores' diets are varied too. Cows munch on short meadow grasses, but bison on the Great Plains prefer beardgrass, which grows to 3 m (10 ft) tall. Even this is small compared to another type of grass, a variety of bamboo that reaches 35 m (115 ft)!

prairie ecosystem

Temperate grasslands such as prairies occur in every continent except Antarctica. The Great Plains of North America are vast prairies covering around 3 million sq km (1.1 million sq miles). Here, enough rain falls to support grasses, but not trees. With nothing to interrupt air flow, the prairie is a windy place. It also has long, hot summers and cold winters. Many rodents and herbivores live on the Great Plains, and these animals are essential for maintaining the grassland ecosystem.

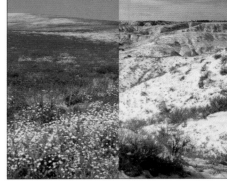

Temperate grasslands are subject to great variations in the weather as seasons change throughout the year. Summer's scorching heat is far removed from the cold winter snow.

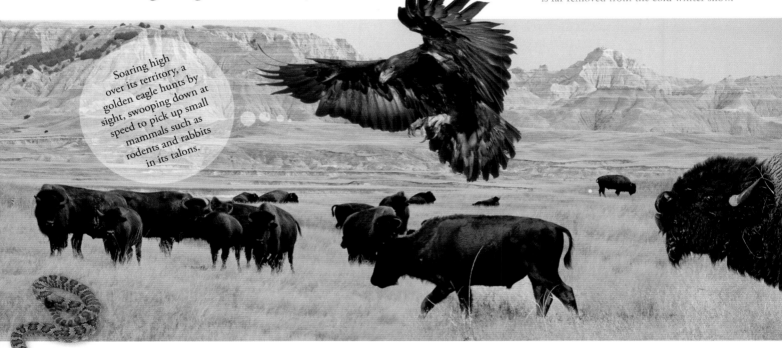

Soaring high over its territory, a golden eagle hunts by sight, swooping down at speed to pick up small mammals such as rodents and rabbits in its talons.

The tall and the short of it Because the Great Plains are so vast, the amount of rainfall they receive varies from place to place, and this difference shows in the vegetation. On the rainier eastern side are the tall grass prairies, where bluegrass stems can reach 2 m (6 ft) tall. In the drier west are short grass prairies, where bunch grass reaches 30–45 cm (12–18 in).

Same difference Temperate grasslands have different names and support very different plants and animals. In South America, they are called pampas; in South Africa, veld; and in south-east Australia, rangeland. Europe's extensive downs, meadows, and pastures were created hundreds of years ago by clearing temperate forest.

GREAT GRASSES

Just as there are different temperate grasslands, there are many varieties of grass too. Clumps of pampas grass, from South America, may reach 3 m (10 ft) tall. It can also survive fire.

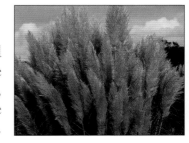

Short grass prairie food chain Both short grass and tall grass ecosystems are based on the vast amount of plant matter that is eaten by herbivores. Plants that are not eaten decompose when they die, which puts nutrients back into the soil.

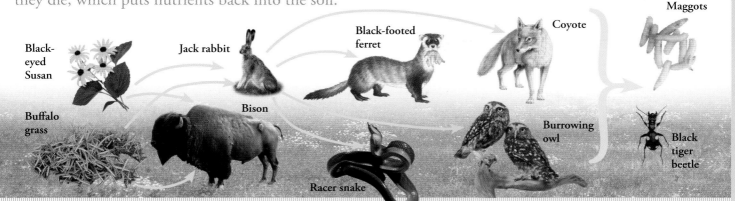

Black-eyed Susan · Buffalo grass · Jack rabbit · Bison · Black-footed ferret · Coyote · Maggots · Racer snake · Burrowing owl · Black tiger beetle

PRODUCERS
Grasses, with their small, green, wind-pollinated flowers, dominate the landscape. Other plants have bright flowers to attract insects.

PRIMARY CONSUMERS
Herbivores (plant eaters) are the leading animals on the prairie. They also help to maintain it.

SECONDARY CONSUMERS
The prairie carnivores feed on invertebrates such as crickets and smaller vertebrates, including jack rabbits. Wolves and other pack animals hunt together to tackle larger prey like deer. Coyotes will also eat carrion, so they scavenge for carcasses as well as hunt for prey.

DECOMPOSERS
All animals and plants eventually die and are broken down and eaten by organisms such as beetles and fly larvae.

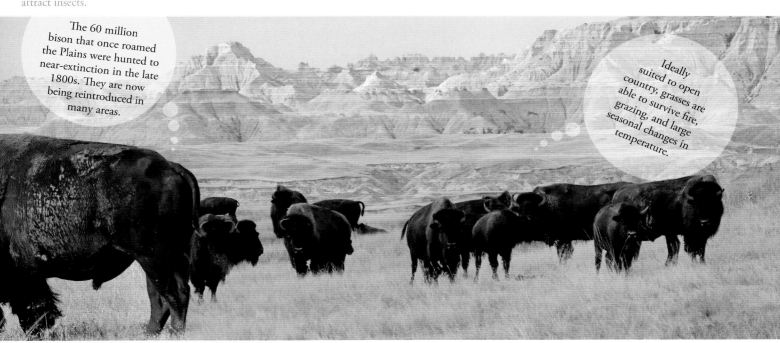

The 60 million bison that once roamed the Plains were hunted to near-extinction in the late 1800s. They are now being reintroduced in many areas.

Ideally suited to open country, grasses are able to survive fire, grazing, and large seasonal changes in temperature.

FLOWER POWER
Grasslands are so-called because the dominant plants are grasses. However, there are plenty of wild flowers growing on the prairie too, such as this coneflower.

PRAIRIE PLANT-EATERS
Mule deer are herbivores. They have broad, flat teeth for chewing plants, strong digestive systems to process grass – and long legs for fleeing from predators on the open prairie.

KEEPING SAFE
Animals have many ways to avoid being eaten. Brightly coloured butterflies are avoided by birds, which know they taste bad. Other animals may use camouflage colours.

NATURE'S GARDENERS
Burrowing animals, such as ground squirrels, are extremely important to the prairie. Their digging allows air into the soil, and also "weeds out" plants, allowing the grass to thrive.

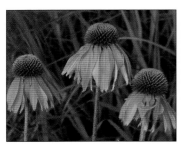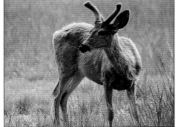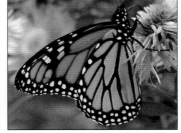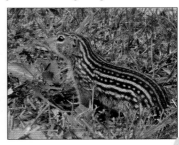

119

prairies under pressure

Across the world, temperate grasslands are disappearing. As much as **90 per cent** of the North American tall grass prairie has been lost, along with three-quarters of the South American pampas and one-fifth of the African veld. As people divide up the land for *farming* or to build on, it becomes impossible for large herbivores to move freely over it. These animals help to maintain the grassland, and the ecosystem **suffers** without them.

Look after your lawn – it's your very own "prairie"! Gardens are home to lots of wildlife. Keep a patch of grass long and see how many animals shelter there.

About 25% of all temperate grassland

Climate change Global warming is causing a problem for short grass prairies. Warmer nights encourage some plants to germinate early, but native grasses germinate late, by which time the weeds have taken over and can successfully compete for the resources the grass needs. As a result, grass is in decline.

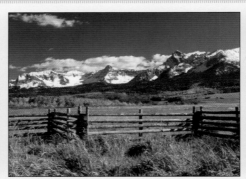

Fencing off When land is divided by fencing, it affects both hunter and prey. In Australia fences designed to keep dingoes off farmland also stop them reaching kangaroos. Without predators, the kangaroos increase in number. This puts more pressure on the land and leads to overgrazing.

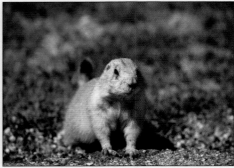

Pest control Prairie dogs are seen as pests: their burrows cause injury to cattle and horses, and they carry diseases. They have been killed in such large numbers that they now occupy only 2% of their original range, and prairie-based carnivores have lost an important food source.

The Dust Bowl The roots of grasses are vital to keeping soil stable and preventing erosion. The Dust Bowl was created between 1930 and 1939 because farmers cleared prairie land for crops. Left exposed to the wind and dried out by drought, the topsoil simply blew away. Huge dust storms swept the land, no crops could grow, and famine was rife. It was a harsh lesson to learn about land clearance, yet the practice still continues.

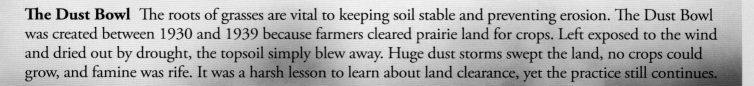

The Dust Bowl occurred in the southern and central Great Plains, in the American states of Texas, Oklahoma, Kansas, Colorado, and New Mexico. Further droughts struck farms here in the 1950s, 1970s, and as recently as 2004.

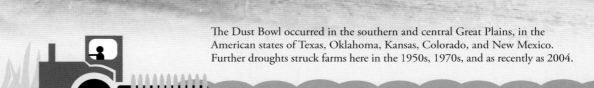

has been lost to urban development.

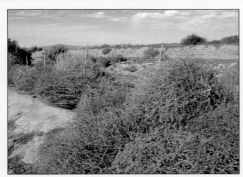

Tough tumbleweed
Introducing alien species to the prairies has altered the balance of plants. Tumbleweed was brought in from Russia to South Dakota in 1877. By 1900, it had taken over whole areas of the west coast, choking out the native vegetation.

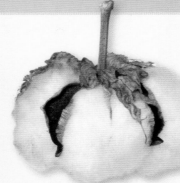

Monoculture Converting temperate grassland to agriculture has destroyed the natural variety of vegetation, replacing it with vast amounts of cotton or wheat. The crops are harvested for sale, so no nutrients can return from the plants to the soil to keep it fertile.

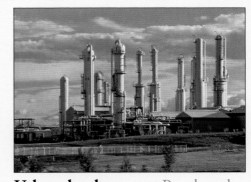

Urban development People today tend to live settled lives and as a result build permanent homes, along with roads, schools, shops, and power stations. Grasslands are easy to build on and have few physical features such as mountains to prevent settlements growing and creating urban sprawl.

super grass

WHAT MAKES THE SMALL, UNASSUMING, LEAFY LAWN PLANT SUCH A SURVIVOR?

Of the thousands of grass species, including cereals, bamboo, and sugar cane, perhaps the most familiar to us are the short grasses found in fields and gardens. These grasses are so common and widespread because, in the natural course of events, they're almost indestructible. Unlike most plants, grass grows from near its base, which is close to the ground – sometimes below the surface – so if the top is mown, eaten, or even burned by wildfire, it won't kill the plant. Small, flexible leaves bounce back even after heavy hooves trample on them, and wind can gust over the leaves without causing damage, which is why grass can survive on windy, treeless plains where taller plants would be too battered by wind to remain upright. Grasses can survive many natural phenomena from grazing to periods of drought – but they often fall victim to human activity.

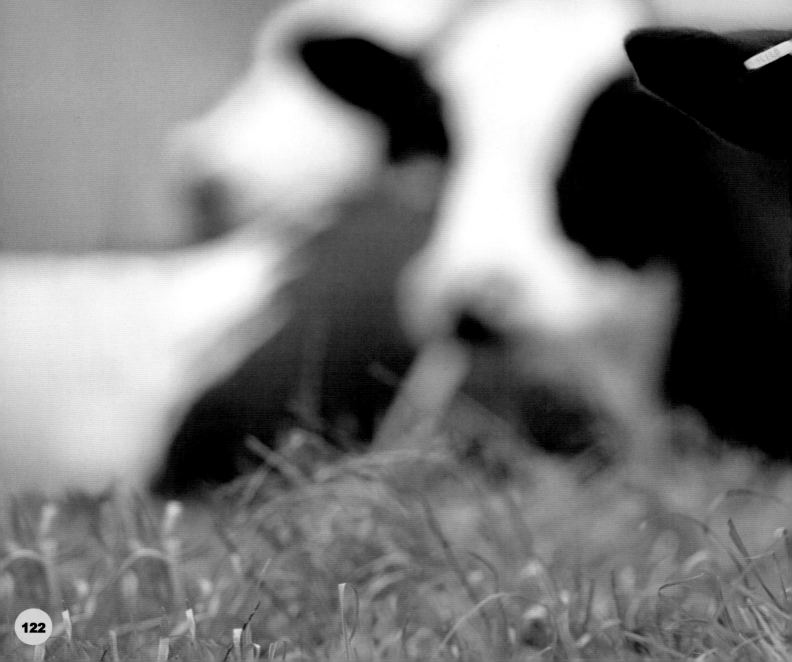

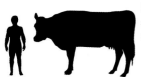

Domestic sheep are ruminants.

Ruminant animals chew the cud to break down the grass they eat. After quickly swallowing a lot of grass, they lie down to rest, "burp" the grass (or cud) back up, and chew it into a pulp.

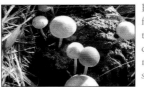

Ruminants don't just take from the grass, they give back too. As their dung is broken down by fungi, nutrients are released into the soil, which supports grass regrowth.

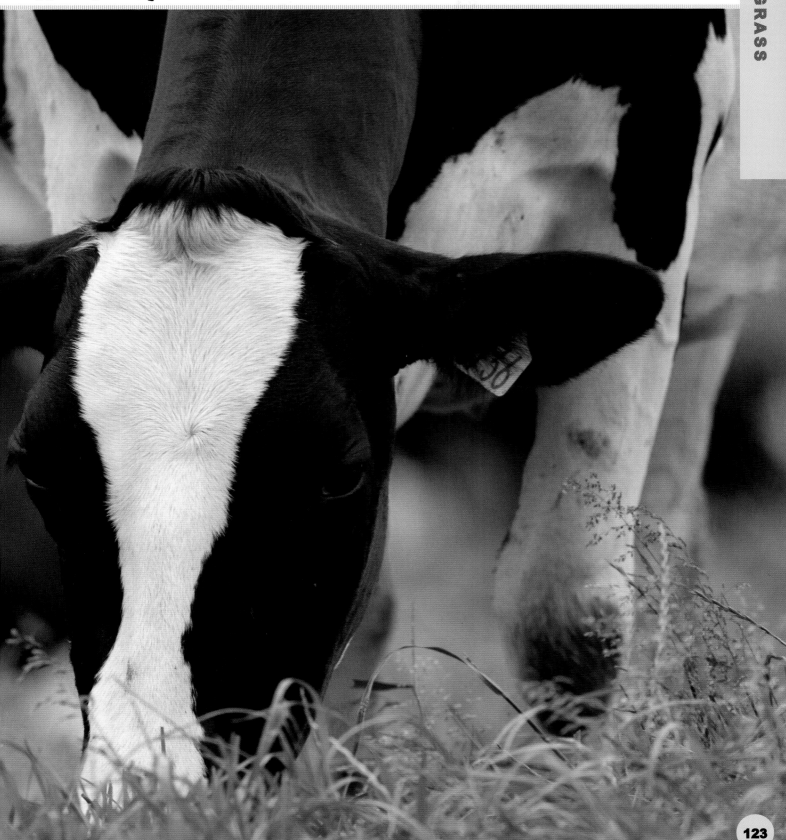

savanna ecosystem

About 40% of tropical land is covered by savanna. These grasslands are hot all year round, but have distinct wet and dry seasons. When rain falls, it is torrential and often accompanied by lightning, which causes many grassland fires. Annual rainfall ranges from 45 cm (18 in) in Australia to more than 1.2 m (50 in) in East Africa. The wetter savanna ecosystems have trees, making the habitat more diverse and supporting a greater variety of wildlife.

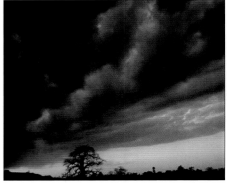

Thick black clouds are the warning sign that comes ahead of a monsoon – the heavy storms that are typical of the savanna wet season. If enough rain falls, trees will be able to grow.

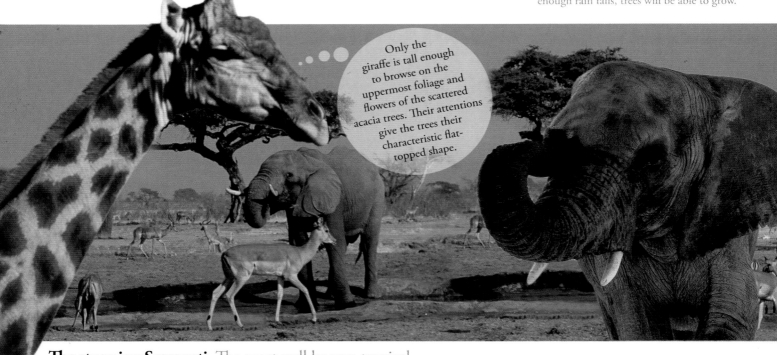

Only the giraffe is tall enough to browse on the uppermost foliage and flowers of the scattered acacia trees. Their attentions give the trees their characteristic flat-topped shape.

The stunning Serengeti The most well known tropical savanna ecosystem is also one of the oldest. The Serengeti is home to a variety of ungulates, or hoofed mammals, some of which occur in vast numbers. Gazelles, zebras, and wildebeest eat different parts of the grasses, and so do not need to compete for food.

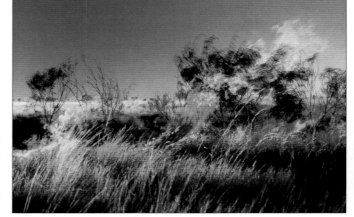

FIRE!

Seasonal fires play a vital role in maintaining savanna. The flames burn off dead plant material, creating ash that washes down into the soil and fertilizes it. After a fire, the landscape quickly recovers. Grass grows fast, more than 2.5 cm (1 in) a day, and soon the large grazing animals that fled the flames can return to feed.

Savanna predators The big cats and dogs of the savanna are expert killing machines. Some live and hunt alone, while others work together to share the work and the reward. There are some predators that supplement hunting with scavenging too.

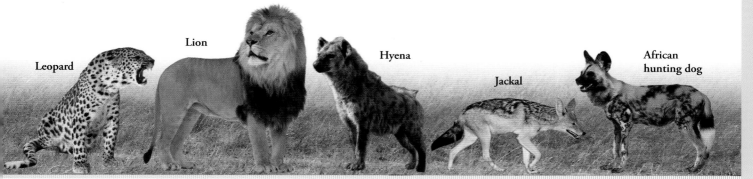

Leopard

Lion

Hyena

Jackal

African hunting dog

LEOPARD

A solitary hunter, the leopard avoids losing its prey to other carnivores by carrying it up into a tree.

LION

Within a lion pride, it is the lionesses that do the hunting. After a kill, the males arrive and take control of the prey. Cubs feed last.

HYENA

The powerful jaws of the hyena make it a formidable hunter as well as a scavenger. It chases its prey to exhaustion and then moves in for the kill.

JACKAL

An opportunist that hunts or scavenges for meat, but also eats fruit and berries, the black backed jackal will eat anything it can catch.

AFRICAN HUNTING DOG

By hunting in a group, African hunting dogs can tackle much larger animals than one dog could attack alone.

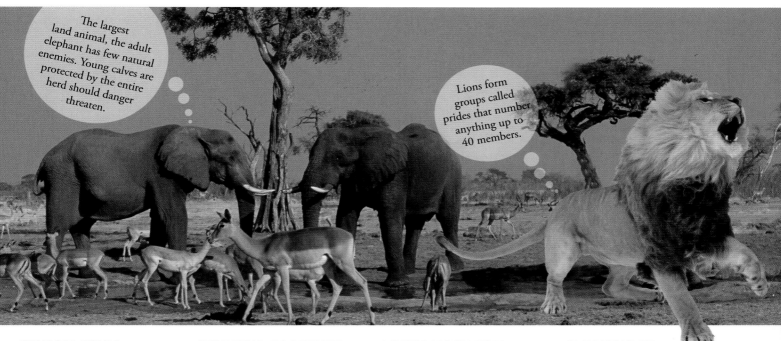

The largest land animal, the adult elephant has few natural enemies. Young calves are protected by the entire herd should danger threaten.

Lions form groups called prides that number anything up to 40 members.

WEAVER BIRDS

Male weaver birds construct elaborate nests out of grass and leaves. Many nests have the entrance at the bottom as a protection from predatory snakes.

WORKING TOGETHER

Oxpeckers are tolerated by animals because they remove irritating ticks, which the birds eat. But they also feed on blood, and have been known to keep their hosts' wounds bleeding.

LIVING TOGETHER

Stinging ants live in the hollowed out thorns of the acacia tree. In return for this safe home, they will emerge and attack any animal that tries to eat the acacia's leaves.

CLEANING UP

Without dung beetles, savannas would disappear under a mountain of animal droppings. They help recycle nutrients by moulding dung into balls and rolling it underground.

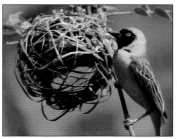

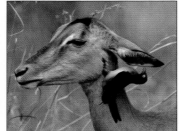

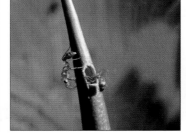

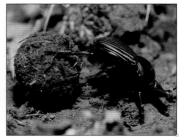

struggling **savannas**

Savannas are vital to keeping Earth's climate stable. They convert as much, if not more, *carbon dioxide* into carbohydrates as **tropical rainforests** do, but they receive far less attention. Losing grassland could eventually have the same effect on global temperatures as felling forests, yet **vast tracts** of tropical grassland are lost each year to agriculture and urban development.

Plants absorb carbon dioxide and turn it into carbohydrates such as glucose for food.

There is a lot of oxygen left over, which is released back into the air.

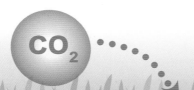

CO_2

O_2

Destroying tropical grasslands could

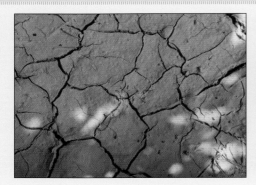

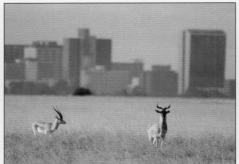

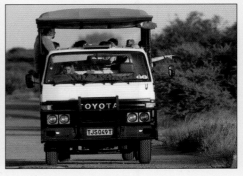

Drying out Global warming may pose a threat to the dry grassland habitat: as temperatures increase, the land could dry out and turn into semi-arid or desert landscape. Clearing grassland makes the problem worse, because it leads to soil erosion, which encourages desertification.

Taking over The human population is growing faster than ever. Everyone needs food and a place to live, but this puts increasing pressure on savanna areas. Cities expand onto some grasslands, while others are cleared for crops. Less and less remains for the savanna wildlife.

Tourism Safaris and other forms of tourism bring in much needed money to poor countries, but it comes at a price as hotels degrade the landscape and increase pollution. Also, animals are developing behavioural problems due to stress from being observed for long periods.

Essential elephants The elephant is a "keystone species", which means it plays a vital part in maintaining its particular habitat. Savanna would eventually turn into scrub if it were not for the elephant, which eats woody vegetation and pushes down trees to gain access to the higher branches. But the elephant is a threatened species.

Don't buy items made of ivory, elephant hair, or elephant skin: no matter how small the object is, an elephant still had to die for it to be made.

POACHING

One of the biggest threats to elephants is poaching. Between 1979 and 1989, 600,000 African elephants were killed for their tusks, halving the population in just 10 years.

CONSERVATION

People pose a threat to both the elephant and its habitat. One of the best ways of conserving elephants is to involve local people and convince them of their worth.

LOSS OF LAND

Elephants roam large distances to feed, but their habitat is shrinking as savanna is built upon or turned into farmland. These developments divide up the remaining savanna, cutting through the elephants' ranges.

RAMPAGING

Elephants may wander on to farmland, where they eat and trample crops. This brings them into conflict with local farmers often with fatal consequences for both sides.

CO_2 .... O_2

be as devastating as felling rainforests.

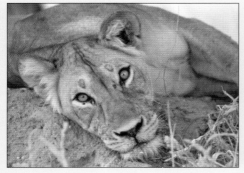

An unfair target The large animals of Africa also attract a different kind of tourist: hunters that kill for sport. The number of African countries offering shooting licences is increasing. The argument for doing this is that it raises money to fund conservation.

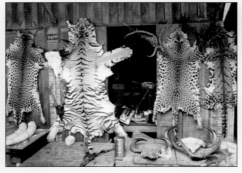

Poaching Although many animals are protected by law, the continuing demand for them leads to poaching. Tigers are killed for their bones and skins, rhinos for their horns, and elephants for their ivory. Some animals are literally worth their weight in gold.

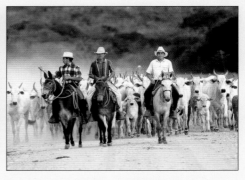

Cattle ranching Many areas of tropical grassland are being used for ranching. Seventy per cent of the llanos, in South America, has been lost over the last 40 years: besides crops, there are now about 15 million cattle there. Very little of the llanos is protected and so the ranching continues to expand.

the wildebeest

FOLLOWING THE MASS MIGRATION OF THE HERBIVORES IN THEIR CONTINUAL SEARCH FOR GRASS SHOOTS

Every year, about one and a half million wildebeest migrate a distance of 1,800 km (1,120 miles) to find food. Wildebeest feed on fresh grass shoots, and spend much of the year moving around to find them. The animals live in the Serengeti during the wet season, from December to March; but come the dry season there is not enough fresh water for them to drink or for new grass shoots to grow, so they must move on. The herds head north to Lake Victoria and then onto the Masai Mara. They spend the dry season that lasts from July to October in the Masai Mara, where occasional rainstorms provide enough moisture for the grass to grow. However, this grass lacks nutrients, so as the wet season commences the herds return south once more to eat the phosphorus-rich grass of the Serengeti.

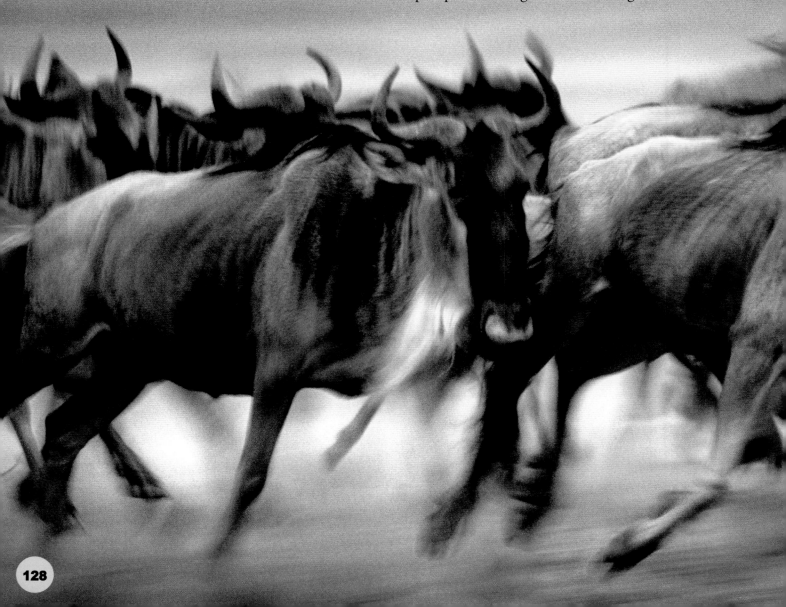

The Serengeti, Lake Victoria, and Masai Mara are all in East Africa. It takes about 3 months to migrate between each place.

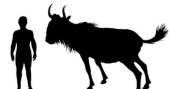

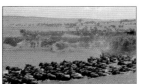

The long migration is not without dangers. Many wildebeest slip down steep riverbanks and drown; others are killed crossing the crocodile-infested waters. Hyenas and jackals are also ready to attack the weak and young.

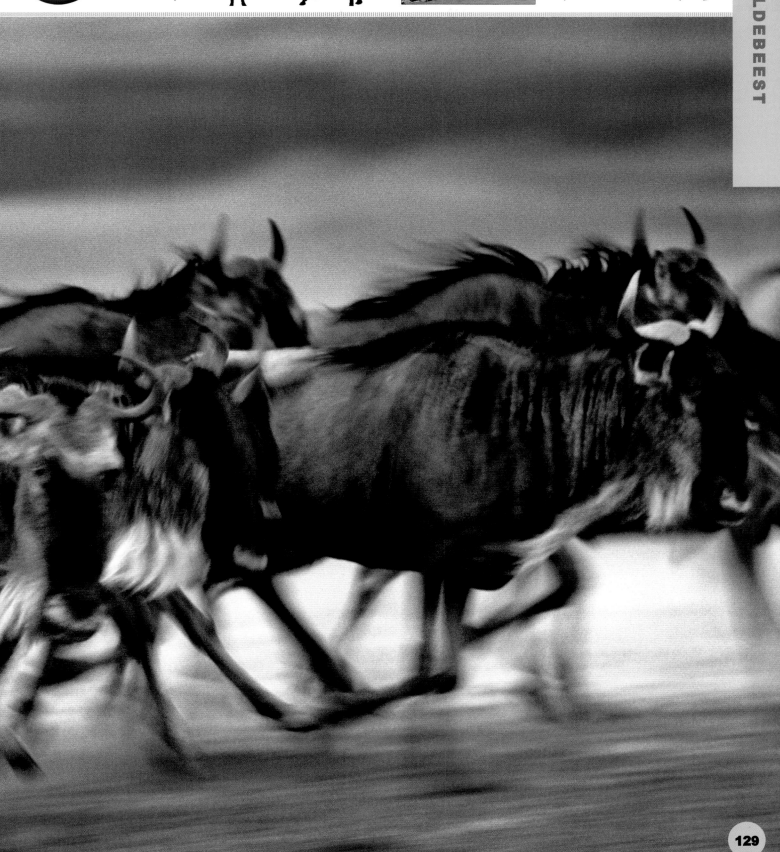

farmland ecosystem

Farmland is not a natural landscape. All land that is used for farming has been converted from another ecosystem, such as prairie, forest, or even desert. Agriculture can change thick woodland to a patchwork of fields that look like they have existed forever – but it's all made by people. In taking over, farming replaces the wild plants and animals with ones that people can control. Most agriculture today is "settled", meaning the soil is fertile enough to support permanent farms.

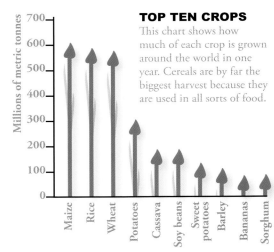

TOP TEN CROPS
This chart shows how much of each crop is grown around the world in one year. Cereals are by far the biggest harvest because they are used in all sorts of food.

Millions of metric tonnes — Maize, Rice, Wheat, Potatoes, Cassava, Soy beans, Sweet potatoes, Barley, Bananas, Sorghum

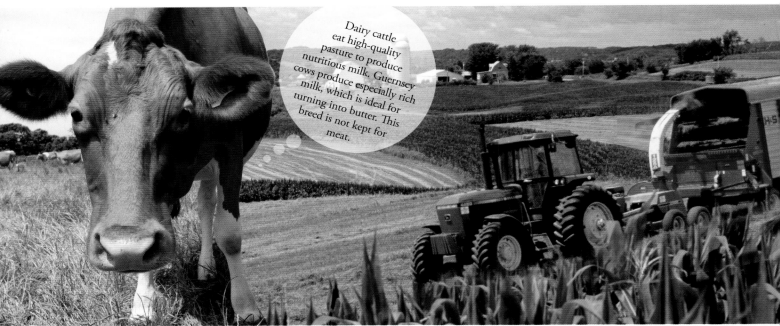

Dairy cattle eat high-quality pasture to produce nutritious milk. Guernsey cows produce especially rich milk, which is ideal for turning into butter. This breed is not kept for meat.

What's growing? Farmland is used for growing crops (arable agriculture) or raising livestock (pastoralism). While the majority of the world's farmland is arable, many farms are mixed, so if harvests are bad the farmer has income from the livestock, and vice versa.

Plantations are large-scale intensive arable farms. Crops such as tea and bananas are grown on trees and bushes, usually for export.

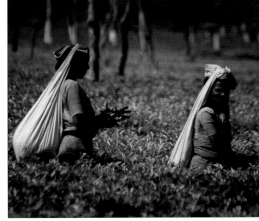

Intensive or extensive?
Farming practices depend on how much land and money are available. Intensive farming puts a lot of work into a small area of land in order to get a good yield. With extensive farming, the same amount of work is spread out over much more land.

Cereal provider Over half the world's food comes from just three sources: maize, rice, and wheat. Like all cereals, these familiar dinner-table crops are actually grasses. The original wild plants were cultivated to produce edible grains.

MAIZE
Also called corn, maize is native to central America. Cultivated maize is totally different to wild maize, which has few, very tough and inedible kernels.

RYE
A close relative of wheat, rye grains are mostly made into flour for bread and crackers. The stalks are also made into corn dollies!

OATS
The most familiar form of oats is as breakfast cereal, including porridge and muesli. Horses and cattle eat crushed raw oats as a main part of their diet.

WHEAT
To get to the edible grain inside the husk, wheat must be winnowed, which is traditionally done by tossing wheat into the air.

RICE
This plant originally comes from Asia and Africa, and today it is the staple food of Asia. Rice is the only crop that can be grown in flooded fields.

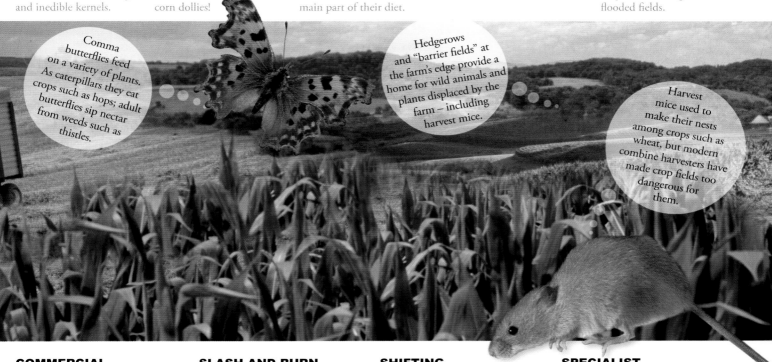

Comma butterflies feed on a variety of plants. As caterpillars they eat crops such as hops; adult butterflies sip nectar from weeds such as thistles.

Hedgerows and "barrier fields" at the farm's edge provide a home for wild animals and plants displaced by the farm – including harvest mice.

Harvest mice used to make their nests among crops such as wheat, but modern combine harvesters have made crop fields too dangerous for them.

COMMERCIAL
Most farms are commercial, with farmers growing crops or raising animals for sale. The biggest are sheep farms, cattle ranches, and those growing cereals.

SLASH AND BURN
A quarter of the world's population relies on slash-and-burn agriculture, where forests are cleared to make room for crops. When the soil gets exhausted, another area will be felled.

SHIFTING
Also called nomadic, shifting farmers keep on the move so their herds can find enough food to eat. This farming occurs where the land isn't fertile enough to support settled farms.

SPECIALIST
Plantations and other farms that focus on one type of produce are specialist. The crop may be dependent on the area's soil and climate: Mediterranean farms are ideal for olives and vines.

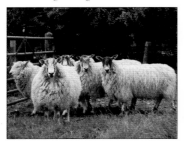

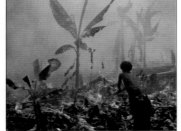

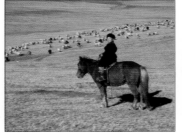

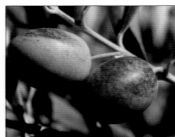

aggressive agriculture

There are **2 million** species of wild animals and plants in the world, but fewer than 30 kinds of animals and 200 kinds of plants found on farms. In order to get the most out of the farms, there are many agricultural practices that affect the environment. As *valuable* sources of food or materials, the domesticated species are given everything they need to grow, and any competition for resources is soon **got rid of**: plants are ploughed up or cut down; animals are fenced off the land; and both may be **poisoned**.

BE AWARE of food miles – know where

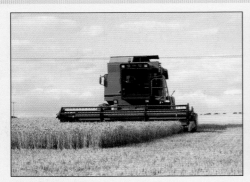

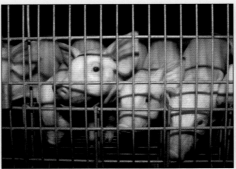

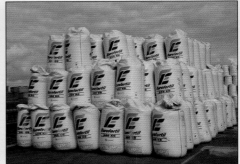

Mechanization Tractors and combine harvesters can process crops more efficiently than a team of people by hand. But machines are large, and fields need to be big enough to accommodate them. Expanding fields destroys hedgerows that provide a safe corridor and a home for wildlife.

Factory farming It is unnatural to force animals to produce lots of meat, milk, or eggs rapidly or to breed every season, but factory farming does just that. Packed into pens with little room to exercise, piglets are fed concentrates and hormones to fatten them up fast so they can be taken to market sooner.

Chemical treatments Pesticides are used to kill bugs that eat crops, but they also kill other wildlife, and pass into the food chain. Fertilizers help crops grow in fields, but when rain washes the fertilizer into rivers, plants spring to life in the water too, choking the river and the wildlife within it.

Chain reaction Land converted from forests and prairies to farmland is not just ideal for fields – it's also a clear, accessible place to build new communities to cope with a growing population. But these extra people need food too, and if housing estates are built on farmland, where will the food come from? More farms will need to be created, and more prairies and forests will be lost.

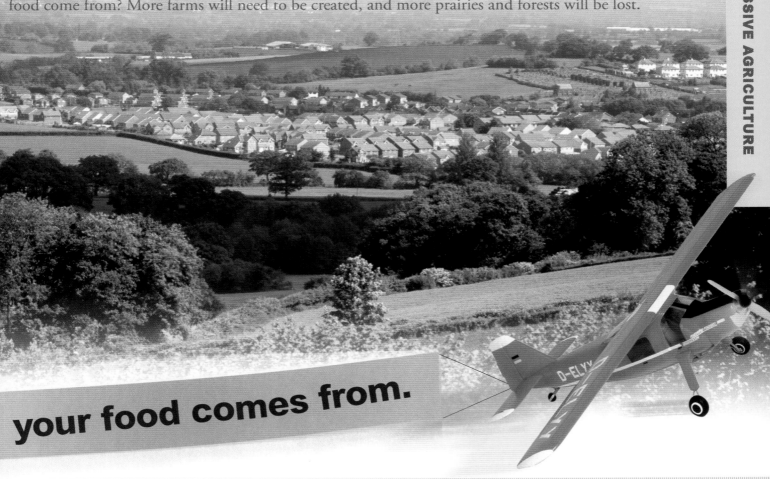

your food comes from.

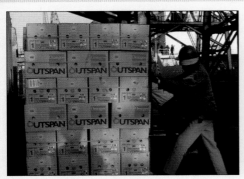

Food miles Importing food such as fruit and vegetables by plane or boat creates pollution. Transporting livestock is also distressing for the animals.

 Look for the "country of origin" label on food. Was your apple grown locally, or has it been flown across the world?

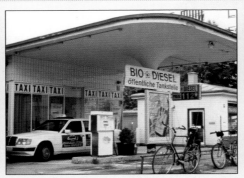

Biofuel There's currently a big demand for "biofuel" – fuel that comes from plant sources rather than minerals such as oil. As fields are given over to rape or soya crops that provide this fuel, there's less land for growing food. So more fields need to be created, taking land from other ecosystems.

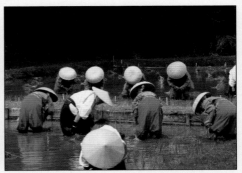

Methane Rice fields, or paddies, are flooded for four months a year. During this time, rice stems rot in the water and release methane into the air. It is thought that wet paddies are the largest man-made source of methane, which is a greenhouse gas that contributes to global warming.

controversial crops

People have always tried to *improve* the food they grow. In the past this was done by taking seeds from only the best plants so that the next year's crops would inherit good qualities. Those that were too small or tasteless or prone to disease wouldn't be used for seeds. **Genetic modification** is different. Scientists alter the actual genes of a plant, perhaps to make them toxic to insects or herbicide-resistant.

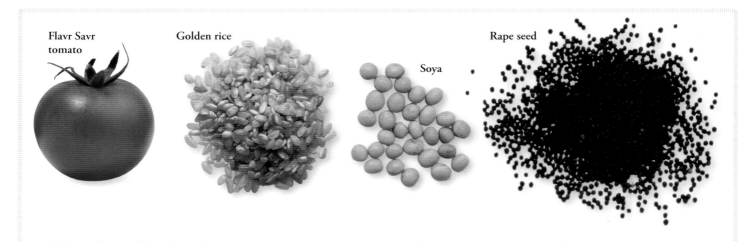

Flavr Savr tomato

Golden rice

Soya

Rape seed

GM gallery The first GM crop grown for sale was the Flavr Savr tomato, made to be resistant to rot so it kept fresh in shops for longer. Today the most widely-grown GM crops are oilseed rape, used in cooking oil and biofuels, and soya, used in lots of processed foods and animal feed. These crops were modified to help the farmer grow them more efficiently, but other crop modifications may be aimed at the consumer: Golden rice has added Vitamin A to boost the diet of people in poor countries.

GM is still quite new – no one can say if

FOR GM

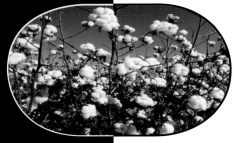

LESS PESTICIDE

"Bt cotton" has been modified to be toxic to bollworms, pests that eat the plant. Now the farmer doesn't have to spray pesticide over the crops to kill the destructive bollworm caterpillars.

BUT...

Over time, bollworms could evolve to have resistance to the toxin, which may also damage beneficial insects, such as the monarch butterfly. The farmer may have to spray pesticides to deal with other pests anyway.

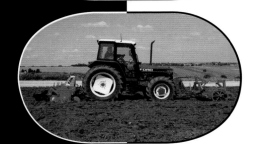

HERBICIDE-RESISTANT CROPS

Fields can be sprayed with very effective herbicides that kill everything but the crop. Without weeds competing for sunlight, water, and nutrients, crop yields will be higher.

BUT...

Growing herbicide-resistant crops is bad for other farmland wildlife. Weeds and their seeds provide vital food for insects and birds. If the food disappears, there will be fewer animals, and this will upset the whole food chain.

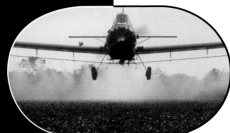

A VARIETY OF FARMS

GM crops can be grown alongside other types of crop and there is no evidence to date that they damage the environment directly.

BUT...

Pollen from GM crops can spread their modified genes into other crops and wild plants. Organic farmers nearby cannot guarantee their food is free from GM genes, so they lose their organic status.

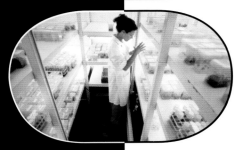

TACKLING CLIMATE CHANGE

Crops can be engineered to cope with harsh, dry, or salty conditions created by climate change, or to increase the health benefits of food to improve the diets of people living in poor countries.

BUT...

Companies that develop GM seeds focus on varieties that will make them the best profit. They are unlikely to help poor farmers in marginal areas.

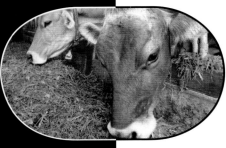

SAFE FOR ANIMALS

Cows, chickens, and pigs are already eating large quantities of GM produce without showing any ill effects. Much of their feed is made from GM soya, which is cheaper to grow than non-GM.

BUT...

We don't know if people will suffer ill effects in the long-term from eating GM foods, either directly or through eating produce from animals fed on GM. Non-GM foods have been proven over centuries to be safe.

it will lead to problems in the future.

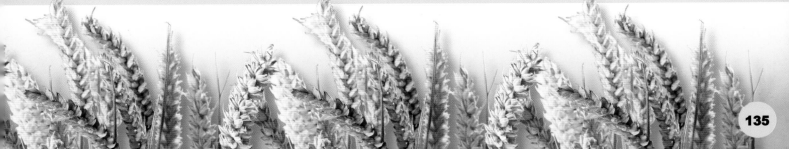

MAKING A DIFFERENCE

How does your GARDEN grow?

★ **Lawns are grasslands too** and it's important not to replace them with paving or tarmac. Avoid using herbicide on the grass so wildflowers can grow and attract wildlife.

★ **Keep a patch of grass long** and watch the wildlife take shelter. You might see insects, birds, frogs, hedgehogs, and even badgers.

★ **Make a compost heap** and use the compost to fertilize flower beds. It's the ultimate in efficient recycling!

Feed your compost with fruit and vegetable peelings, used teabags, and lawn clippings.

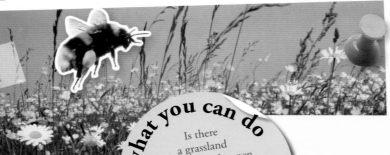

Wild flowers love long lawns

what you can do

Is there a grassland (such as a park, open space, or Green Belt land) in your area that's under threat? Start or join a campaign to protect it.

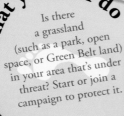

Dear Mrs Smith, MP

I have seen in my local newspaper that developers want to build houses on an area of Green Belt grassland. I am writing to ask that you do not let this happen.

Grassland needs to be protected. Some species of animals and plants will die out if this land is lost, and people will also lose their breathing spaces outside of town.

Grass also helps to combat global warming because it helps to absorb CO_2. If grasslands are destroyed, we lose this benefit, and the problem is made worse because the new houses would create even more pollution. Please preserve our natural open spaces.

Yours sincerely

Sam Green

Write a letter

Write a letter to your Member of Parliament to show that you care!

From providing animals with homes and food to helping combat global warming, grasslands are the planet's unsung heroes.

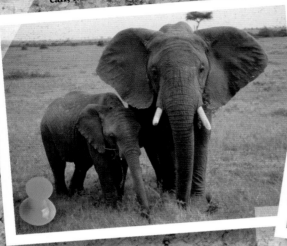

African elephant mother and calf, Masai Mara, Africa

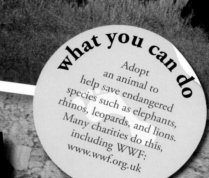

what you can do

Adopt an animal to help save endangered species such as elephants, rhinos, leopards, and lions. Many charities do this, including WWF: www.wwf.org.uk

Black rhino mother and calf, Tanzania, Africa

what you can do

Think about where you buy your food. Support local shops and cut down on pollution by walking or taking the bus rather than the car.

KNOW THE DEBATE:

local food

- **Local food never has to travel very far,** so it doesn't use much energy in transport. This helps cut down on pollution.
- Because it takes less time to get from field to shop, **local food is likely to be fresher,** and so there is less need for large amounts of refrigeration or packaging to protect it, which take a lot of energy to produce.
- Buying locally **supports your local economy and provides jobs for local farmers.**
- Local food helps you learn about **where your food comes from and what your own country can produce.**
- **BUT local food may be produced using environmentally polluting farming methods,** such as herbicides, pesticides, and fertilizers.

organic food

- Grown in harmony with the environment, organic food has **no pesticides, herbicides, or other chemical fertilizers.**
- **These chemicals take a lot of energy to manufacture.** By not using them, organic farming uses a lot less energy overall than conventional food production.
- **Organic farms support more birds, mammals, insects, and wild flowers.**
- **Organic farms are kinder to their animals** – cows are cared for, pigs are not packed into pens, and chickens are uncaged. They are never given hormones or unnecessary drugs to boost production.
- **BUT not many farms produce organic food, so it often has to be imported from far-away countries to meet demand. This creates extra "food miles", and increases carbon emissions.**

TROPICAL FORESTS

Tropical **forests** grow near the *Equator.* The constant **heat** and high rainfall helps *trees* grow tall.

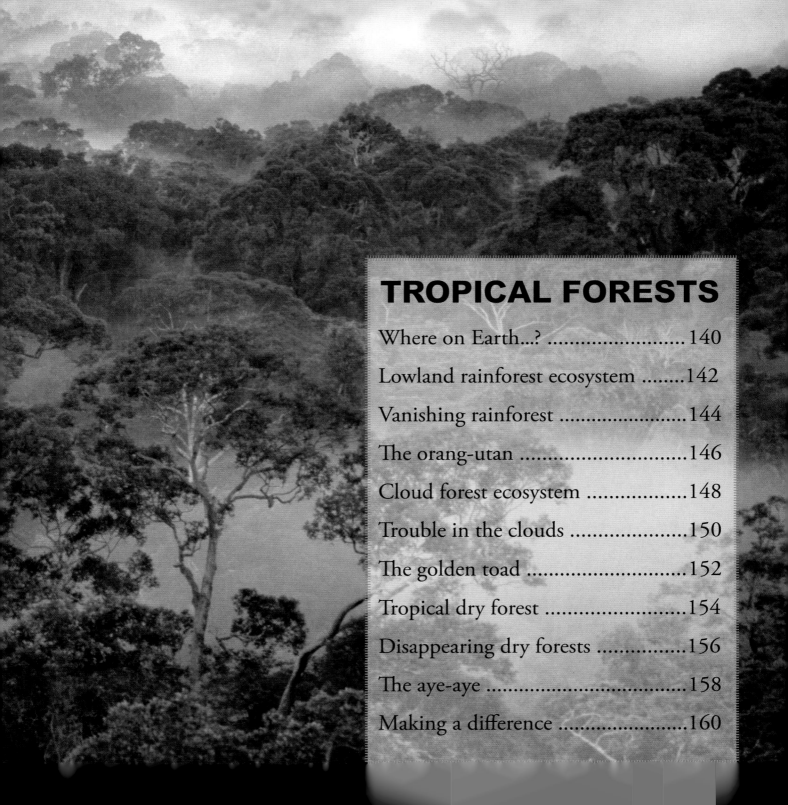

Some forests have rain all year. Some are only wet for part of the year. Others get the moisture they need from clouds. They are all shrinking, as humans cut them down for timber, or to open up the land beneath the trees. Changing climate could cause even more problems.

TROPICAL FORESTS

where on earth...?

Tropical forests grow throughout the tropical zone close to the Equator, wherever it is wet enough for trees to grow (savanna grasslands or deserts are found in drier areas). The type of forest depends on how much it rains and how often.

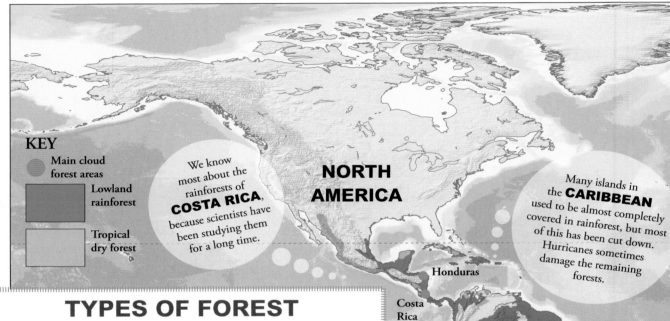

KEY

- Main cloud forest areas
- Lowland rainforest
- Tropical dry forest

We know most about the rainforests of **COSTA RICA**, because scientists have been studying them for a long time.

NORTH AMERICA

Many islands in the **CARIBBEAN** used to be almost completely covered in rainforest, but most of this has been cut down. Hurricanes sometimes damage the remaining forests.

Honduras

Costa Rica

Equator

Amazon rainforest

SOUTH AMERICA

Tropic of Capricorn

Atlantic cloud forest

The **AMAZON** rainforest is the largest in the world. It covers an area just a little smaller than Australia.

TYPES OF FOREST

● **LOWLAND RAINFOREST**

These forests grow in low-lying areas where lots of rain falls in every month of the year. They get at least 180 cm (70 in) of rain in a year. The hot, wet conditions are perfect for plants to grow, and many animals enjoy the rich food supply.

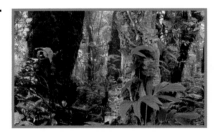

● **CLOUD FOREST**

These rainforests are up in the mountains where conditions are cooler. Where winds off the sea meet high mountains, dense clouds form. The trees in the cloud forest get the moisture they need from these clouds, as well as from rain.

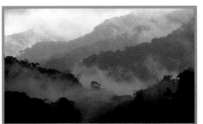

● **TROPICAL DRY**

These forests grow in parts of the tropics where a little less rain falls. In parts of Asia, heavy rain falls during the monsoon season. The rest of the year is much drier. Here the trees lose their leaves during the dry season.

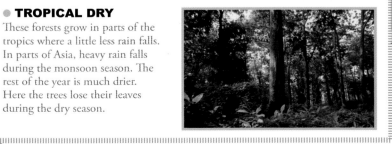

Rainforests are the richest places on Earth for plants and animals. Trees grow well and their leaves and fruits provide plentiful food. However, plants cannot grow if their leaves are eaten as soon as they appear, so many

WHERE'S THE JUNGLE?

Rainforests and other tropical forests are sometimes called jungles, but thick "walls" of plants only appear along the riverbanks. Inside, the forest can be quite open.

ALWAYS SUMMER

In rainforests and cloud forests, it is warm and wet all year. In these conditions plants can grow and produce fruits and flowers right through the year. This ensures a constant supply of food for animals.

LOSING THEIR LEAVES

In monsoon forests, the trees only produce flowers and fruit in the wet season. When the dry season comes, most trees shed their leaves to stop them losing water.

AIR FRESHENER

The many trees and other plants of the tropical forests give out huge amounts of oxygen. All animals rely on oxygen to live and these forests have been described as the "lungs of the world".

VANISHING FORESTS

Many tropical forests produce valuable timber, so people cut them down. In the future, more rainforests will die if climate change leads to less rain falling on them.

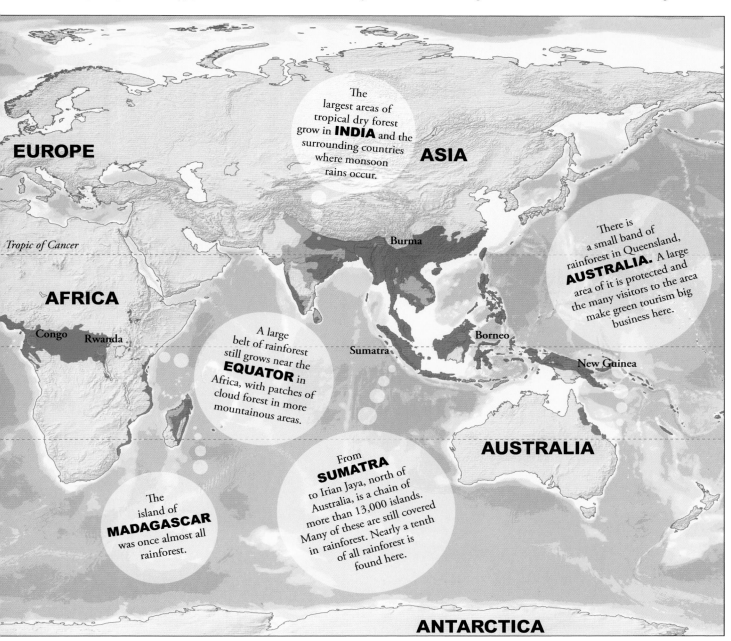

EUROPE

ASIA

The largest areas of tropical dry forest grow in **INDIA** and the surrounding countries where monsoon rains occur.

Tropic of Cancer

Burma

There is a small band of rainforest in Queensland, **AUSTRALIA.** A large area of it is protected and the many visitors to the area make green tourism big business here.

AFRICA

Congo   Rwanda

A large belt of rainforest still grows near the **EQUATOR** in Africa, with patches of cloud forest in more mountainous areas.

Sumatra

Borneo

New Guinea

AUSTRALIA

The island of **MADAGASCAR** was once almost all rainforest.

From **SUMATRA** to Irian Jaya, north of Australia, is a chain of more than 13,000 islands. Many of these are still covered in rainforest. Nearly a tenth of all rainforest is found here.

ANTARCTICA

rainforest plants have leaves containing nasty chemicals to stop animals eating them. Some animals have developed clever means of getting round these defences – and to stop other animals eating them! Over thousands of years, this constant battle to eat or be eaten has made plants and animals change, as they have found new ways to live. Many changed so much they became new species. This battle for life is why so many different kinds of plants and animals are found here.

lowland rainforest

Lowland rainforest is the largest tropical rainforest ecosystem. It is hot all year round and more than 180 cm (70 in) of rain falls during the year. In the warm, wet climate trees grow very tall. The forest forms three layers – an evergreen canopy in the middle, a layer of smaller plants on the forest floor, and scattered taller trees towering above the canopy.

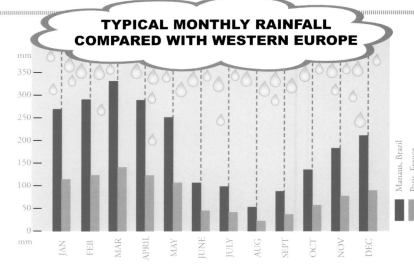

TYPICAL MONTHLY RAINFALL COMPARED WITH WESTERN EUROPE

Manaus, Brazil
Paris, France

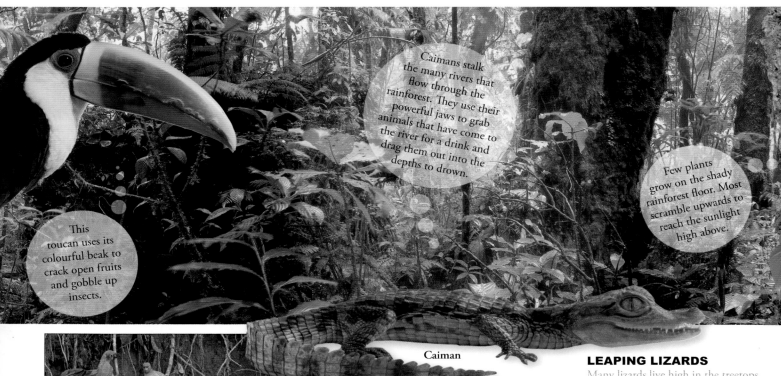

This toucan uses its colourful beak to crack open fruits and gobble up insects.

Caimans stalk the many rivers that flow through the rainforest. They use their powerful jaws to grab animals that have come to the river for a drink and drag them out into the depths to drown.

Few plants grow on the shady rainforest floor. Most scramble upwards to reach the sunlight high above.

Caiman

Chemical warfare With so many grazing animals around, many trees have developed poisons in their leaves to stop animals from eating them. However, some animals, like these mealy parrots, get round this by eating clay from riverbanks. The clay lines their stomach and absorbs the poisons from the leaves.

LEAPING LIZARDS
Many lizards live high in the treetops and some of them have flaps of skin along their body. They can spread these out to glide from tree to tree.

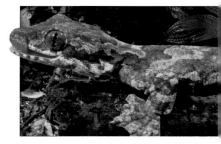

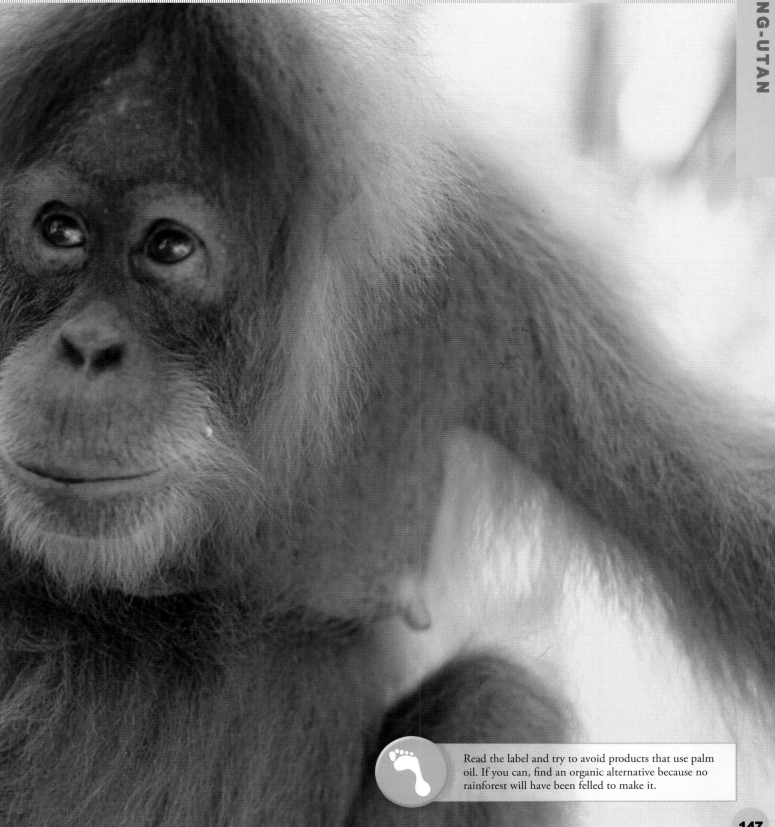

Orang-utans live in rainforests on the islands of Sumatra and Borneo. Scientists think these are two different species.

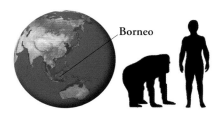

Borneo

Since 1980, large parts of the forests where orang-utans live have been felled by people in order to plant oil palms. Oil from the fruits of these palm trees is used to make many popular goods such as ice cream, chocolate, crisps, biscuits, margarine, toothpaste, soap, and cosmetics.

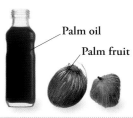

Palm oil

Palm fruit

Read the label and try to avoid products that use palm oil. If you can, find an organic alternative because no rainforest will have been felled to make it.

cloud forest ecosystem

Cloud forest is a form of rainforest that grows between 2,000 and 3,500 m (6,500–11,500 ft) up in tropical mountains. Winds full of moisture from the sea are forced upwards when they hit the mountains. As it is cooler higher up, moisture comes out of the air to form clouds. The clouds make the forest dripping wet, even when it is not raining, but they also hide the Sun.

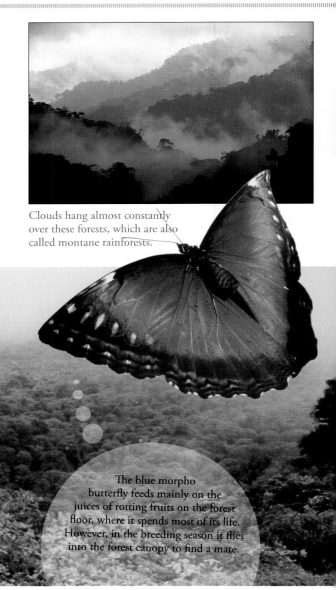

Clouds hang almost constantly over these forests, which are also called montane rainforests.

The emerald toucanet uses its large bill to dig holes in trees for its nest and to eat berries.

The blue morpho butterfly feeds mainly on the juices of rotting fruits on the forest floor, where it spends most of its life. However, in the breeding season it flies into the forest canopy to find a mate.

Mountain gorillas, like this baby, live in cloud forests in the mountains of central Africa.

Forest-covered mountains in Democratic Republic of Congo and Rwanda are the home of the mountain gorilla. A male gorilla weighs twice as much as a human, yet this big beast lives entirely on leaves, shoots, and stems gathered from the forest floor. He is too heavy to climb trees.

GORILLA GROUP

Family groups of gorillas move into clearings in the forest to feed. Younger animals climb trees to find fruit. A big male can eat 30 kg (66 lbs) of plants a day.

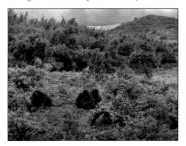

Richness in numbers The Monteverde cloud forest in Costa Rica, Central America, has been studied in detail by many scientists. They have found amazing numbers of plants and animals there.

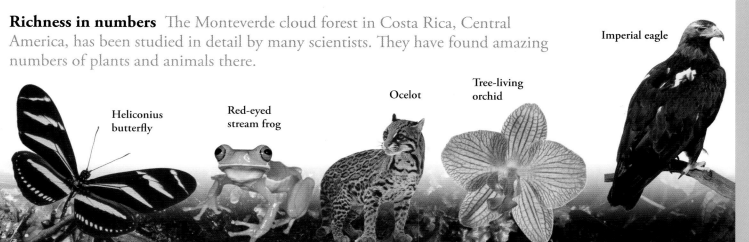

Heliconius butterfly

Red-eyed stream frog

Ocelot

Tree-living orchid

Imperial eagle

BUTTERFLIES
Scientists have found more than 500 different species of butterflies living in the 50 sq kms (19 sq miles) of protected nature reserve in Monteverde.

AMPHIBIANS
The damp conditions on the forest floor suit amphibians perfectly. Monteverde is home to 120 species of amphibians and reptiles.

MAMMALS
There are 100 species of mammals in Monteverde, including the ocelot. This shy cat hunts small mammals on the forest floor at night.

PLANTS
The ever-damp conditions support 2,500 plant species, including this orchid that lives on forest tree branches high above the ground.

BIRDS
Many birds pass through Monteverde as they migrate between North and South America. More than 400 species of birds have been recorded.

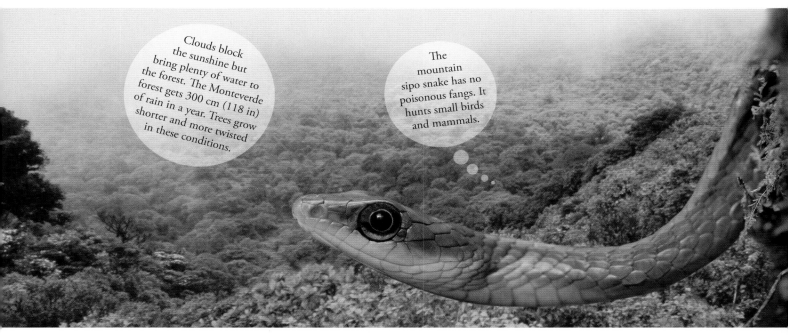

Clouds block the sunshine but bring plenty of water to the forest. The Monteverde forest gets 300 cm (118 in) of rain in a year. Trees grow shorter and more twisted in these conditions.

The mountain sipo snake has no poisonous fangs. It hunts small birds and mammals.

VOLCANIC LIVING
Mountain gorillas live above 3,000 m (10,000 ft) in protected cloud forest on the slopes of volcanoes that lie between Rwanda and Uganda in central Africa.

RIVER RUNNER
The plumed basilisk lizard lives beside cloud-forest ponds. When danger threatens, it can run across the water, helped by the hairy fringes on its toes.

MOSSY WORLD
Cloud-forest trees grow shorter and more twisted than those in rainforests. In the constant dampness, lichens and mosses flourish.

POKEY COATI
The coati is a mongoose-sized animal from South America. It uses its long, flexible nose to poke around among the dead leaves on the forest floor to find worms and other insects.

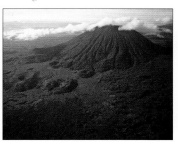
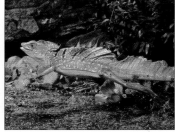
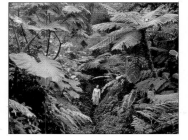
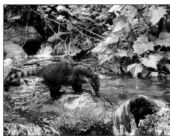

trouble in the clouds

Cloud forests are under threat. In areas where people are *poor* and short of food, they have cut down the trees to make cheap fuel and to create space to grow crops, especially on islands in the **Caribbean** like Cuba and Trinidad. Today cloud forests survive mainly on *higher, steeper* slopes that are not easily accessible.

Fruit bats move around the forest to find ripe fruits. If climate change affects fruiting times, it may cause problems for bats feeding.

Cloud forests are being cut down, and

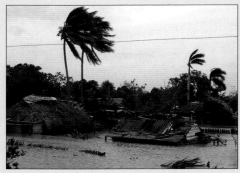

Hurricane alley Scientists think that climate change is causing bigger hurricanes to happen more often. The shape of cloud forests generally protects them from hurricanes, but, where they have been opened up by felling, the winds can cause serious damage.

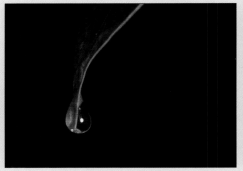

Drip tip Many leaves of cloud-forest trees end in a long point called a drip tip, which allows rain to run off and stops damaging fungi growing all over their surface. This adaptation shows how well designed they are for ever-wet conditions, but it makes them very sensitive to dry weather.

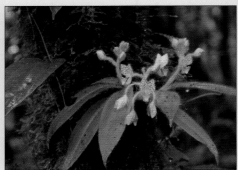

Tree hitchhiker Many plants, like this orchid, grow perched on the branches of cloud-forest trees. They get the moisture and nutrients they need from clouds and rain. Climate change may cause them real problems as nine out of ten plants in the Monteverde cloud forest cannot stand being dry for long periods.

EL NIÑO

Every 3–5 years, the cold current off the coast of South America is replaced by unusually warm water at the sea surface. This event is called *El Niño* ("the boy child") as it happens at Christmas time. Although *El Niño* arises off the coast of Peru, its effect is widespread in the Pacific. In Central America, the winds off the sea die away, so no clouds form over the mountains. The wet season becomes shorter and drier, many plants cannot flower, and animals fail to breed. *El Niño* is a natural event and the forest survives, but climate change is making *El Niño* events more severe and possibly more frequent.

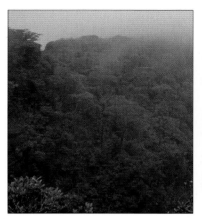

LIFE-GIVING CLOUDS
Cloud forests rely on winds off the sea. These bring clouds to the mountains during the dry season, when it rains very little, and torrential storms during the rainy season. In *El Niño* years, the clouds and rain disappear (right) and the forest becomes drier. Toads and other wet-loving creatures suffer from the dry conditions.

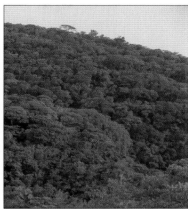

The forest can cope with these changes, provided they do not happen too often.

climate change affects the forests that are left.

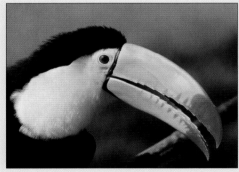

Lowland invader Some lowland species are already moving upwards into the cloud forest as it becomes drier and warmer in the mountains. Birds like this keel-billed toucan could not breed in the forest when it was always wet, but have now begun breeding higher up in the mountain forests.

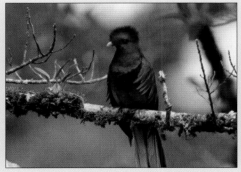

Locals in trouble As lowland birds become more frequent visitors to the cloud forest, they eat up large quantities of fruit and other food. That leaves much less for the native birds, like this colourful quetzal. It relies so much on fruit that it moves through the forest to catch trees as they start fruiting.

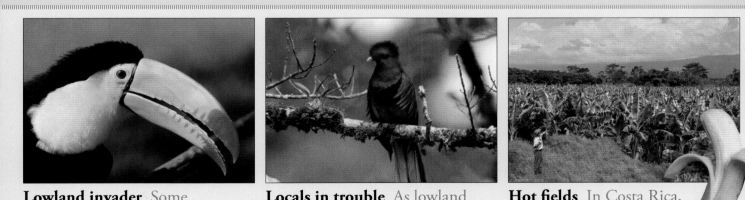

Hot fields In Costa Rica, more and more wild countryside is being made into farmland. This makes the land warmer as dark soil absorbs heat and there are no cooling trees. The warming land forces drier winds higher up the mountains, reducing the thickness of cloud cover.

the golden toad

NO-ONE WILL EVER SEE A SIGHT LIKE THIS AGAIN AS HOTTER, DRIER CONDITIONS HAVE WIPED OUT THE GOLDEN TOAD

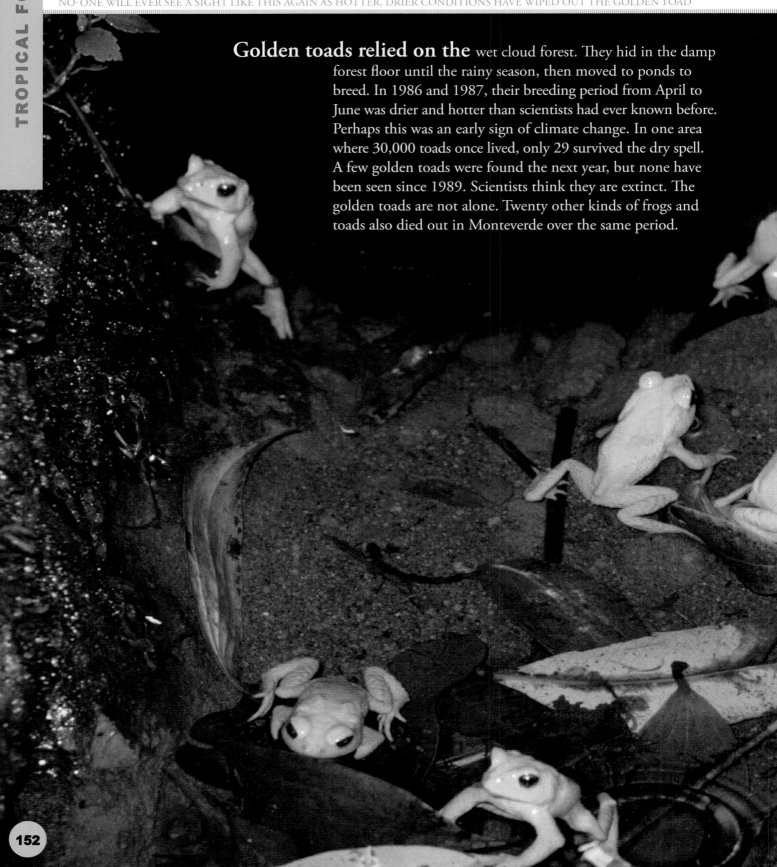

Golden toads relied on the wet cloud forest. They hid in the damp forest floor until the rainy season, then moved to ponds to breed. In 1986 and 1987, their breeding period from April to June was drier and hotter than scientists had ever known before. Perhaps this was an early sign of climate change. In one area where 30,000 toads once lived, only 29 survived the dry spell. A few golden toads were found the next year, but none have been seen since 1989. Scientists think they are extinct. The golden toads are not alone. Twenty other kinds of frogs and toads also died out in Monteverde over the same period.

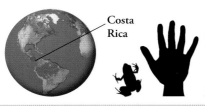

Costa Rica

The golden toad was only ever found at about 2,000 m (6,500 ft) in the Monteverde cloud forest of Costa Rica.

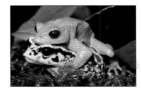

Female golden toads were dark brown, marked with red and orange blotches. At the start of the rainy season, they gathered round ponds to lay eggs. A golden-coloured male hopped on top of the female to fertilize her eggs, so they could become tadpoles. The eggs were then left in the ponds to hatch.

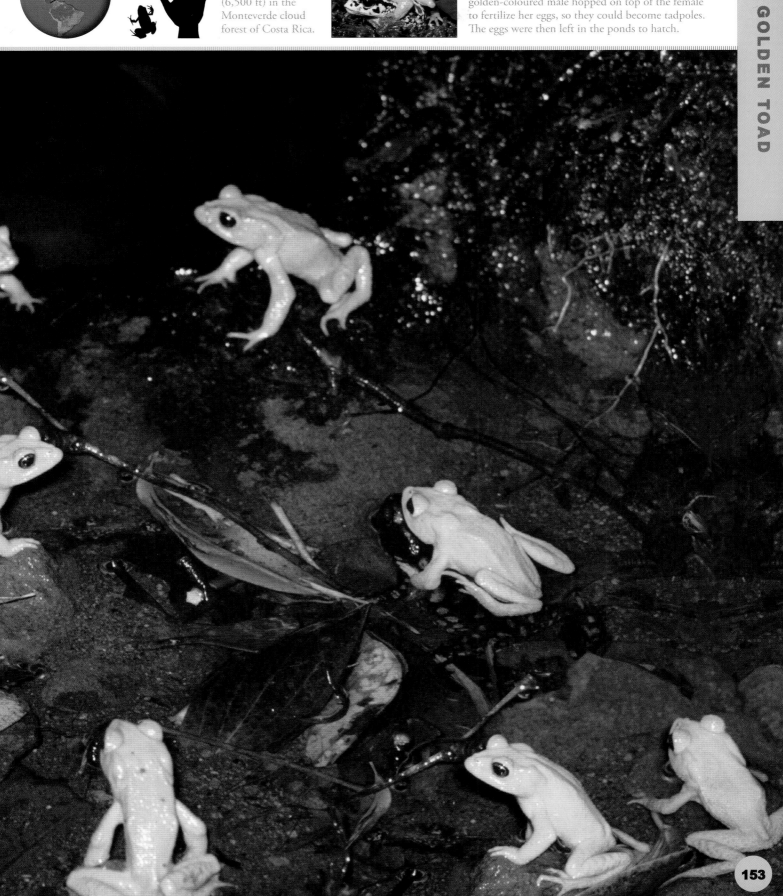

tropical dry forest

Many tropical dry forests are dry only in comparison with rainforests. Monsoon forests have regular thunderstorms with heavy rain during the wet season, when moisture-laden winds blow off the sea. But for part of the year they are very dry. Other forests in southern Africa and South America are truly dry, with little rainfall all year.

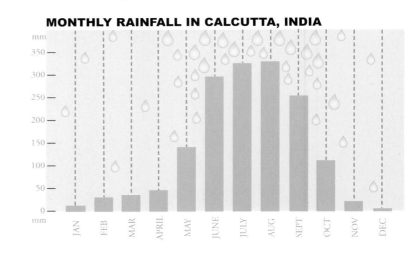

MONTHLY RAINFALL IN CALCUTTA, INDIA

mm
350
300
250
200
150
100
50
mm

JAN FEB MAR APRIL MAY JUNE JULY AUG SEPT OCT NOV DEC

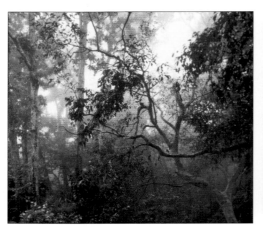

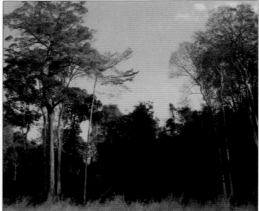

Monsoon seasons In summer, strong winds blow from the cool sea towards the hot land carrying lots of rain into the forest (far left). When winter comes, the land cools down and the wind blows off it, so it becomes very dry. Little rain falls and the trees begin to shed their leaves (left).

A monsoon forest food chain Food is abundant during the wet season, but scarce during dry times.

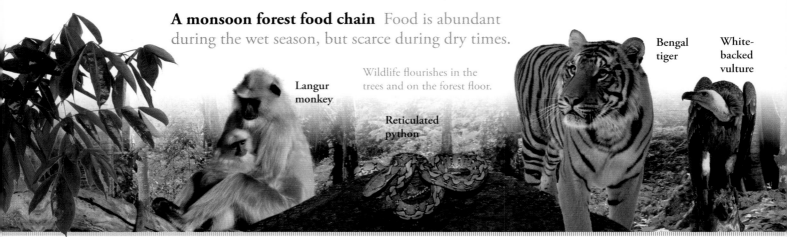

Langur monkey

Wildlife flourishes in the trees and on the forest floor.

Reticulated python

Bengal tiger

White-backed vulture

PRODUCERS
Plants grow lushly through the monsoon season. They produce flowers and then fruits, so there is plenty of food for animals.

PRIMARY CONSUMERS
Many monkeys, like these langur monkeys, live in the monsoon forest. They eat leaves off the trees and fruits when available.

SECONDARY CONSUMERS
Reticulated pythons are tree-top hunters. They coil up on a branch and wait for a small monkey to come too close.

TOP CARNIVORES
Pigs, deer, and antelopes are the main food of the tiger, but it will hunt monkeys if they come to the ground – and even an occasional python.

SCAVENGERS
Vultures are the forest dustbin men, clearing up the remains of all dead animals. They sit in trees or glide above the forest, looking out for their next meal.

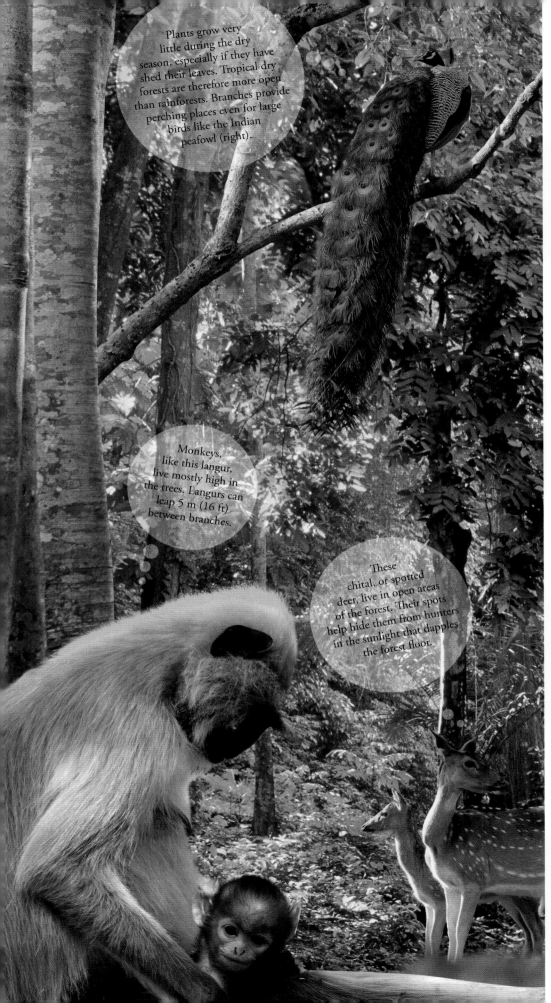

Plants grow very little during the dry season, especially if they have shed their leaves. Tropical dry forests are therefore more open than rainforests. Branches provide perching places even for large birds like the Indian peafowl (right).

Monkeys, like this langur, live mostly high in the trees. Langurs can leap 5 m (16 ft) between branches.

These chital, or spotted deer, live in open areas of the forest. Their spots help hide them from hunters in the sunlight that dapples the forest floor.

WET "DRY" FORESTS
Some monsoon forests get 3.5 m (11 ft) of rain in just four months of monsoon. That means 3 cm (1.2 in) of rain falls in a day, mostly in torrential showers.

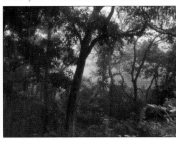

DRY FLOWERING
Some monsoon forest trees flower during the dry season when they have no leaves. This timing lets them spread their seeds in the wet season, when they will grow best.

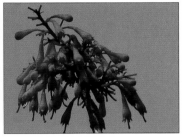

ELEPHANTS IN MOPANE
Elephants are at home in the Mopane forest, which covers a huge area in drier parts of Africa, near the Equator. This open, scrubby woodland is halfway to savanna.

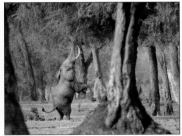

AFRO-MONTANE FOREST
Other kinds of tropical forest are dry all year round, but get just enough rain or mist for trees to grow. Afro-montane forest like this is found in upland areas of Africa.

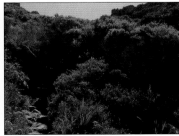

disappearing dry forests

Almost all tropical dry forest is found where **people** are desperately poor and struggle to survive. In *African* forest areas, many people rely on wood to cook food and boil water to **drink**, but that means the **trees soon disappear**. In the monsoon forests of Asia farming began many centuries ago. Great areas have been *burnt* and *cleared* to make way for fields.

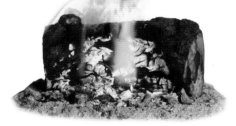

Burning logs helps people live, but soon kills the forest.

Support charities in Africa that are helping people plant trees, so they can grow firewood for the future.

The greatest threat to tropical dry forests

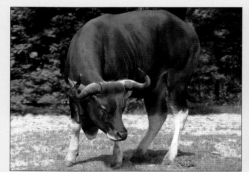

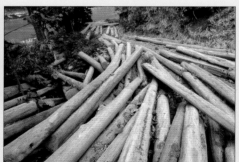

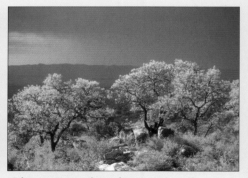

Ox in danger A forest ox called the kouprey was discovered by scientists in the monsoon forests of eastern Asia in 1937. It is greatly in danger because of hunting and clearance of its forest home. None have been seen in the wild since 1988.
A few kouprey, like this one, live in zoos.

Valuable timber Teak trees produce the finest timber in the monsoon forests. The hard and long-lasting wood is very valuable and many teak trees are still felled illegally. It can take more than a century for a new tree to grow, so we need to value teak as much as we do gold and protect its forests carefully.

Chopping the chaco The chaco, or Great Thorn Forest, once covered vast areas of South America but much of it has been destroyed. Trees were used for building or as fuel for sugar refineries. Cattle ranching destroyed more trees and now more chaco is being cleared for soya farming.

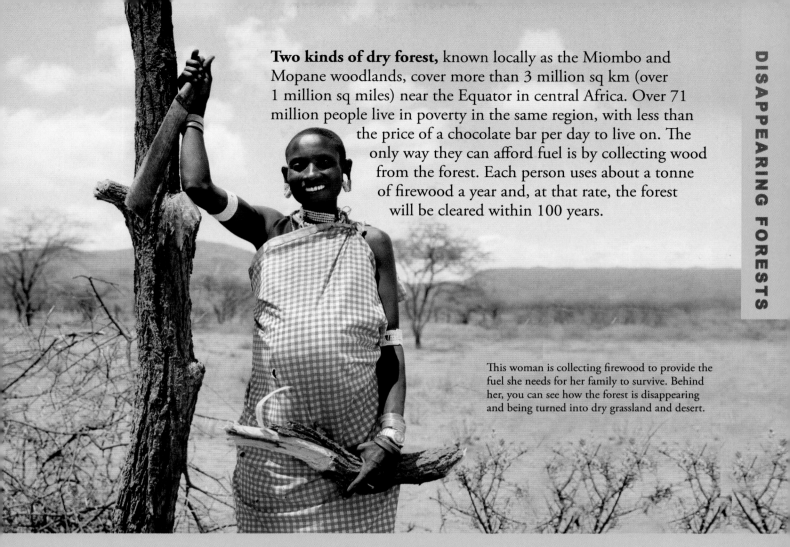

Two kinds of dry forest, known locally as the Miombo and Mopane woodlands, cover more than 3 million sq km (over 1 million sq miles) near the Equator in central Africa. Over 71 million people live in poverty in the same region, with less than the price of a chocolate bar per day to live on. The only way they can afford fuel is by collecting wood from the forest. Each person uses about a tonne of firewood a year and, at that rate, the forest will be cleared within 100 years.

This woman is collecting firewood to provide the fuel she needs for her family to survive. Behind her, you can see how the forest is disappearing and being turned into dry grassland and desert.

around the world is human poverty.

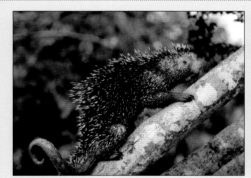

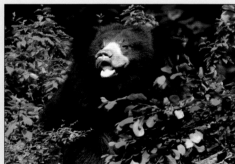

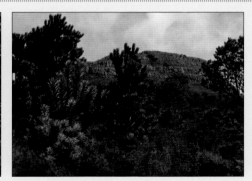

Spiny climber As the chaco disappears, its animals, like the Brazilian prehensile-tailed porcupine, have fewer places to live. It uses its specially-adapted tail to wrap around a branch so it can hang as it feeds on leaves and bark. It often moves over 700 m (half a mile) a night in search of food.

Not so much sloth The sloth bear lives in tropical dry forests in India and Nepal. It feeds on insects called termites, honey, and birds' eggs. The destruction of forests means that today only a tenth of India's forests are large enough to offer it a safe home, and only 6,000–11,000 sloth bears remain.

Silver survivor The silver tree is one of the special species found in the Afro-montane forest. It grows only on the slopes of Table Mountain and Lion's Head, a neighbouring hill, right on the outskirts of Cape Town in South Africa. It is now a protected species – although that does not save it from fires.

the aye-aye

THE SPOOKY-LOOKING AYE-AYE LIVES IN THE FORESTS OF MADAGASCAR, BUT THESE ARE DISAPPEARING FAST

Although Madagascar is close to Africa, it has been separate for a long time, so many animals living there are found nowhere else. The aye-aye is a kind of lemur or early monkey. It hunts at night for insects, using its big ears to track them down and its long fingers to winkle them out from beneath the bark of trees. Sometimes it uses its extra-long middle finger to scoop the flesh out of coconuts or other fruits, like we would use a long ice-cream spoon. As forests are destroyed, the aye-aye is becoming extremely rare. Nobody knows how many are left, but there are probably fewer than 2,500 of them.

A few zoos are trying to breed aye-ayes in cages to make sure some survive. Find out if you can visit one of these zoos. Your entry fee will help their work.

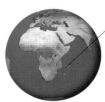

Madagascar

Madagascar is the fourth biggest island in the world. It is a bit larger than France.

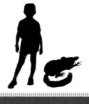

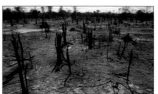

Many people live on Madagascar and its forests are being cut and then burnt to clear land for farming. Three-quarters of the forest has already gone, and the rest could be destroyed within 50 years, along with all the animals that live there, including the aye-aye.

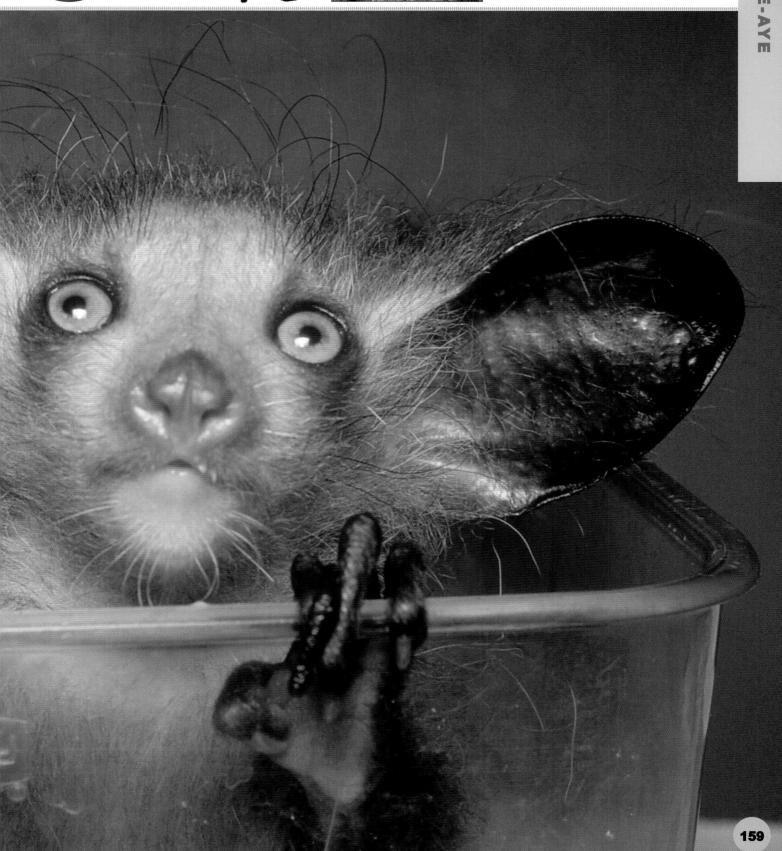

MAKING A DIFFERENCE

FRIENDS OF THE FOREST

* **The Fairtrade Association** makes sure small farmers in third-world countries get fair prices for their products.
* **World Wide Fund for Nature** works to protect tropical forests and rare species like the Bengal tiger.
* **Forest Stewardship Council** helps people to buy tropical timber wisely.

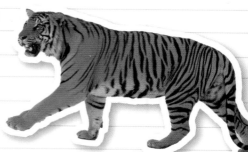

Save the Bengal tiger

Bird-friendly coffee

Coffee was once grown beneath trees. Many new kinds are grown in open sunshine, so trees go and birds lose their homes. Buy shade-grown coffee to help the birds.

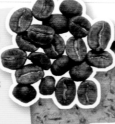

Shade-grown coffee beans

what you can do

ADOPT-AN-ACRE
Sponsor an acre of rainforest for yourself to help keep it safe.
www.worldlandtrust.org

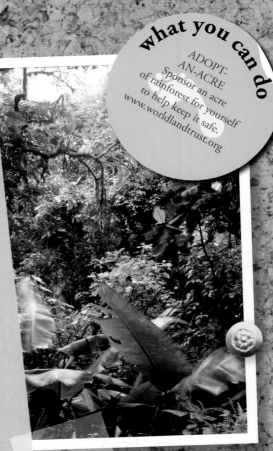

GARDEN FURNITURE FOR SALE

 BUY WISELY
FSC APPROVED

NOT CHEAP BUT NOT TEAK
HARD WEARING AND ECO-FRIENDLY

EXTRA COMFORT AT AFFORDABLE PRICE
NO RAINFOREST DESTROYED

MADE FROM SUSTAINABLE FOREST

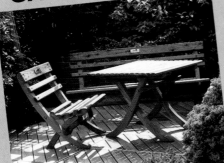

Rainforest-friendly furniture

Teak and mahogany from tropical forests offer long-lasting timber for garden furniture. But if buy them unwisely, we contribute to the

Look for furniture with the Forest Stewardship Council logo, showing it has come from forests that are being looked after for the future. Over 2 million hectares (5 million acres) of forest in Bolivia have become FSC certified. This helps to protect important areas of the Amazon rainforest. Certified wood from these forests is

Green tourism shows local people the value of their forest. If you get a chance, take a jungle holiday and explore the rainforest.

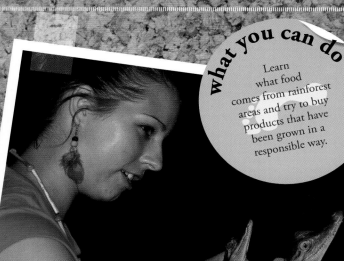

what you can do

Learn what food comes from rainforest areas and try to buy products that have been grown in a responsible way.

Along the Amazon, local people earn cash taking tourists out to photograph caimans at night. The animals are later released.

RAINFOREST-FRIENDLY SHOPPING

- Fairtrade coffee
- Fairtrade chocolate
- local meat
- organic palm oil products
- organic soya

Oil palm

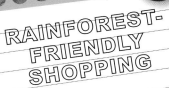

Organic crisps

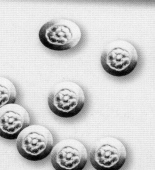

HELP PROTECT MOUNTAIN GORILLAS

Mountain gorillas are one of the rarest cloud-forest animals; there may only be 700 of them left in the wild. Several conservation charities have got together as the International Gorilla Conservation Programme to help save them. They are working with the governments of the Democratic Republic of Congo, Rwanda, and the Congo, together with local people, to look after the forest. They employ rangers to guard the animals from poachers, and to welcome visitors who come to see the gorillas. Visit www.igcp.org for the latest news about the gorilla programme.

what you can do

Help protect orang-utans by supporting the WWF's "Heart of Borneo Programme". Go to www.panda.org

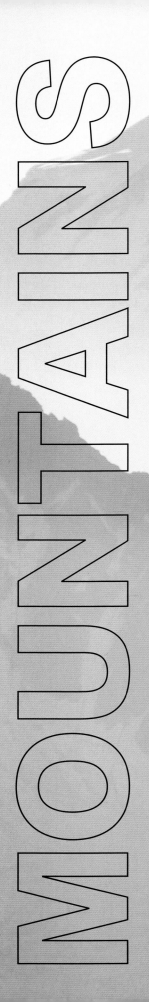

MOUNTAINS

Mountains and highlands are *tough places* to live. They have severe weather and **poor**, *rocky* soils.

In many ways they are like the polar regions. Temperatures drop very low at night and in winter. Winds are strong, and often bring snow. Only plants and animals that are specially adapted can survive such bitter conditions.

MOUNTAINS AND HIGHLANDS

where on earth...?

Mountains are high hills rising well above the surrounding land. There is no exact height at which land becomes a mountain, although generally high land is more than 500 m (1,640 ft) above sea level and most mountains are above 2,000 m (6,560 ft).

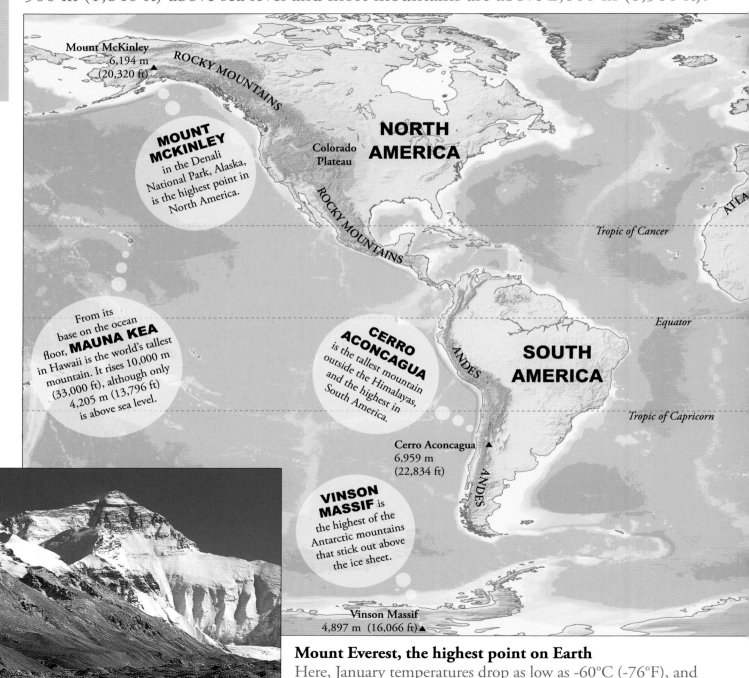

Mount McKinley
6,194 m
(20,320 ft) ▲

ROCKY MOUNTAINS

MOUNT MCKINLEY in the Denali National Park, Alaska, is the highest point in North America.

NORTH AMERICA

Colorado Plateau

ROCKY MOUNTAINS

ATLA

Tropic of Cancer

From its base on the ocean floor, **MAUNA KEA** in Hawaii is the world's tallest mountain. It rises 10,000 m (33,000 ft), although only 4,205 m (13,796 ft) is above sea level.

Equator

CERRO ACONCAGUA is the tallest mountain outside the Himalayas, and the highest in South America.

ANDES

SOUTH AMERICA

Tropic of Capricorn

Cerro Aconcagua
6,959 m
(22,834 ft) ▲

ANDES

VINSON MASSIF is the highest of the Antarctic mountains that stick out above the ice sheet.

ANDES

Vinson Massif
4,897 m (16,066 ft) ▲

Mount Everest, the highest point on Earth
Here, January temperatures drop as low as -60°C (-76°F), and the warmest daytime temperature in July is around -16°C (3.2°F). Winds commonly reach over 160 km/h (100 mph). No animal lives at its summit, although a few birds may visit in summer.

ARCTIC LINKS

Mountain plants and animals face weather that's very similar to the Arctic. Some plant species are found in both areas – scientists and gardeners call these plants "arctic-alpines". Some mountain animals also live in the Arctic.

WEATHER EFFECT

Mountain weather depends on the climate of the surrounding area. Mount Kilimanjaro is close to the Equator where it is hot. There trees grow at 3,000 m (9,800 ft). In Scandinavia, where it is cold, mountains that high are snow covered all year.

HIGH LIVING

Plants and animals live at different heights up a mountain depending on the weather. So a plant that lives at 3,000 m (9,800 ft) in the warmth of the Alps, lives a third as high in the Scottish mountains, and beside the sea in Alaska or Greenland.

SPOT THE HEIGHT

The exact height of a mountain is difficult to measure. In 1953 Mount Everest was estimated at 8,848 m (29,028 ft) high. In 1999, Americans using satellites decided it was seven feet taller, but a later survey reduced it to 8,844 m (29,016 ft).

LONE PEAK

Although Mount Everest is the world's highest point, it rises from an area of high land. If you think of a mountain as a cone shape lying on a flat plain, then Mount Kilimanjaro is the tallest mountain, rising 4,600 m (15,990 ft) from the plains below.

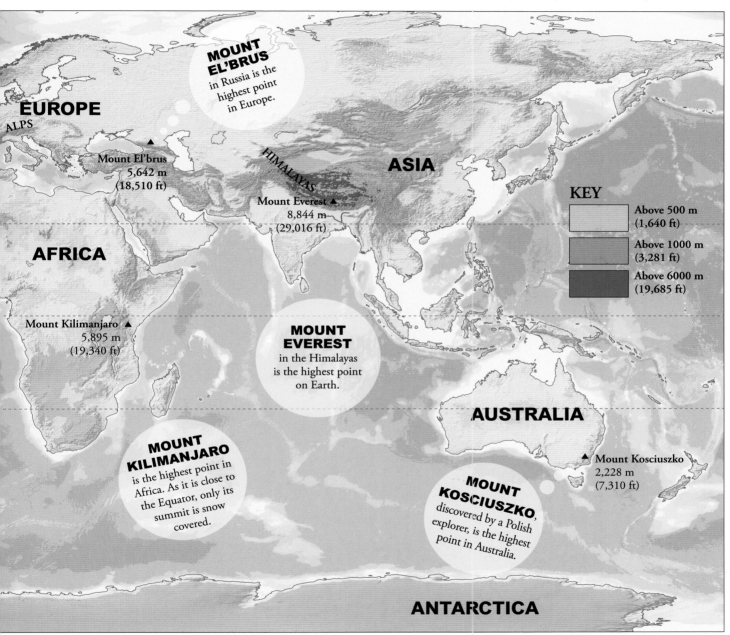

MOUNT EL'BRUS in Russia is the highest point in Europe.

EUROPE

ALPS

Mount El'brus
5,642 m
(18,510 ft)

HIMALAYAS

ASIA

Mount Everest ▲
8,844 m
(29,016 ft)

AFRICA

KEY

	Above 500 m (1,640 ft)
	Above 1000 m (3,281 ft)
	Above 6000 m (19,685 ft)

Mount Kilimanjaro ▲
5,895 m
(19,340 ft)

MOUNT EVEREST in the Himalayas is the highest point on Earth.

AUSTRALIA

MOUNT KILIMANJARO is the highest point in Africa. As it is close to the Equator, only its summit is snow covered.

▲ Mount Kosciuszko
2,228 m
(7,310 ft)

MOUNT KOSCIUSZKO, discovered by a Polish explorer, is the highest point in Australia.

ANTARCTICA

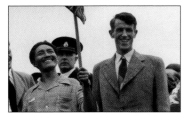

In 1953 Edmund Hillary and Sherpa Tenzing Norgay were the first to reach the top of Mount Everest.

Mountains and highlands are upland areas that have harsh weather, with strong winds, cold temperatures at night and in winter, and often ice and snow. Since mountains rise more steeply and to greater heights than highlands, they have the worst weather.

mountain ecosystem

In the mountain valleys, plants and animals thrive, but life is very different on the high mountain slopes. Here it is icy cold in winter, and bitterly cold at night. During the day, the Sun warms the slopes, but at night the thin air above the peaks lets heat escape quickly. In winter, when the Sun is furthest away and wind and snow whip the icy ground, very few plants and animals survive.

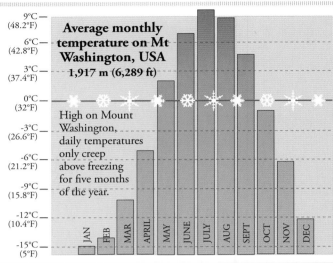

Average monthly temperature on Mt Washington, USA 1,917 m (6,289 ft)

High on Mount Washington, daily temperatures only creep above freezing for five months of the year.

9°C (48.2°F)
6°C (42.8°F)
3°C (37.4°F)
0°C (32°F)
-3°C (26.6°F)
-6°C (21.2°F)
-9°C (15.8°F)
-12°C (10.4°F)
-15°C (5°F)

JAN FEB MAR APRIL MAY JUNE JULY AUG SEPT OCT NOV DEC

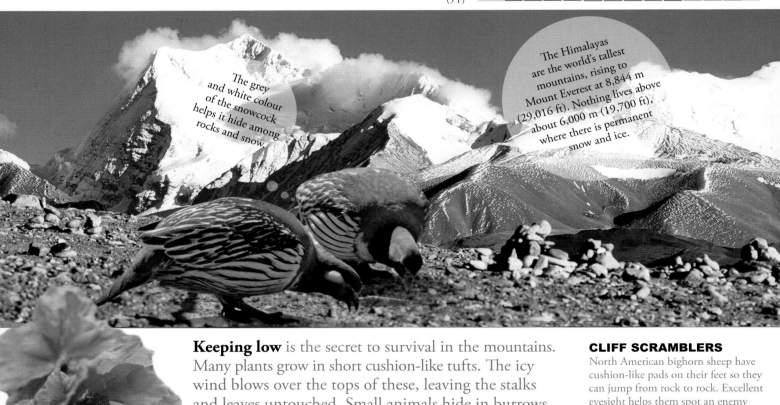

The grey and white colour of the snowcock helps it hide among rocks and snow.

The Himalayas are the world's tallest mountains, rising to Mount Everest at 8,844 m (29,016 ft). Nothing lives above about 6,000 m (19,700 ft), where there is permanent snow and ice.

Keeping low is the secret to survival in the mountains. Many plants grow in short cushion-like tufts. The icy wind blows over the tops of these, leaving the stalks and leaves untouched. Small animals hide in burrows or under rocks. Large animals move to find shelter and places to feed.

Himalayan poppies grow 4,000 m (13,100 ft) above sea level in the mountains of Nepal and China. Although the flowers die at the end of summer, their roots stay alive under the soil. The blanket of snow protects the roots from winter ice, so they can sprout again in spring.

CLIFF SCRAMBLERS

North American bighorn sheep have cushion-like pads on their feet so they can jump from rock to rock. Excellent eyesight helps them spot an enemy up to 1 km (0.6 miles) away.

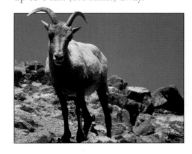

As you travel up a mountain, the average temperature falls by about 1°C for every 150 m (1°F for every 300 ft) you climb. It gets windier the higher you go, and there is more snow and ice. Fewer living things can cope with this increasingly harsh weather, so there are different – and fewer – plants and animals living high up.

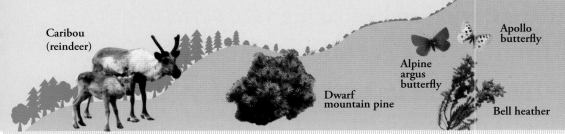
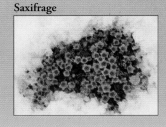

Caribou (reindeer)

Dwarf mountain pine

Alpine argus butterfly

Apollo butterfly

Bell heather

Saxifrage

LOW FORESTS

Trees grow in valleys, but cannot cope with the cold and wind higher on the mountain. Caribou live on the edges of the forests.

MONTANE SCRUB

Some trees and shrubs can grow a little way above the forest. They have low, twisted shapes and are called montane scrub.

MOUNTAIN HEATH

Above a height called the scrubline, no trees can grow. Here different heathers are the main plants. A few insects visit their flowers.

ICY TOPS

On the highest tops, snow and ice take over completely. In pockets where snow melts in summer, tough mountain flowers briefly appear.

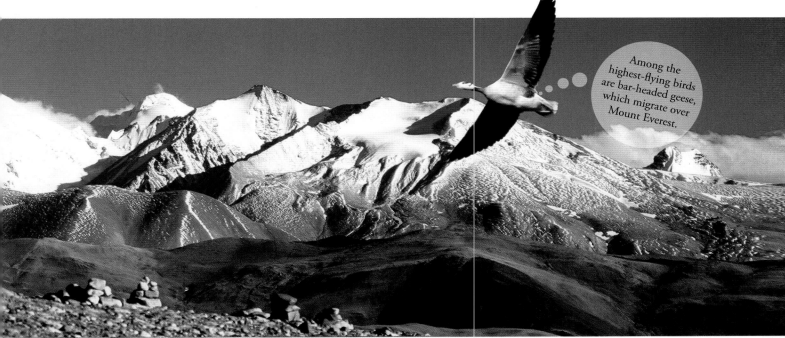

Among the highest-flying birds are bar-headed geese, which migrate over Mount Everest.

SNOW BLOSSOMS

In early spring, snowbells grow under the snow. They heat the snow and melt tiny spaces around themselves. When the snow melts, they are already in flower.

TINY MOUNTAINEER

Insects avoid the Sun by hiding in holes or under leaves. The world's most abundant insects – springtails – live in all habitats including 6,000 m (19,700 ft) up mountains.

HIGH LIVING

This chubby relative of the hare is called a Mount Everest pika. It makes its home 6,125 m (20,100 ft) up in the Himalayas. That's higher than any other mammal.

FLOWER SHOW

The glacial buttercup is Europe's highest-living flowering plant. It has been seen in flower 4,275 m (14,026 ft) up in the Swiss Alps. It often grows close to glaciers.

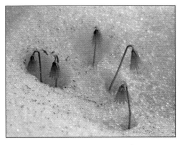
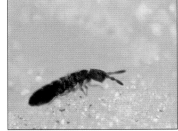
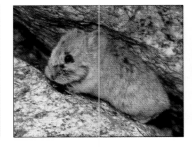
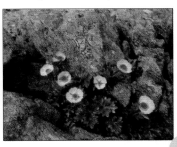

the *shrinking* mountain

Climate change is generally making *temperatures rise.* Although it is **difficult to be certain,** scientists think world temperatures in 2100 could be up to *6.4°C (11.5°F) higher* than they are today. That means mountain **plants** and **animals** would have to move higher to find the *climate* they need, and to escape from *lowland species* moving in to their home from the lower slopes.

Mountain habitats are shrinking as

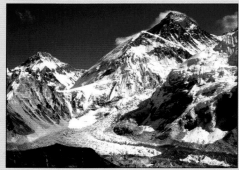

Melting the ice

The world has been getting warmer since the end of the last Ice Age around 11,000 years ago. But now greenhouse gases are changing temperatures more quickly. As a result, some glaciers in the Himalayas are shrinking by 30–40 m (100–130 ft) a year.

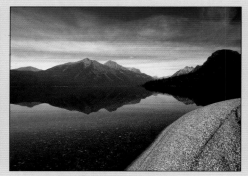

Disappearing glacier

Since the Glacier National Park was set up in Montana, USA, in 1910, glaciers have melted so much that today they only cover a quarter of the area they once occupied. If they go on melting, it could be No-glacier National Park by 2030!

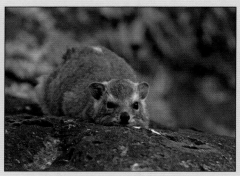

Rocky future

The rock hyrax lives in rocky places throughout Africa. One kind lives 3,500–4,700 m (11,500–15,500 ft) up on Mount Kenya. Eagles are its main enemy there. If the climate gets warmer, it might gain a new hunter as leopards move up the mountain.

As temperatures rise, animals and plants can move up the mountain. In the Himalayas, bharal sheep and yak will be able to move upwards, although there will be less space as they go higher. But the chiru antelope on the highest peaks might simply run out of mountain.

The living zones on the mountain for bharal, yak, and chiru antelope will shift with changing climate.

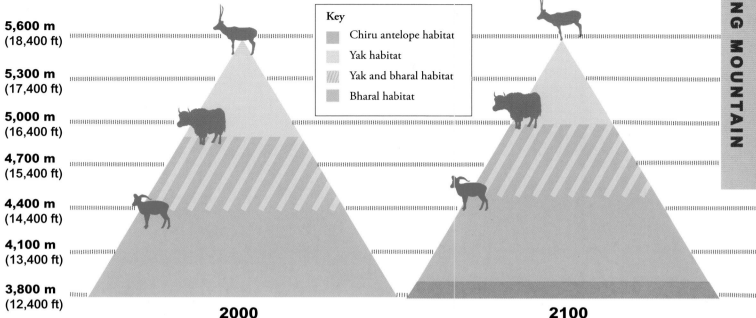

Key
- Chiru antelope habitat
- Yak habitat
- Yak and bharal habitat
- Bharal habitat

5,600 m (18,400 ft)
5,300 m (17,400 ft)
5,000 m (16,400 ft)
4,700 m (15,400 ft)
4,400 m (14,400 ft)
4,100 m (13,400 ft)
3,800 m (12,400 ft)

2000   **2100**

global temperatures continue to rise.

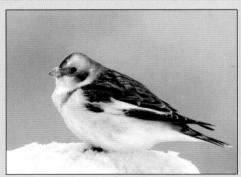

Snowless bunting
Snow buntings breed high in the Scottish mountains, above 900 m (2,900 ft). A 3°C (5°F) increase in temperature would force their habitat up to 1,350 m (4,430 ft). But there are no mountains that high in the UK, so there would be no place left for the buntings.

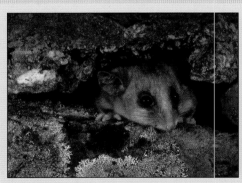

Pygmy-possum problem
The tiny mountain pygmy-possum lives up to 2,200 m (7,200 ft) in the mountains of south-east Australia. In winter it hibernates in a burrow under the snow. A slight temperature rise could cut snow cover, leaving it with nowhere to hibernate.

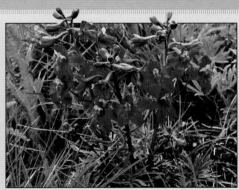

Bad timing
In the Rocky Mountains, USA, the two-lobe larkspur is pollinated by hummingbirds. Warmer weather would make the larkspur flower early. As hummingbirds only visit the mountain on long summer days, they might arrive too late to pollinate the flowers.

the snow leopard

ALTHOUGH AN ENDANGERED ANIMAL, THE SNOW LEOPARD IS STILL HUNTED BY HUMANS

The snow leopard is known for its pale, spotted fur, which helps it hide on its snowy hillside home. The animal is prized by hunters – its fur is used to make expensive coats and rugs, and its bones are used in Chinese medicine. Snow leopards were never common because few other animals live in these high mountains, so food is scarce. Now there may be only 2,500 adults left in a home range three times the size of France.

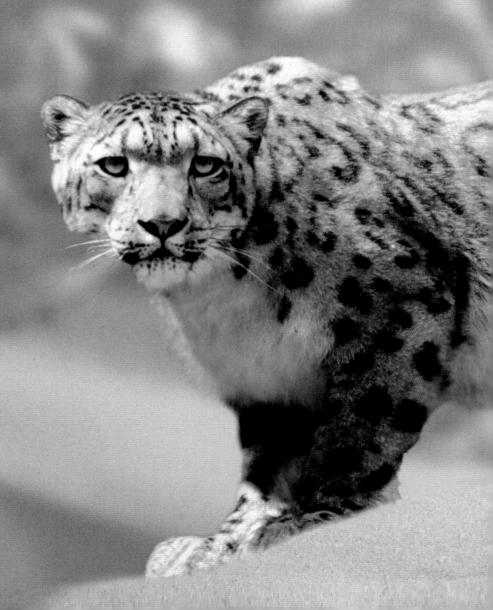

Snow leopards live in the mountains of central Asia. They are mostly found above the forest zone, and go as high as 6,000 m (19,700 ft) in the Himalayas.

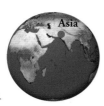

The snow leopard is 60 cm (2 ft) from shoulder to ground.

On the bare hillsides, snow leopards hunt wild sheep, deer, and pikas, as well as goats, like the markhor. The markhor lives in herds of up to 35 animals. Both males and females have large corkscrew-shaped horns.

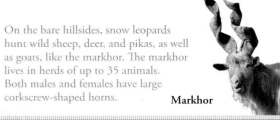

Markhor

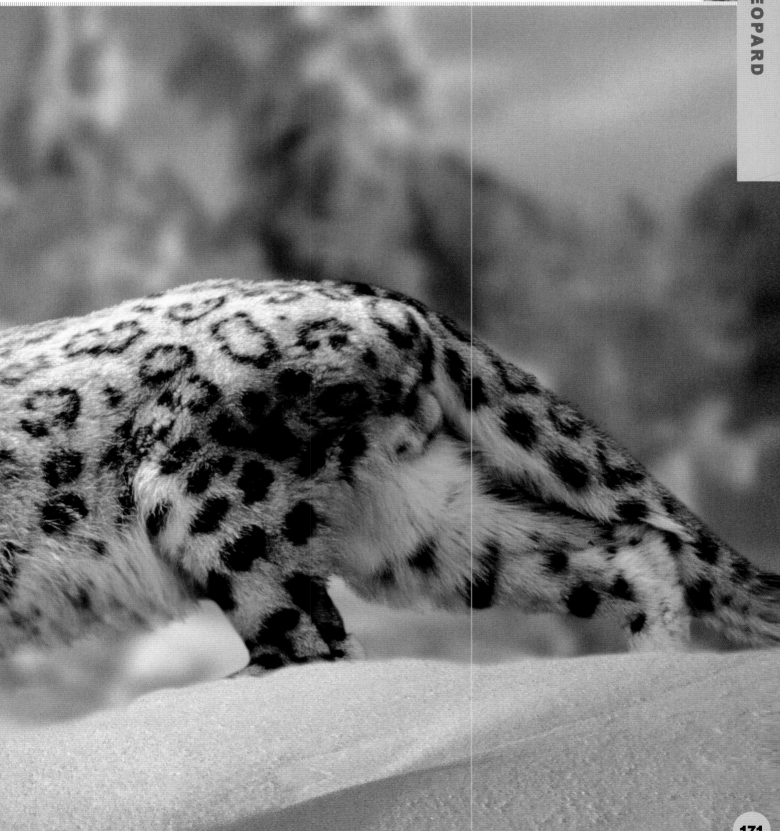

highland ecosystem

Highlands are flat, or gently sloping, upland areas. They are lower than mountains, but like mountains are very cold in winter. Some animals visit these highlands only in summer, when the Sun bakes down and warms them. However, a few, tough animals live there all year round. The Altiplano is a highland area in the Andes mountains, South America. It is a vast, high-level plain, lying 3,600 m (11,800 ft) above sea level.

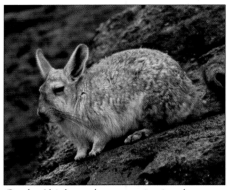

On the Altiplano, the mountain viscacha survives extreme temperature changes – from a warm daytime 20°C (68°F), to a freezing -20°C (-4°F) at night.

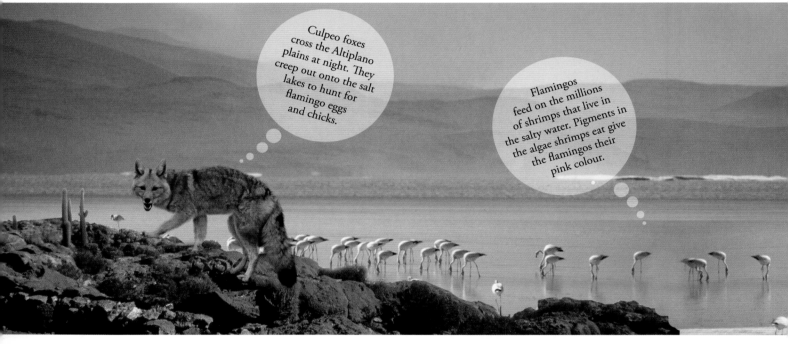

Culpeo foxes cross the Altiplano plains at night. They creep out onto the salt lakes to hunt for flamingo eggs and chicks.

Flamingos feed on the millions of shrimps that live in the salty water. Pigments in the algae shrimps eat give the flamingos their pink colour.

High-level salt lakes 10,000 years ago, a huge lake covered the Altiplano. It has gradually dried out, leaving behind smaller lakes. No rivers run out of these lakes – they simply dry up in the Sun. Salt washed in from rocks makes their water very salty.

High plateau The Drakensburg Plateau in South Africa was raised up as one block of land by earth movements 200 million years ago. It looks like a massive castle, 1,290 km (800 miles) long and rising to 3,482 m (11,420 ft).

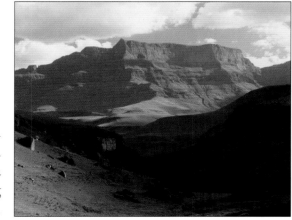

Altiplano food chain Tough grasses and spiny shrubs are the commonest plants on the Altiplano. They are difficult for animals to eat and do not provide much goodness, but they form the base of the entire food chain for the area.

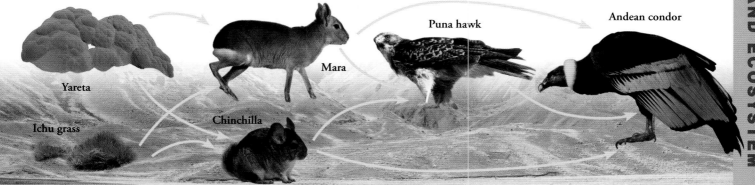

Yareta

Ichu grass

Chinchilla

Mara

Puna hawk

Andean condor

PRODUCERS
The rounded, cushion-like yareta bush can survive cold, dry conditions. Ichu is a tough grass found nowhere else in the world.

PRIMARY CONSUMERS
Maras are long-legged relatives of rats. Chinchillas live in South American mountains and highlands. Both animals eat any plants they can find.

SECONDARY CONSUMER
Maras and chinchillas are tempting food for hunters like the puna hawk. In fact, maras and their relatives, called cavies, make up a fifth of the hawk's food.

TOP PREDATOR
The Andean condor is a giant vulture whose wings reach 3 m (10 ft) from tip to tip. It feeds mainly on dead animals, but can kill using its powerful beak.

Very little rain or snow falls on the Altiplano. Most plants here are desert species, such as this cactus.

Vicuñas are wild relatives of llamas. Their fine wool keeps them warm on cold nights.

JEWEL IN THE CLOUD
The slopes of the Drakensberg are often hidden in cloud, so they get lots of rain. Some flowers, including this Drakensberg agapanthus, thrive in the wet climate.

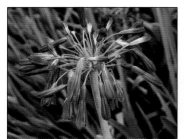

FRENCH TOPS
The Massif Central in France is a flat highland area, reaching 1,886 m (6,187 ft) above sea level. Because it is higher than the surrounding land, it has its own weather and wildlife.

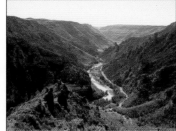

WOOLLY JUMPERS
Few crops can be grown on highland farms because of cold or wet weather, so fields are usually grazed by sheep and cattle, as on this farm in Northumberland, England.

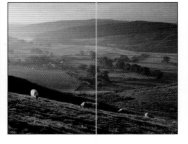

HEATHER EATER
Many upland areas have been changed by humans. In the Scottish Highlands, purple heather is grown to provide food for the red grouse, which people then hunt for sport.

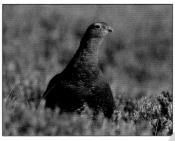

Highlands in danger

There are more people than ever in the world and they all need somewhere to live and work. To fit them in, more *land* is being **used up**, even in many *highland* areas. The city of La Paz, Bolivia, for example, lies in a canyon in the Altiplano. The **city** has now filled the canyon, and a huge suburb called El Alto (the Heights) is spreading onto the highlands above the canyon. El Alto has *taken over* land where wild *plants* and *animals* once lived.

People need houses, so towns have to spread. But we can still make space for wildlife in parks, and provide bird-nesting boxes and food in our gardens.

In 1900, no one lived in El Alto.

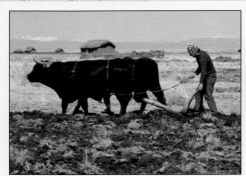

Farming the highland
Life is healthier in the highlands of the Altiplano than on the hot, wet plains below, so many people moved up there to farm. However, farming destroys natural plant cover and places where wild animals live. Also, nearby towns get bigger to supply the farmers.

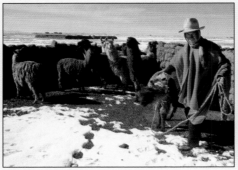

Taming the wild
The best animals to farm on the Altiplano are the ones that belong there naturally. Around 4,000 years ago, people tamed two South American relatives of camels – llamas and alpacas. More than three million of each are now kept on farms there.

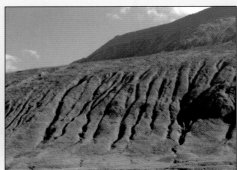

Stripping hills
Overgrazing causes problems in highland areas all round the world. Farmers keep as many sheep and cattle as they can on the hillsides. The animals eat all the natural plants. The bare soil and rocks then get washed away in rainstorms.

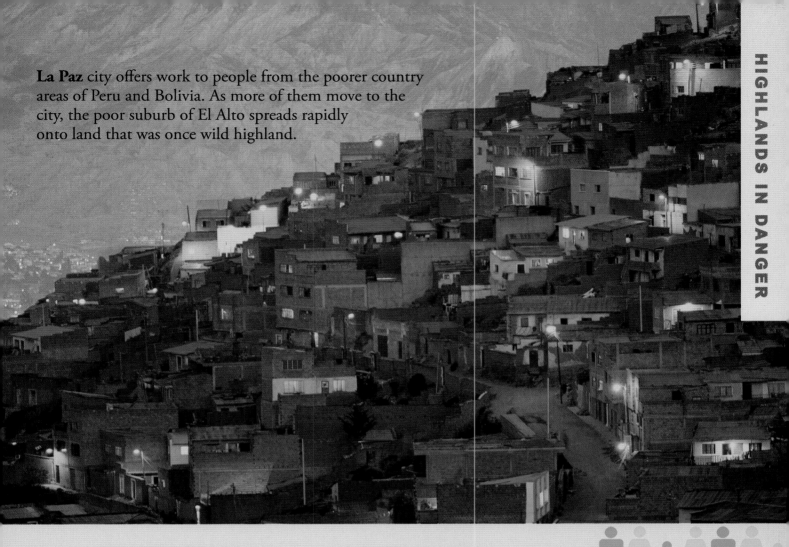

La Paz city offers work to people from the poorer country areas of Peru and Bolivia. As more of them move to the city, the poor suburb of El Alto spreads rapidly onto land that was once wild highland.

Now 650,000 people live there.

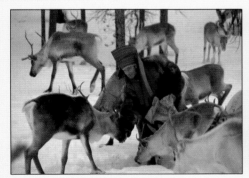

Too many hooves
In Scandinavia, local people herd semi-wild reindeer for use as food and clothing. By the end of the 1990s, the number of herded reindeer had increased to around 750,000. In winter, their many mouths and feet destroy the natural cover of lichens.

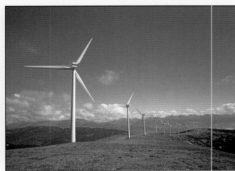

Hilltop wind factories
On hilltops, huge turbines use wind to make electricity. As they do not burn fossil fuels, they help slow climate change. However, windfarms spoil the wild appearance of highlands, and birds flying past are sometimes killed by the giant blades.

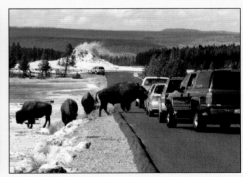

Popular place
Three million people a year visit Yellowstone National Park in the Rocky Mountains, USA. There they enjoy the highland scenery and wild animals. But too many people spoil the feeling of wildness and chase away animals. Visitor numbers are now strictly limited.

fragile roof of africa

THE ETHIOPIAN HIGHLANDS ARE AN OUT-OF-THE-WAY HABITAT IN A WAR-TORN REGION OF AFRICA

Few people visit the rocky Ethiopian highlands. As a result many wild animals, such as these gelada baboons, still live there. Fossils show the baboons were once much more common in Africa, but they were forced back into the hills as humans took over the lowlands. Their home needs protection – but this is not a high priority in a country troubled by famines, armed rebellions, and war, and where some people are desperately poor.

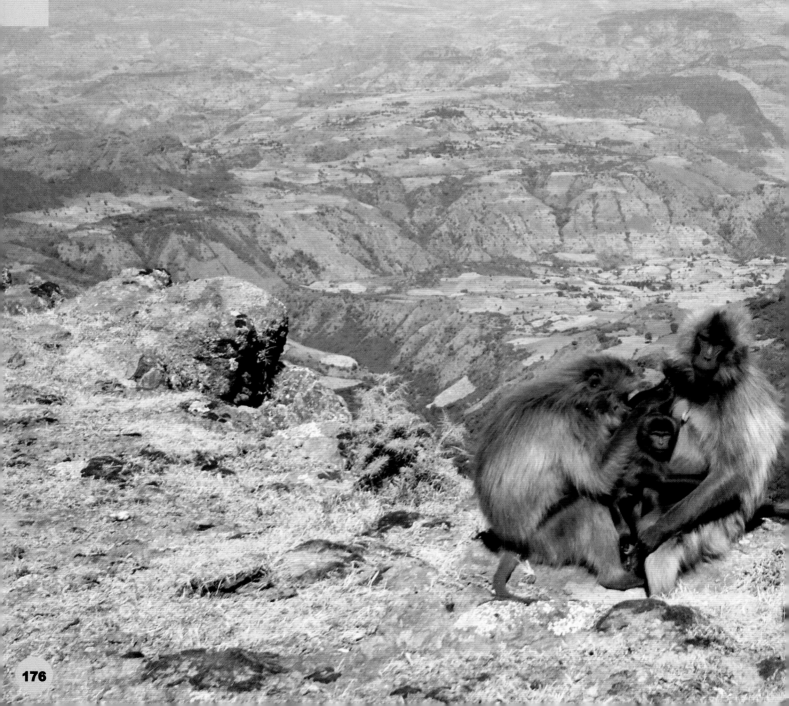

The Ethiopian Highlands lie in northern Africa. They form a vast dome of high land 1,000 km (620 miles) across and rising to 4,620 m (15,160 ft).

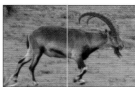

Ethiopian highlands

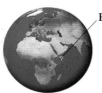

The gelada baboon's head and body are up to 76 cm (30 in) long.

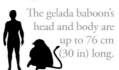

The walia ibex is a type of mountain goat. Its soft, flexible hooves help it pick its way across rock ledges to nibble grasses and herbs. Although rare, it is still hunted for meat by local people who are short of food.

Charities like Oxfam help Ethiopian people make a living without hunting wild animals. Find out more at www.oxfam.org.uk/coolplanet/kidsweb/world/ethiopia/

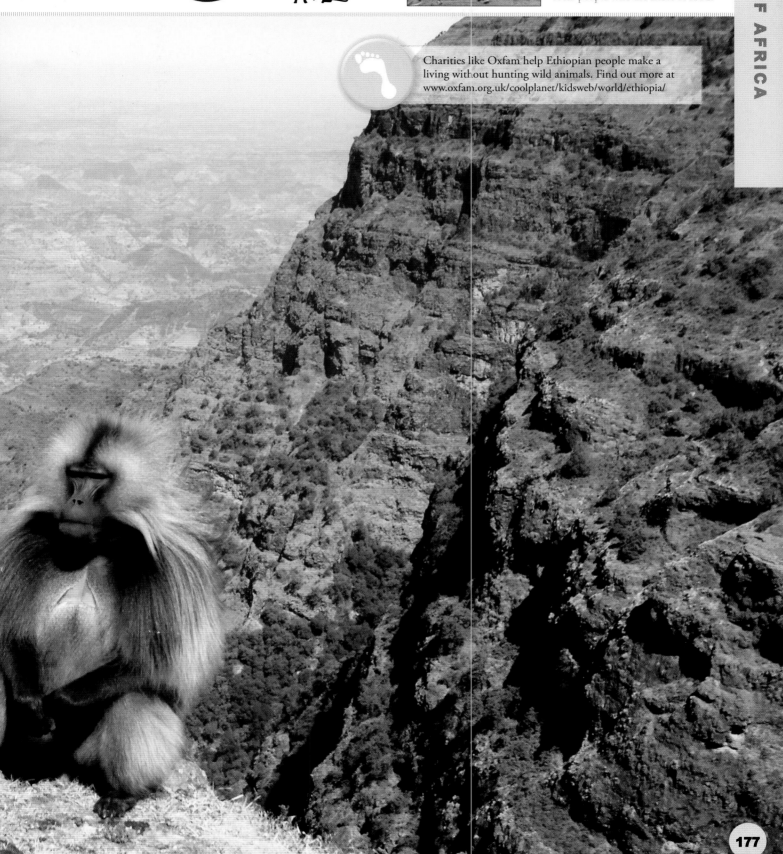

mountain valleys

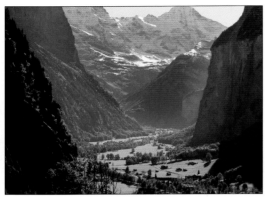

Lauterbrunnen Valley in Berner
Oberland, Switzerland

Valleys were formed when ancient rivers cut deep paths through the mountains. They wore away the rock, washing tiny pieces of it – called silt – down to the bottom of the river. Floods spread the silt across the valley floor, creating a rich, fertile soil. Now flowers and trees grow in the soil, sheltered from wind and cold by high valley walls. These plants provide homes and food for animals, birds, and humans.

Food chain The valleys are warmer and more sheltered than the mountaintops and have a richer food chain.

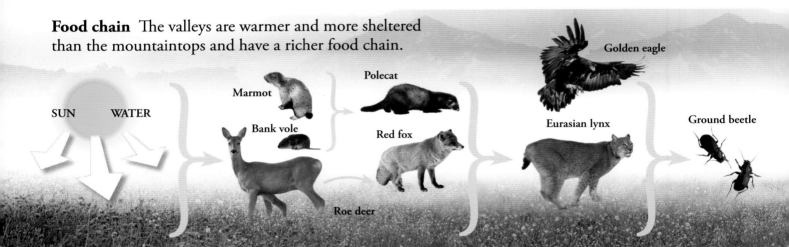

SUN   WATER

Marmot

Bank vole

Roe deer

Polecat

Red fox

Golden eagle

Eurasian lynx

Ground beetle

PRODUCERS
Sunshine and regular rain help plants to grow well. These form the base of the valley food chain, providing food for all the animals further up the chain.

PRIMARY CONSUMERS
Marmots are common grazers in mountain areas. Voles, deer, and wild sheep also graze the valley slopes and shelter in the woods.

SECONDARY CONSUMERS
Foxes, polecats, and other small hunters go after marmots, voles, and mice. Foxes kill young roe deer if they get the chance.

TOP CARNIVORES
Although top hunters such as eagles and lynxes prefer to hunt large prey, like deer or wild sheep, they will kill a red fox or a polecat if it crosses their paths.

DECOMPOSERS
Ground beetles are common in mountain valleys. They clean up droppings and the remains of dead animals, helping to put goodness back into the soil.

Return of the Rocky Mountain wolves The last grey wolves in the Rocky Mountains, USA, were killed by human hunters about 40 years ago. Wolves keep down numbers of deer, sheep, and goats and stop them eating all the young trees. In 1995, scientists released 14 wolves back into the Yellowstone National Park. They settled down and began breeding. Today around 250 wolves live in the area.

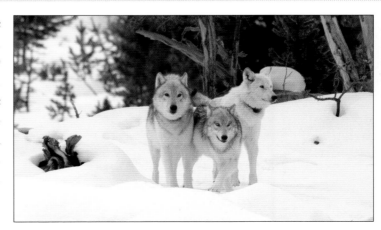

Mountain valleys Most plants and animals live in the shelter of the valley floor and on the lower slopes. As you climb, it gets colder and windier, so the higher you rise, the fewer species you will find.

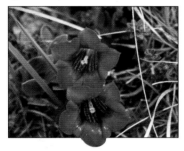

SLOPES

High up in the mountains, no trees and shrubs grow because it is too cold. A few tough plants, called alpines, survive to flower in summer, like this gentian. Its roots are a favourite food for voles.

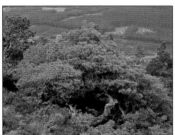

SCRUB

At slightly lower levels, a few trees and shrubs begin to grow. Ice and wind kill off many of their branches, giving them a low and twisted shape. Birds like ptarmigan and bluethroats live there.

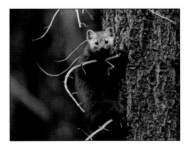

WOODS

Below the scrub, trees grow tall as they have more shelter. The level where they start growing, called the treeline, varies with local climate. Woodpeckers feed in the trees, hunted by pine martens (left).

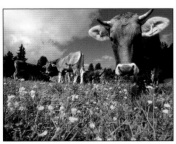

MEADOWS

In summer, meadow flowers bloom on the valley floor and farm animals graze on the rich grass. A blanket of snow protects the meadows through the winter, while insects hibernate in the soil.

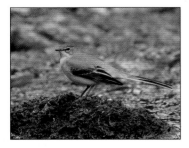

RIVERS

Mountain rivers are clean, fresh, and fast-moving. Young insects, called larvae, live among stones on the river bottom. They are food for river birds like the grey wagtail (left) and dipper.

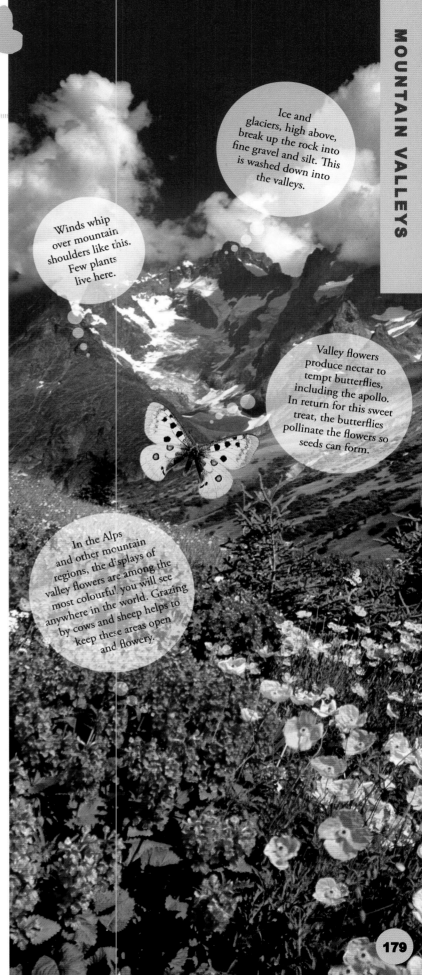

Ice and glaciers, high above, break up the rock into fine gravel and silt. This is washed down into the valleys.

Winds whip over mountain shoulders like this. Few plants live here.

Valley flowers produce nectar to tempt butterflies, including the apollo. In return for this sweet treat, the butterflies pollinate the flowers so seeds can form.

In the Alps and other mountain regions, the displays of valley flowers are among the most colourful you will see anywhere in the world. Grazing by cows and sheep helps to keep these areas open and flowery.

mountain valleys

MOUNTAINS

Mountain valleys are great places to visit as tourists. In winter, we can **ski** there. In summer, they offer *walks* or places to go *mountain biking* among lovely scenery. Tourism provides a **living** for local people. This helps to protect the valleys, because it shows that wild countryside can *bring in money*. But too many people can damage the countryside, and **climate change** might alter the environment for ever.

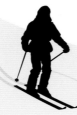
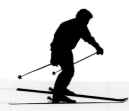

Lots of people have fun in mountain

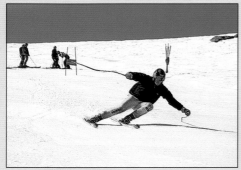

Going downhill
People want to enjoy skiing holidays in the mountains, but this means that trees have to be cut down to make ski runs. And when people crowd into skiing areas, wild animals run away. They hide in places where it is difficult for them to live, so they die.

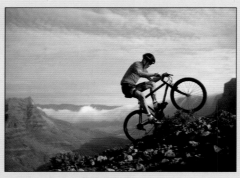

Mountain biking
Mountain walkers leave paths bare, so soil washes away. The tyres of mountain bikes do even more harm to paths. Proper bike tracks and good walking trails allow visitors to explore mountain valleys without causing damage.

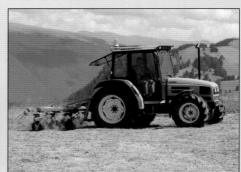

Modern farming
Old-fashioned farming helps maintain flower-rich meadows. The problem is that mountain farming is hard work and does not pay well, so farms are being bought up, joined together, and farmed with big, modern machines that destroy the meadows.

under threat

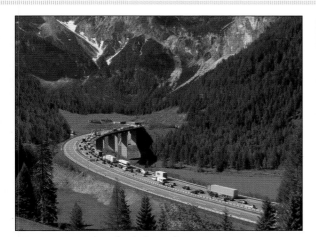

Mountain roads The Alps mountain range once stopped people moving between northern Europe and the Mediterranean. But now roads cut through the valleys, including this 192 km (119 mile) route south from Salzburg, Austria.

More and more cars In the early 1970s, 600,000 vehicles a year drove through the Brenner Pass in the Alps. In 1999, 6.5 million cars and lorries drove along this route. The road blocks the movement of wild animals, and traffic fumes damage forests and plants.

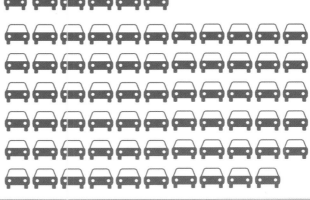

🚗 = 100,000 cars

1970 🚗 🚗 🚗 🚗 🚗 🚗

1999 🚗 🚗 🚗 🚗 🚗 🚗 🚗 🚗 🚗 🚗
🚗 🚗 🚗 🚗 🚗 🚗 🚗 🚗 🚗 🚗
🚗 🚗 🚗 🚗 🚗 🚗 🚗 🚗 🚗 🚗
🚗 🚗 🚗 🚗 🚗 🚗 🚗 🚗 🚗 🚗
🚗 🚗 🚗 🚗 🚗 🚗 🚗 🚗 🚗 🚗
🚗 🚗 🚗 🚗 🚗 🚗 🚗 🚗 🚗 🚗

valleys, but they're easily damaged.

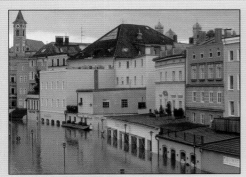

Flooding the lowlands
Scientists are worried that climate change will increase rain and snow fall in some areas. More snow and warmer winters might cause more avalanches. In spring, snow will melt quickly, rushing down rivers and causing floods in the flat plains below.

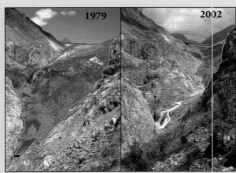

Shrinking glaciers
Although a few glaciers are still growing (because climate change is making more snow fall on them), most are shrinking in the warmer weather. They are melting faster than ever before. The picture above shows the dramatic shrinking of the Altsch glacier in the Swiss Alps.

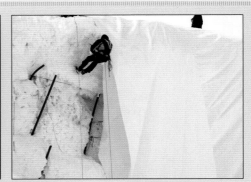

Wrapping a mountain
This glacier, above the Swiss ski resort of Andermatt, is melting. If it disappears, the local ski industry will suffer and people will lose their jobs, so the local government wrapped it in plastic foam during the summer to try to stop it melting away.

MAKING A DIFFERENCE

MOUNTAINS NEED OUR HELP!

Mountains around the world are protected as national parks and nature reserves – but some are protected in name only. They are marked on maps, but little is done to keep them safe.

Who's helping?

International organizations are helping local people make a living today, while caring for the environment to help people in the future. The United Nations works for a safe and peaceful future for people worldwide. The World Conservation Union is trying to do the same for plants and animals. It is trying to:

- **teach people** just how important mountains are for our future
- **celebrate** mountains, the wildlife, and people who live there
- develop **new ways of farming** that respect the land and keep it safe
- **protect** mountain habitats and wildlife

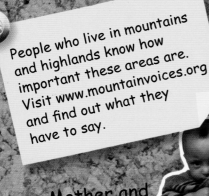

People who live in mountains and highlands know how important these areas are. Visit www.mountainvoices.org and find out what they have to say.

Mother and child from the Ethiopian highlands.

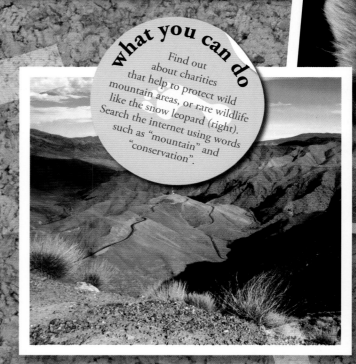

what you can do

Find out about charities that help to protect wild mountain areas, or rare wildlife like the snow leopard (right). Search the internet using words such as "mountain" and "conservation".

Mountains are incredibly useful — they provide more than half our fresh water, as well as timber and minerals, and their rivers make electricity.

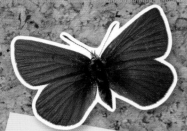

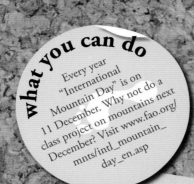

what you can do

Every year "International Mountain Day" is on 11 December. Why not do a class project on mountains next December? Visit www.fao.org/mnts/intl_mountain_day_en.asp

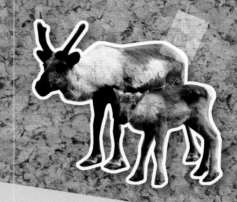

As the climate changes, butterflies are on the move. Help to record where they live now at www.butterfly-conservation.org

TAKE A MOUNTAIN HOLIDAY
Tourism helps to support the economies of mountain areas. If local people know that it is scenery and wildlife that attract people there, then they will try harder to look after them. By taking a holiday in the mountains, you are playing your part in helping them.

VISIT A RESERVE
When you are in the mountains, try to visit any nature reserves that are open to the public. If lots of people go to them, it is much easier to argue that they should be looked after — and anyway they're great places to visit!

SUPPORT THE MOUNTAINS!

KEEP YOUR EYES OPEN

If you do go walking in mountain areas, watch where you are going! Make sure you keep to the paths so you don't damage plants or disturb wildlife that

is not used to visitors. Only ride a mountain bike on routes that are specially marked out for mountain bikers.

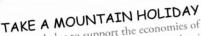

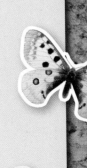

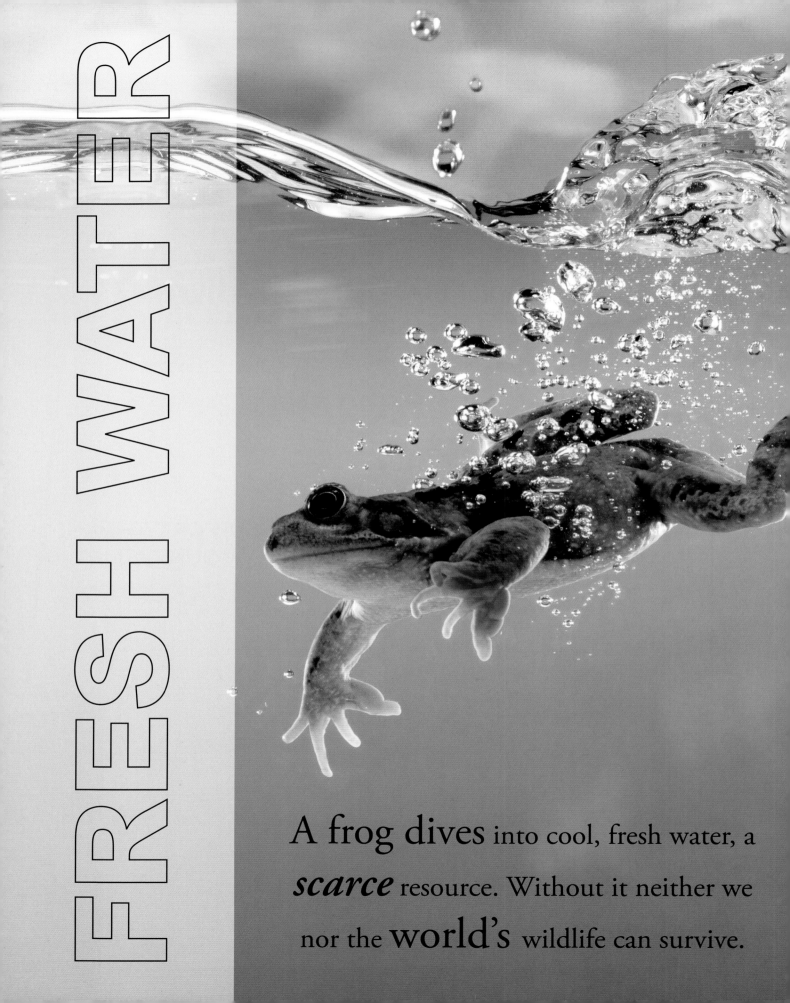

FRESH WATER

A frog dives into cool, fresh water, a *scarce* resource. Without it neither we nor the world's wildlife can survive.

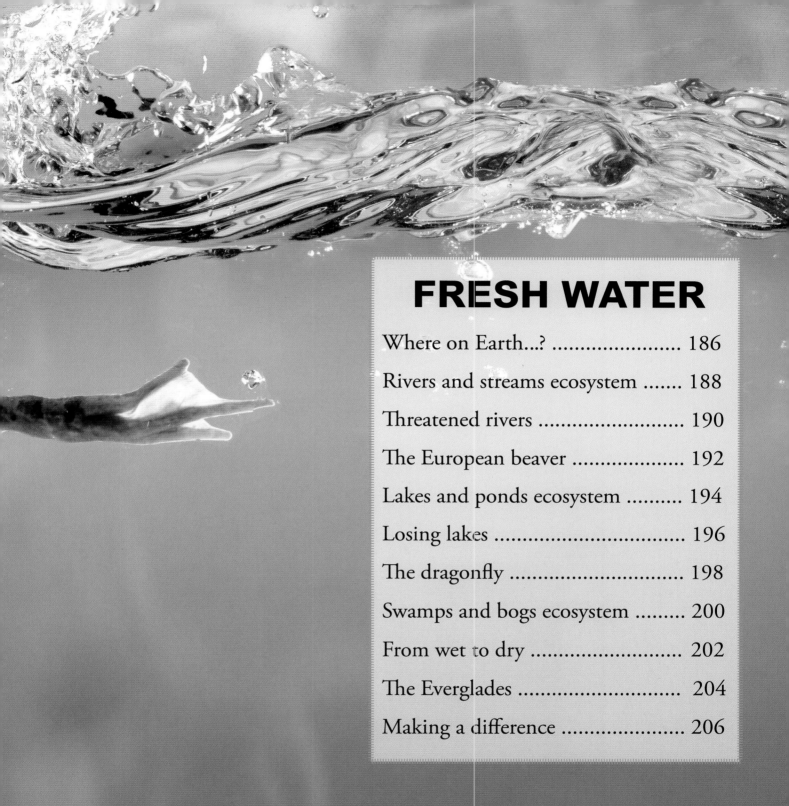

FRESH WATER

Still, clear water looks soft and inviting, but rushing water is powerful enough to carve out deep canyons and caves. Hidden beneath the surface of almost every body of water – large or small, still or rough – live many different animals and plants. Only the most polluted waters have no life at all.

where on earth...?

Fresh water is in short supply on Earth. Most is hidden away underground as groundwater or locked up in ice. What we see in rivers, lakes, and wetlands is less than one per cent of the total. That tiny amount is vital to us and to Earth's wildlife.

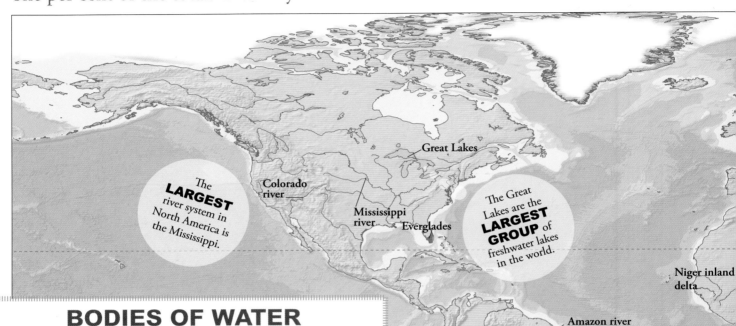

Great Lakes

Colorado river

Mississippi river

Everglades

The **LARGEST** river system in North America is the Mississippi.

The Great Lakes are the **LARGEST GROUP** of freshwater lakes in the world.

Niger inland delta

Amazon river

The Amazon is the **GREATEST** river with the largest basin and volume of water.

Pantanal wetlands

The Pantanal in Brazil also extends to Bolivia and Paraguay and is the **LARGEST** freshwater wetland covering 129,500 sq km (50,000 sq miles).

BODIES OF WATER

● LAKES AND PONDS
Some lakes are millions of years old but most are relatively young. They formed after the last ice age when water collected in hollows gouged out by ice. Eventually, most will shrink and disappear, especially those not fed by rivers and streams.

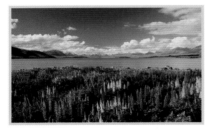

● RIVERS AND STREAMS
Every continent is criss-crossed by a network of rivers and streams that carry water from mountains and hills down to the sea. Dry continents like Australia have only a few large rivers, and Antarctic rivers flow for just a few weeks each summer.

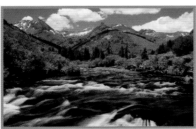

● WETLANDS
Bogs and fens have wet, peaty soils and are common in temperate regions like much of Europe and North America where rainfall is high. Swamps (wetland forests) are common in the tropics, while marshes (wet grasslands) are found worldwide.

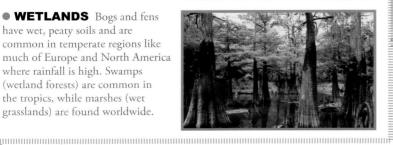

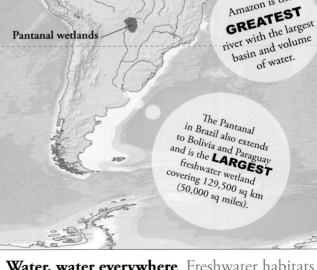

Water, water everywhere Freshwater habitats occur all over the world. There are even freshwater springs under the sea along the coast! Exactly what occurs where depends on geology and climate, especially rainfall.

GLACIERS

Glaciers hold nearly three quarters of the world's fresh water. They form when layers of snow fall in the same place. As they pile up, they turn into a lump of ice. Some glaciers end up in lakes where they slowly melt, adding more water to the lake.

HARDNESS

When it falls, rainwater is almost pure, but streams and rivers absorb minerals as they flow over and through the ground. Rivers in chalky areas pick up calcium and are said to have hard water. Rivers flowing over granite or peat have soft water.

NUTRIENTS

Mountain rivers and lakes are cold and contain little nitrogen and phosphorus so not much can grow in them. But too many nutrients from sewage or farm runoff can cause problems too. A healthy ecosystem needs the right balance of nutrients.

TEMPERATURE

The temperature of rivers and lakes depends on the climate, the depth, and the flow of water. Many rivers in or near the Arctic Circle freeze over during the winter. Some rivers and lakes in hot climates dry up and disappear in summer.

OXYGEN

A rushing bubbling stream picks up a lot more oxygen than a still lake. Stormy waves on large lakes also help to mix up the water and oxygenate it, but in summer deep lake bottoms can become stagnant and animals must move out or die.

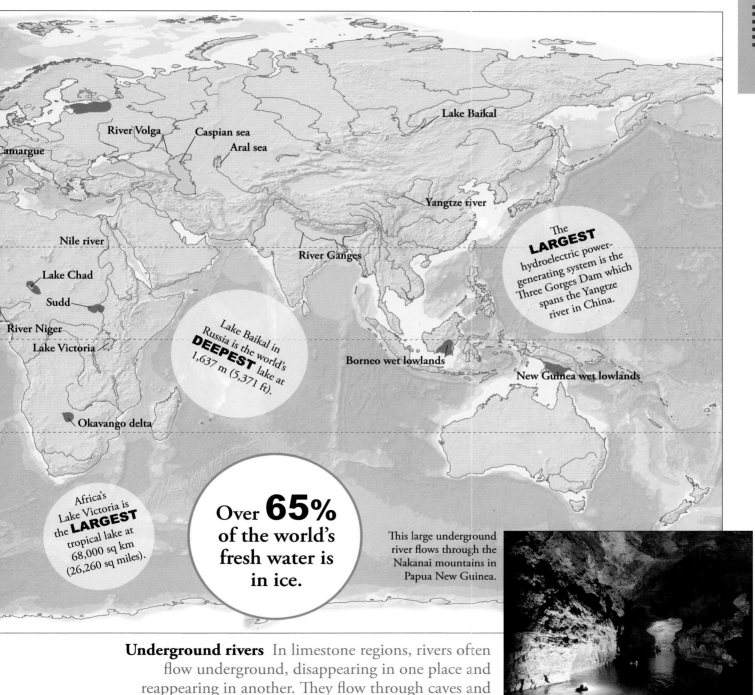

Lake Baikal

River Volga

Caspian sea

Aral sea

Camargue

Yangtze river

Nile river

River Ganges

Lake Chad

Sudd

River Niger

Lake Victoria

Okavango delta

The **LARGEST** hydroelectric power-generating system is the Three Gorges Dam which spans the Yangtze river in China.

Borneo wet lowlands

New Guinea wet lowlands

Lake Baikal in Russia is the world's **DEEPEST** lake at 1,637 m (5,371 ft).

Africa's Lake Victoria is the **LARGEST** tropical lake at 68,000 sq km (26,260 sq miles).

Over **65%** of the world's fresh water is in ice.

This large underground river flows through the Nakanai mountains in Papua New Guinea.

Underground rivers In limestone regions, rivers often flow underground, disappearing in one place and reappearing in another. They flow through caves and passages formed over time as the limestone is slowly dissolved by slightly acidic water.

rivers and streams

Much of our landscape as we know it today was shaped by rivers. The source (beginning) of a river may be a small spring, a lake, or melting ice. As the water flows downhill it collects into small rivulets in cracks and gullies. These merge together forming streams and eventually rivers. A river system with its many tributaries distributes water to a wide area giving life to plants, animals, and people.

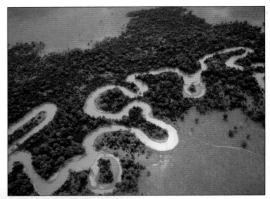

The natural winding course of this river in Kenya provides space for a wide variety of wildlife.

1 MELTING ICE

Melting ice and snow provide the starting point for many rivers. Meltwater is also important for sweeping away silt that has built up in rocky canyons.

The water in streams and rivers comes originally from rain and snow. Rainfall upstream affects river flow downstream.

3 DELTAS

Huge amounts of river silt are carried downstream, building up fertile land in large deltas.

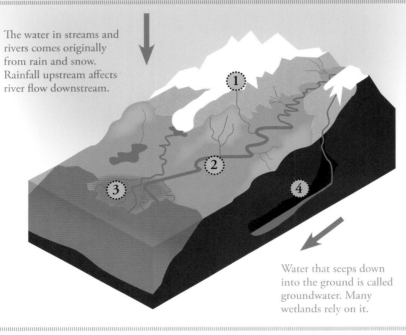

2 RIVERS AND STREAMS

Many small streams collect surface water from a wide area called a drainage basin. Then they join up to make bigger rivers.

Water that seeps down into the ground is called groundwater. Many wetlands rely on it.

4 UNDERGROUND RIVERS

Some rivers in limestone areas disappear underground to flow through caves and tunnels, then surface again further down.

Changing shape Rivers in lowland areas meander or curve across flatter ground. The water on the outside of a bend usually flows faster, cutting away the bank. Water on the inside of a bend flows slowly and drops its load of silt. That's how each curve gets bigger with time.

An ox bow lake is formed when the two ends of a river loop join and the loop gets pinched off.

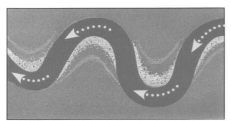

today

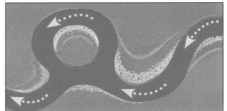

10 years

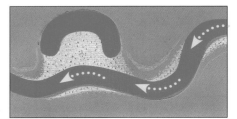

50 years

ecosystem

River flow The flow of a river changes along its length, and this affects both its landscape and wildlife. Fast water wears down rocks and is a challenging place to live. Slow water drops silt, but is full of nutrients.

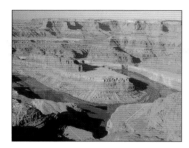

WATER SCULPTURE
Over millions of years, the Colorado River, USA, has cut down through layers of colourful rocks to form more than 1,600 km (1,000 miles) of canyons including the Grand Canyon.

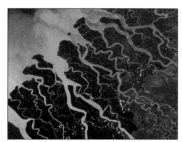

RIVER'S END
The Ganges, like most rivers, finishes its journey slowly through a wide delta. The river divides into a network of channels – like the veins in a hand – as it flows into the Bay of Bengal.

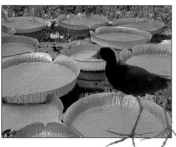

RIVER HUNTERS
Giant water lilies in Amazon backwaters provide stepping stones for the jacana, or lily trotter, as it probes for water insects. Predators lurk both above and below the slow-flowing, murky water.

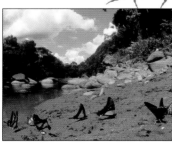

ALONG THE EDGE
River banks appear and disappear with the water flow rather like ocean shores with the tide. When the water is low, Amazonian butterflies suck up vital minerals from the mud. Other animals come to hunt and drink.

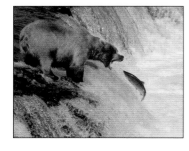

IN THE FAST LANE
Brown bears enjoy a feast of salmon as the fish fling themselves up waterfalls to reach the gravelly headwaters where they lay their eggs. Tumbling water provides these energetic fish with plenty of oxygen.

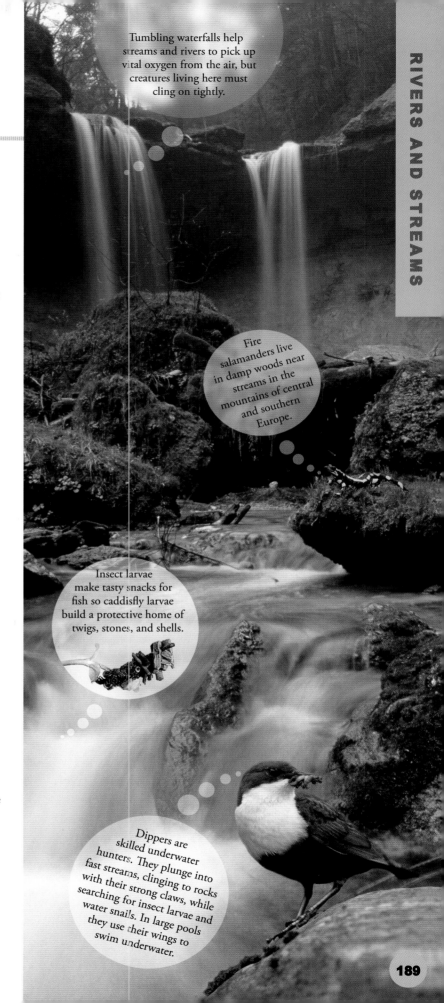

Tumbling waterfalls help streams and rivers to pick up vital oxygen from the air, but creatures living here must cling on tightly.

Fire salamanders live in damp woods near streams in the mountains of central and southern Europe.

Insect larvae make tasty snacks for fish so caddisfly larvae build a protective home of twigs, stones, and shells.

Dippers are skilled underwater hunters. They plunge into fast streams, clinging to rocks with their strong claws, while searching for insect larvae and water snails. In large pools they use their wings to swim underwater.

189

threatened rivers

There are very few natural rivers left in the world. The flow and *course* of most rivers have been altered by dams and engineering works, which provide water and stop flooding. Changing or **polluting** one part of a river can affect wildlife and people living many miles downstream. Some rivers, such as London's River Thames, have been successfully cleaned up.

Just 21 out of 177 of the world's longest rivers

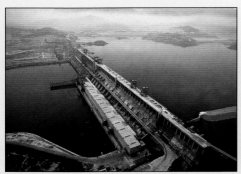

Damming rivers China's Three Gorges dam across the Yangtze River is one of the world's largest dams. It was built to prevent flooding and to generate clean, renewable hydroelectric power. Above the dam, small streams are now deep rivers and many people have lost their homes.

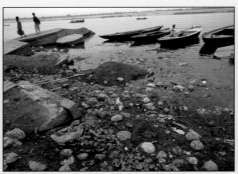

Polluted rivers Many rivers around the world are polluted with sewage, industrial waste, and farm runoff. In some stretches of India's River Ganges fish and other wildlife are dying due to low oxygen levels, and the water is dirty enough to make swimming dangerous.

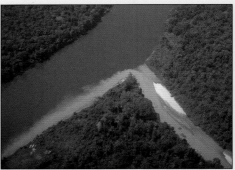

Muddied rivers Silt carried by rivers is important for building up fertile floodplains and deltas downstream. But too much silt smothers plants and makes it difficult for fish and birds to hunt. Here, soil washes into the Amazon River as a result of rainforest trees being cut down.

Abstraction in the River Nile Ten countries depend on water from the 6,700 km (4,160 miles) of the world's longest river. The White Nile and Blue Nile branches flow through Uganda, Ethiopia, Sudan, and Egypt, and the river basin also drains water from Tanzania, Burundi, Rwanda, Republic of Congo, Kenya, and Eritrea. The river flow reduces along its route, as water is taken out (abstracted) by each country.

Egypt Egypt is the largest user of Nile water, mainly for crop irrigation. International agreements help to make sure upstream countries allow enough Nile water to reach Egypt. But higher evaporation due to climate change and greater use of water by other developing Nile-basin countries will reduce the flow and may cause further conflict.

Other countries By 2025, the population of all the Nile-basin countries is expected to be double what it was in 1995. Each country will need more water so less will be left for wildlife and people in each downstream country.

Sudan The White Nile and Blue Nile join at Khartoum in Sudan. Much of Sudan is desert but by building irrigation dams, Sudan grows cotton for export, a vital source of revenue.

Uganda The River Nile begins at the northern end of Lake Victoria in Uganda. Many other streams and rivers from surrounding countries flow into the lake.

Ethiopia The Blue Nile provides much of the water used by Sudan and Egypt in the summer. Seasonal rainfall in the Ethiopian highlands feeds into Lake Tana, the source of this major Nile tributary.

Nile

White Nile

Blue Nile

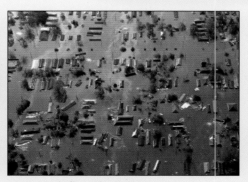

still flow freely from source to sea.

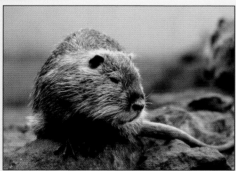

Alien invasion Coypu are dog-sized rodents from South Africa. A few escaped from fur farms in East Anglia, UK, in around 1929 and invaded nearby rivers and fens. They damaged river banks and destroyed reed beds for 50 years before they were finally exterminated.

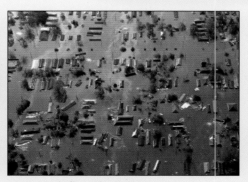

Natural flood plains Rivers flow along channels they have carved out, but spill over onto natural flood plains after heavy rain. New Orleans, built on a low-lying flood plain, suffered terrible flooding when its flood defences gave way during Hurricane Katrina in 2005.

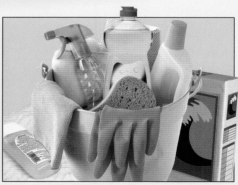

Household impact Many cleaning products contain hard-to-break-down chemicals called phosphates. These find their way into rivers causing a great deal of damage.

 Encourage your parents to shop for ecologically friendly cleaning products with no phosphates.

the european beaver

CONSERVATIONISTS ATTEMPT TO RETURN BEAVERS TO THEIR NATURAL HABITAT AFTER DECADES OF EXTINCTION IN THE WILD

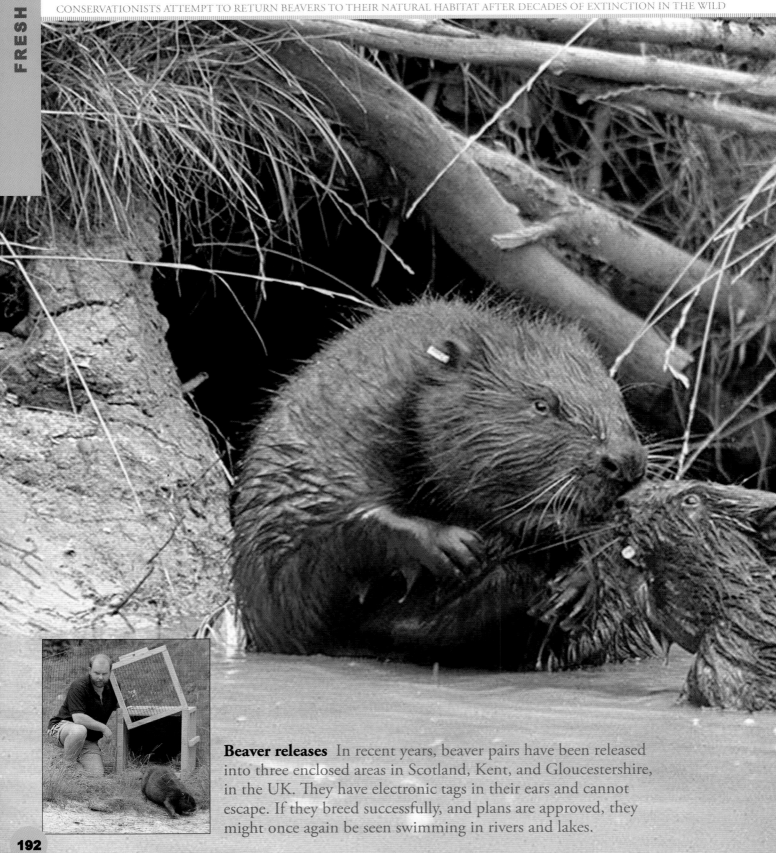

Beaver releases In recent years, beaver pairs have been released into three enclosed areas in Scotland, Kent, and Gloucestershire, in the UK. They have electronic tags in their ears and cannot escape. If they breed successfully, and plans are approved, they might once again be seen swimming in rivers and lakes.

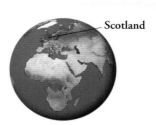

If trials succeed, Scotland may be the next European country to re-introduce beavers into the wild.

Scotland

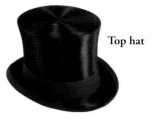

Top hats made from beaver skin came into fashion in Europe and America in the 1780s.

Top hat

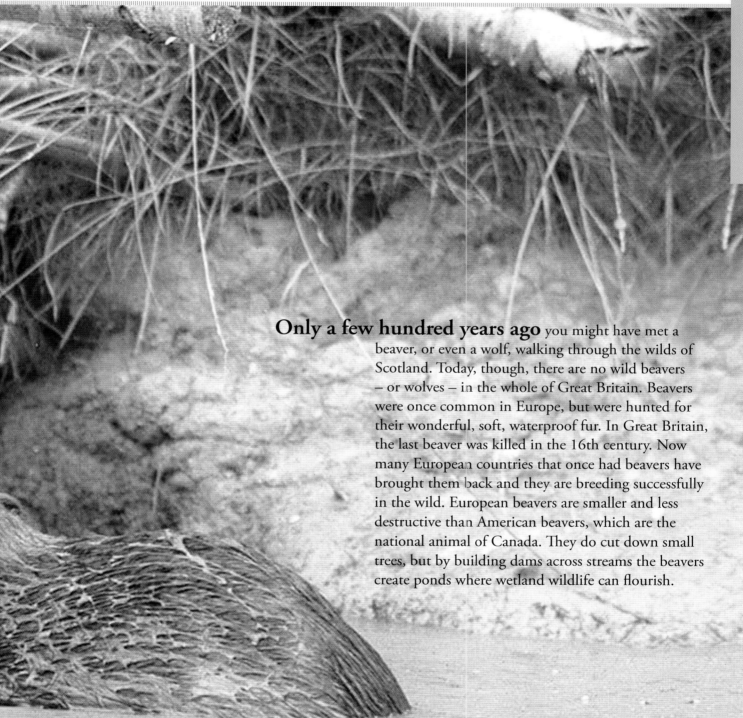

Only a few hundred years ago you might have met a beaver, or even a wolf, walking through the wilds of Scotland. Today, though, there are no wild beavers – or wolves – in the whole of Great Britain. Beavers were once common in Europe, but were hunted for their wonderful, soft, waterproof fur. In Great Britain, the last beaver was killed in the 16th century. Now many European countries that once had beavers have brought them back and they are breeding successfully in the wild. European beavers are smaller and less destructive than American beavers, which are the national animal of Canada. They do cut down small trees, but by building dams across streams the beavers create ponds where wetland wildlife can flourish.

lakes **and** ponds

Lakes and ponds are bodies of still, fresh water that are home to a huge variety of wildlife. Millions of people also rely on lakes for drinking water, fishing, and fun. They vary in size from the immense Lake Superior in North America to tiny pools. Small ponds and lakes in lowland areas are often muddy and full of nutrients from the surrounding land. Some fish survive in stagnant water by gulping air into special air sacs.

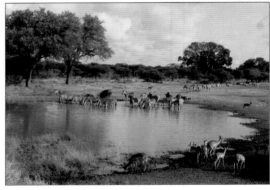

A spring-fed pool in the Kruger National Park, South Africa, draws animals in to drink, wallow, and hunt.

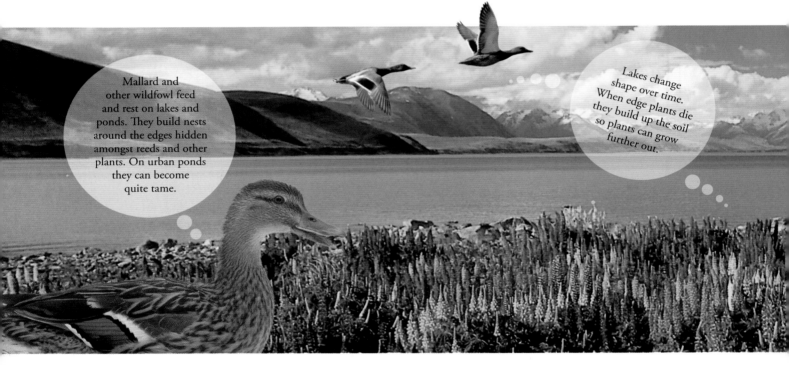

Mallard and other wildfowl feed and rest on lakes and ponds. They build nests around the edges hidden amongst reeds and other plants. On urban ponds they can become quite tame.

Lakes change shape over time. When edge plants die they build up the soil so plants can grow further out.

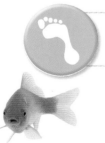

Don't release any pet fish, turtles, or terrapins into the wild where they can upset the fragile ecosystem.

LAKE BAIKAL
Lake Baikal in the heart of Siberia, Russia, at 1,637m (5,371 ft) deep, is the deepest lake in the world. It also holds around a fifth of the Earth's surface fresh water.

Special seals Baikal seals are unique in living permanently in fresh water. They are endemic (unique) to Lake Baikal and cannot be found anywhere else. Nearly half the fish in Lake Baikal are also endemic. The number of seals is going down because people hunt them for their meat and fur. Disease and pollution add to their problems.

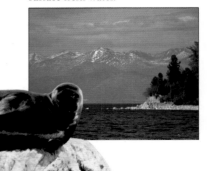

ecosystem

SUN

OSPREYS
Ospreys hunt over lakes, snatching up pike and other fish.

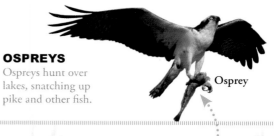

Osprey

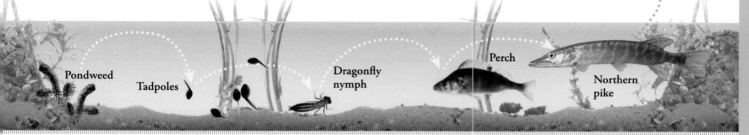

Pondweed

Tadpoles

Dragonfly nymph

Perch

Northern pike

PLANT LIFE
Submerged plants grow lushly in shallow, well-lit water where they form the basis of the food chain. Plant plankton also provide food.

AMPHIBIANS
Young tadpoles graze on soft plant material and debris and, when older, eat injured tadpoles and other animals. Adult newts eat tadpoles.

POND NYMPHS
Many types of insects, including dragonfly nymphs, eat tadpoles. These predators hunt underwater for years then change into flying adults.

COARSE FISH
Young perch feed on tiny plankton animals and later grow fat on insect larvae. As they get bigger they eat other small fish, sometimes even their own young.

TOP PREDATORS
Pike are experts at stalking perch and other fish. They have hundreds of small teeth and can also snap up frogs, voles, and even ducklings.

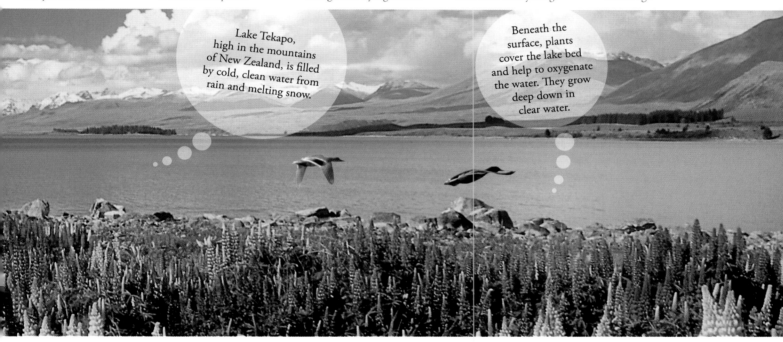

Lake Tekapo, high in the mountains of New Zealand, is filled by cold, clean water from rain and melting snow.

Beneath the surface, plants cover the lake bed and help to oxygenate the water. They grow deep down in clear water.

STILL LIFE
Pond snails living in stagnant water have no gills. Instead, they come to the surface and breathe air using a simple lung. They also absorb oxygen from the water through their skin.

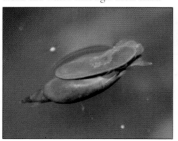

SALT LAKES
Salt Lake in Utah, USA is saltier than the sea! Water with mineral salts flows in but not out of the lake, and the Sun evaporates the water. In winter the lake freezes as shown here.

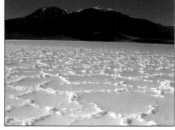

HERE TODAY GONE TOMORROW
Fairy shrimps appear as if by magic in temporary pools. They hatch from tiny eggs that are so tough they can survive for years in dried out mud.

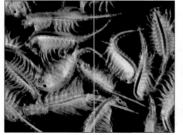

LAKE TITICACA
The Peruvian Uros people live on Lake Titicaca 4,000 m (13,000 ft) above sea level. They build their homes on floating islands and fish from boats crafted entirely from reeds.

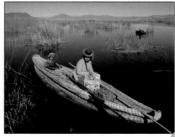

losing lakes

Many towns and cities around the world have **grown** up around lakes, which provide a ready *supply* of water and food, especially *fish*. Taking **too much** water out of the lakes for **industry** and farming, and putting too much **waste** back in affects both people and wildlife. Climate change can cause lakes to shrink or *dry up* if there is less rainfall. Shrinking lakes can also become more salty as minerals in the water are *concentrated.*

Reducing water use in homes, industry,

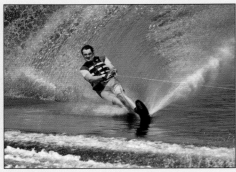

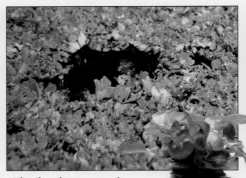

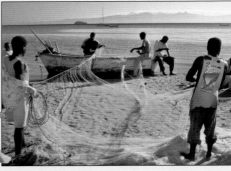

Water sports Lakes are great places for holiday activities. Lake Geneva in Switzerland used to be very polluted from nearby industrial cities. Tourists complained and eventually the lake was cleaned up. But sewage from tourist boats and hotels can still pollute lakes.

Choked up 19th-century travellers to Brazil admired the lovely water hyacinth and took plants back to grow at home. Some escaped into the wild. Now in Africa many lakes are choked by this fast-growing invader.

Fishing problems Many people live around the shores of Lake Malawi in Africa. They take water and fish to eat from the lake. But as the human population goes up, they need more fish, so fish numbers are going down. Birds that feed on fish are also becoming scarce.

ecosystem

In the past, wetland areas provided a living for local people. They caught fish, shot wildfowl, dug peat for fuel, and cut reeds.

Wetland use Today wetland areas are more likely to be used for walking, sailing, and watching wildlife, but reeds are still cut for thatching houses.

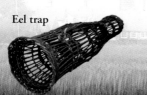
Eel trap

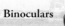

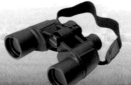
Binoculars

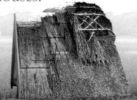
House made of reeds

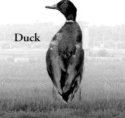
Duck

EEL FISHING
Eels are common in wetland pools and waterways. They are caught in special traps and fyke nets. Bait tempts the eels into these tunnel-shaped structures.

RECREATION
Wetlands are excellent for bird watching. In summer, bitterns, harriers, and warblers nest in the tall reeds, while in winter ducks and geese feed in flooded areas.

REEDS FOR THATCHING
Tall, flexible stems of Norfolk reed are ideal for thatching houses. Reeds harvested from wetland nature reserves re-grow quickly and help fund conservation work.

WILDFOWL FOR FOOD
In the past, people in wetland areas ate ducks, geese, and even swans. Today wildfowl are hunted for sport while farmed birds provide us with food.

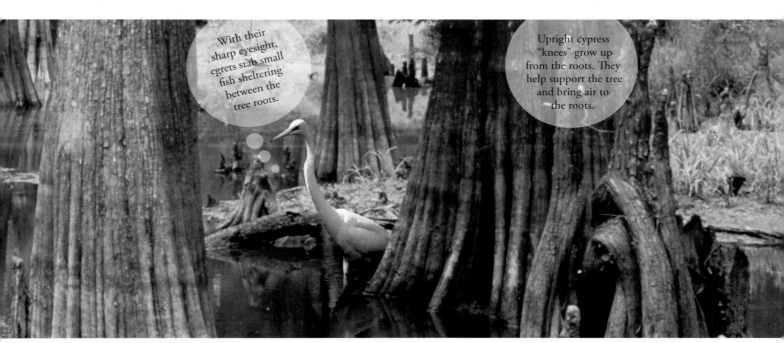

With their sharp eyesight, egrets stab small fish sheltering between the tree roots.

Upright cypress "knees" grow up from the roots. They help support the tree and bring air to the roots.

BOGGED DOWN
In 1984, peat cutters at a moor in Cheshire found the remains of 2,000-year-old "Lindow man". He had been killed and thrown into a bog, where acidic water preserved him.

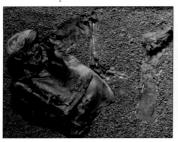

CARNIVOROUS PLANTS
Plants living in boggy places can get extra nutrients from insect prey. The leaves of the Venus fly-trap snap shut when a fly lands on them. The prisoner is dissolved and absorbed.

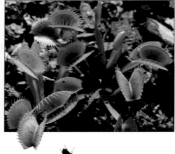

CAMARGUE HORSES
Herds of white horses have lived in the French Camargue for centuries. This vast plain of marshlands, lakes, and reedbeds is one of Europe's most important wetlands.

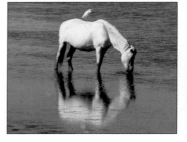

COASTAL WETLANDS
Tropical-island wetlands are rich in wildlife. The Caroni swamp in Trinidad has freshwater marshes, tidal mangroves, and lagoons where scarlet ibis and howler monkeys live.

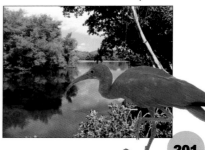

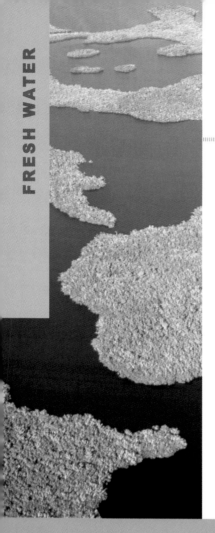

Wet and wild areas support a huge variety of wildlife from birds to frogs.

from wet...

Wetlands are often thought of as wasteland – and many have been drained, transforming them from wild, **wet** areas to tame, rich farmland. Recently, developed countries have begun restoring

What has happened?
As the world's population increases, more and more land is needed for housing, agriculture, and industry. Wetland areas are drained and dams are built to store water for irrigation and to prevent flooding.

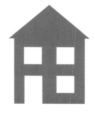

Building homes on floodplains and deltas has destroyed many wetlands.

Farming areas of fen and marsh has turned these wetlands into dry land.

The world has lost as much as 50%

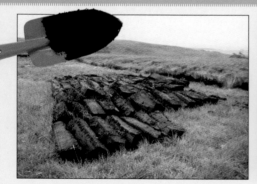

Peat cutting Peat compost helps gardeners to keep their soil moist and plants grow well in it. But demand for peat compost has encouraged commercial cutting, and entire peat bogs and their wildlife are being destroyed.

Encourage your parents to buy peat-free compost, which does not contribute to the destruction of wetlands.

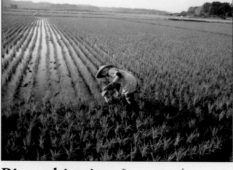

Rice cultivation In central California, USA, large areas of wetland have been drained to grow wheat and oats. But now some farmers are growing rice in wet fields. Flooding the fields in the winter after harvest provides a temporary home to migrating ducks and geese.

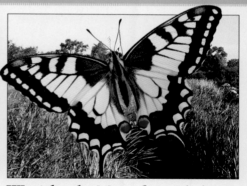

Wet islands Many formerly huge European wetlands are now only small islands dotted among dry farmland. In the UK, the rare swallowtail butterfly has been stranded in the lakes and marshes of the Norfolk Broads. Now there are plans to re-create some larger wetland areas.

...to dry

Once people move in, the water must be drained or contained.

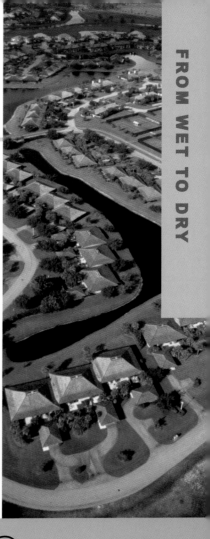

them by re-flooding drained **farmland**. This can prevent flooding elsewhere, as storm water is soaked up. Also, as in the Florida Everglades of the USA, restored wetlands benefit *wildlife* and tourism.

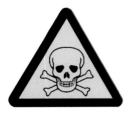

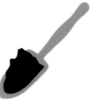

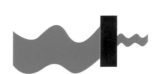

Pollution from homes and industry is spread by rivers and streams.

Dams prevent seasonal floods essential for many wetland areas.

Peat excavation has destroyed bogs that took thousands of years to form.

# of its wetlands in the last 100 years.

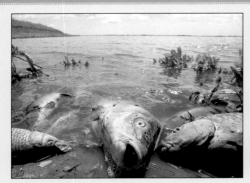

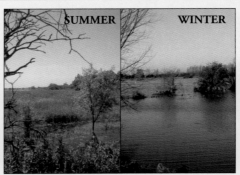

SUMMER WINTER

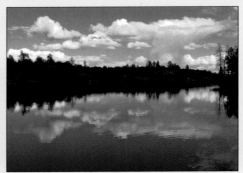

Polluted wetlands Important wetlands need a wide buffer zone around them to prevent pollution. In 1998 a mining dam broke in Spain. Millions of tonnes of toxic waste flooded into nearby rivers and was carried into the Donana nature park, where it killed many fish.

Dry to wet In summer, cattle graze, hay is made, and birds nest in the Ouse Washes, UK. In winter, water from rivers on each side is pumped into the area to save farmland from flooding. Thousands of swans, geese, and ducks fly into this seasonal wetland.

Constructed wetlands Large wetlands can purify water, a very useful service. At Show Low in northeastern Arizona, lakes and marshes are the final part of a big natural scheme to clean waste water. The resulting wetland is very attractive to wildlife – a double benefit.

the everglades

MORE THAN HALF THE EVERGLADES WETLANDS HAVE BEEN LOST TO AGRICULTURE AND DEVELOPMENT

Imagine finding an alligator in your swimming pool! That's a problem faced by some residents of Florida, USA. Alligator numbers have grown since hunting ended in 1967, but the human population has risen too – bad news for the Everglades that cover most of southern Florida. This wet wilderness depends on water flowing from Lake Okeechobee in the north towards the Gulf of Mexico in the south, a flow now interrupted by land drainage for housing, flood prevention, and city water supplies.

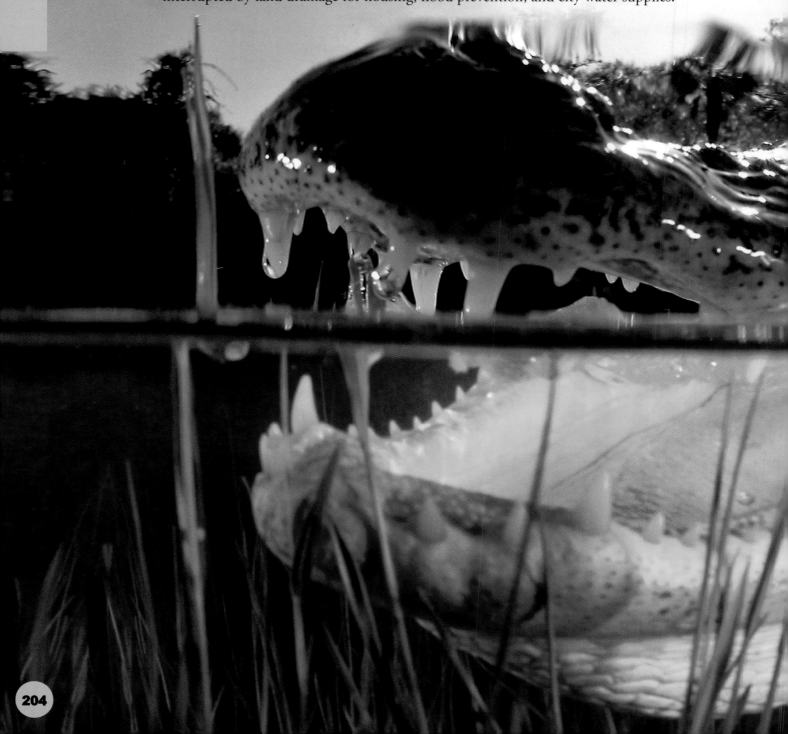

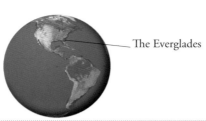

The restoration plan for the Everglades (CERP) covers a much wider area than the Everglades themselves.

The Everglades

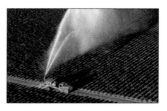

Tomatoes need a lot of water to grow. In southern Florida, crops are often irrigated with huge amounts of water pumped out of wells. But diverting this well water onto the fields reduces the natural flow of water heading towards the Everglades.

Now an ambitious plan is underway to help both people and wildlife. The Comprehensive Everglades Restoration Plan (CERP) aims to improve the flow of water to the Everglades, provide people and farms with water, and prevent flooding. It will cost billions of dollars and take at least twenty years to complete, but the funding for this ambitious project is already starting to dry up.

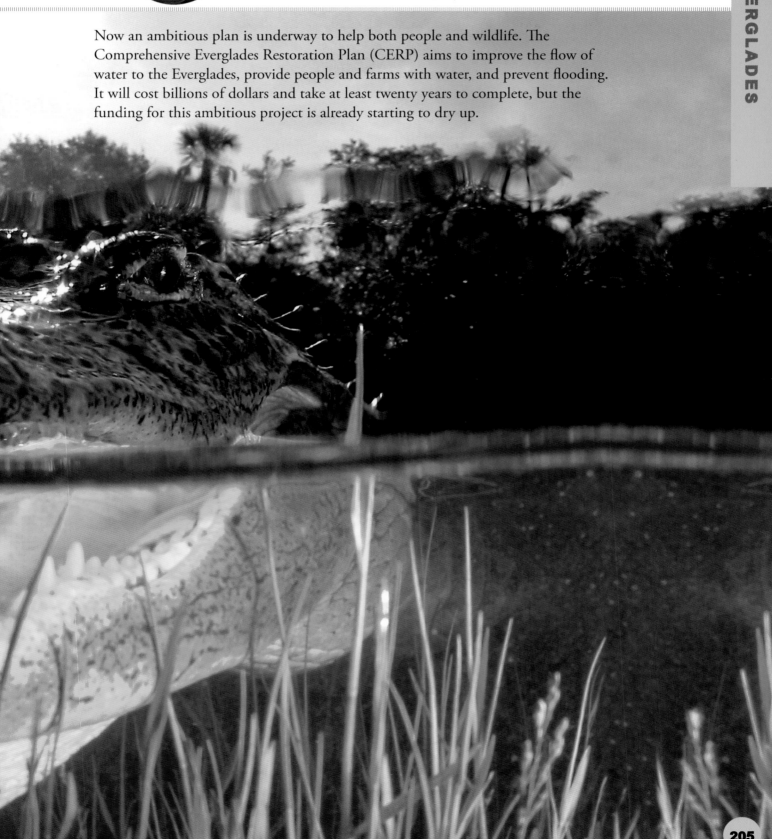

MAKING A DIFFERENCE

Who's helping and how

* Governments The USA's Clean Water Act (1977) set out to stop factories and farms polluting lakes and rivers. It has been regularly updated and improved ever since.

* Local governments Inner-city rivers are being cleaned up. London's River Thames, once highly polluted, is home to salmon and other wildlife once more.

* Construction companies Some new houses are built with the technology to recycle "grey" (dirty) water or rainwater so it can be used to flush the toilet.

* Inventors Removing the salt from seawater so it can be used for drinking takes a lot of energy, but inventors are finding ways to do this using the power of the Sun.

what you can do
Some toads and frogs return to the lake where they were born to mate and lay their eggs. Join a wildlife group that helps these creatures reach their destination safely.

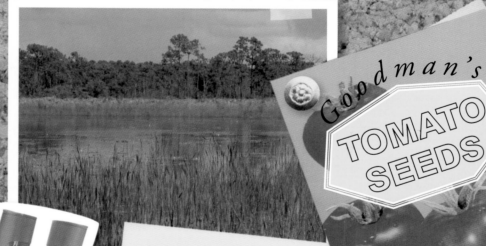

SHOPPING

- Washing-up liquid *
- Washing powder *
- Shower gel *
- Toilet cleaner *
- Fish for supper
(from sustainable source)
- Boots for community
clean-up day

*= eco-friendly

Arrange to visit a nature reserve.

Goodman's TOMATO SEEDS

It's not all bad news. Take action in your own home and neighbourhood. If everyone did this, the Earth would be much healthier.

what you can do
Instead of buying a bottle of water when you're out and about, get into the habit of carrying a re-useable flask or bottle.

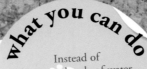

TERRIFIC TOILET
Only £150
It's terrific!

Uses only 6 litres per flush
(Some toilets use a massive 13 litres)

When you need a new loo, get one that uses less water. Meanwhile, put a brick in the cistern to save water.

Friends of Wimble Lake
Wimblebury-on-the-Water
Northeasterham
England

Invitation

Dear neighbour,

Let's make Wimble Lake sparkle!

Please join us on Saturday 7th July at 1pm for a community clean-up of the lake, followed by a barbecue at 6pm.

See you there!

what you can do
Build a pond in your back garden to attract frogs, insects, and plants whose habitats are being destroyed.

TURN FRONT GARDEN INTO A DRIVEWAY?

PROS	CONS
- No more parking problems - No need to mow lawn - Easier to unload shopping	- Lose flowers and apple tree - Less pretty view from living room - No more playing in front garden - Need good drainage as rain won't be able to drain into lawn

Don't do it!

Get some peat-free compost to plant seeds.

what you can do
Visit a wetlands nature reserve. You enjoy the wildlife, and your entrance fee will help to protect the creatures and maintain the environment.

4   THE DAILY NEWS
16th April 2007

AMAZON SWIMMER
THE WORLD NEEDS CLEAN RIVERS

On 8th April 2007, Slovenian marathon swimmer Martin Strel became the first person to swim the entire 6,400 km (4,000 miles) of the Amazon. Of his epic 66-day feat, the swimmer said "My aim was to promote a message of clean rivers, clean water and friendship, because these rivers and water have to stay clean, otherwise the world will surely collapse. The Amazon river is still very clean, local people use it as a natural resource and I believe it should stay clean forever."

Water shortage predicted for summer
Scientists working at the Meteorological Office are predicting an unusually dry summer. River levels have already dropped. Spring

Environment minister Jo Smith hinted hosepipe bans were

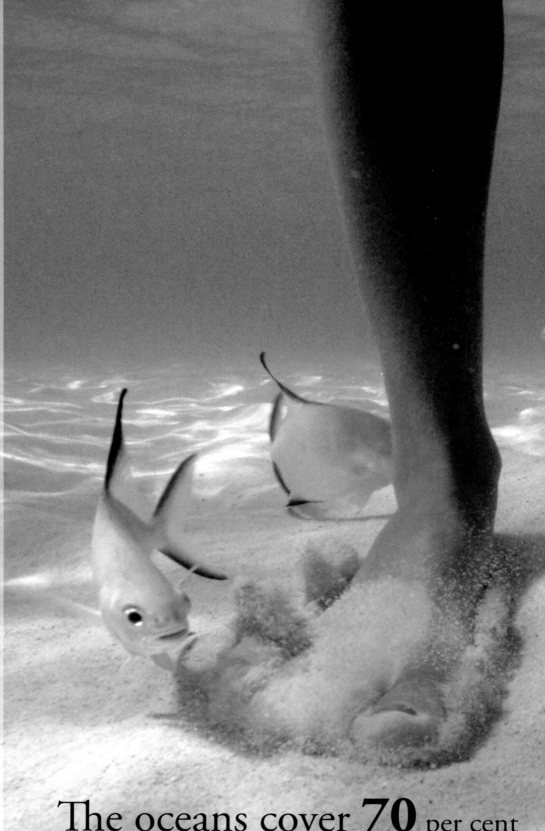

OCEANS

The oceans cover **70** per cent of our planet. Yet they are the most *mysterious* and unexplored part of it.

Global conveyor belt

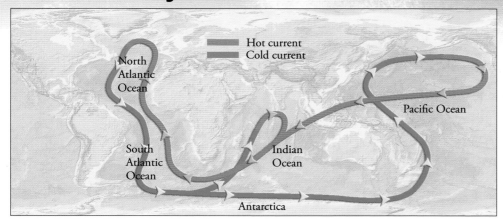

Hot current
Cold current

North Atlantic Ocean

Pacific Ocean

South Atlantic Ocean

Indian Ocean

Antarctica

Water circulates slowly through the ocean like a giant factory conveyor belt. Heavy cold water sinks deep into the North Atlantic and flows south towards Antarctica. It then flows east and north into the Indian and Pacific oceans, then back west into the Atlantic.

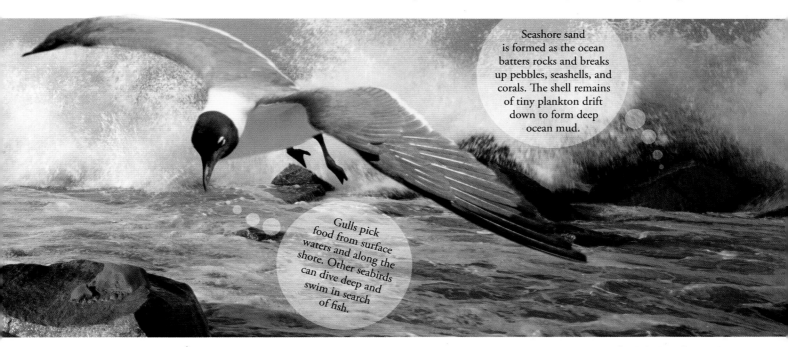

A mass of seawater takes 1,000 years to complete a lap.

Seashore sand is formed as the ocean batters rocks and breaks up pebbles, seashells, and corals. The shell remains of tiny plankton drift down to form deep ocean mud.

Gulls pick food from surface waters and along the shore. Other seabirds can dive deep and swim in search of fish.

VERTICAL CURRENTS
When warm and cold ocean currents meet, they push water down or up. Upwelling brings nutrients from the seabed to the surface. This causes plankton to grow, producing food for fish and other creatures.

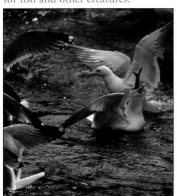

ATLANTIC CONVEYOR
The Atlantic Conveyor is a system of currents that includes the Gulf Stream. It keeps western Europe, including the west coast of Ireland (below), warm by carrying warm water north from the tropics.

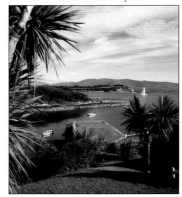

OCEAN FOOD
Life in the ocean is fuelled by floating plant plankton. A complex food web links animals at all depths to the plankton at the surface. Plant plankton makes food using the Sun's energy.

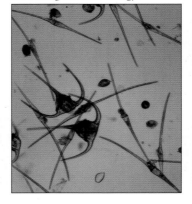

TIDAL CURRENTS
Tides are the regular in-and-out movements of the ocean from the shore. They are caused by the pulling effect (gravity) of the Moon and Sun. Whirlpools can form when water is pulled through narrow channels.

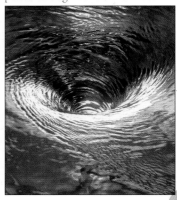

using the ocean

The way we use the ocean has *changed* over centuries. More people now live on the coast and there is more **industry** there too. In the developed world, *traditional* fishing has mostly

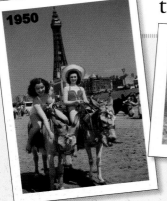
1950

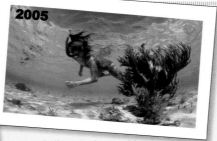
2005

Snorkelling in the Caribbean is no longer just a dream.

"I do like to be beside the seaside..."
Seaside holidays became very popular in Britain after 1938, when workers were first entitled to paid holidays. People visited seaside towns such as Blackpool to stroll along the beach in the bracing air. Now cheap air travel has changed all this.

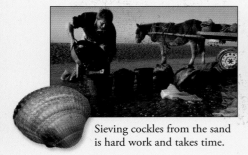

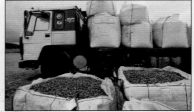

Sieving cockles from the sand is hard work and takes time.

Harvesting machines can destroy cockle beds if collecting is unrestricted.

Food for free People all over the world have collected wild shellfish since early times. Shellfish were traditionally dug out by hand leaving small ones behind to grow and reproduce. Modern commercial machines dig or suck out huge numbers.

Empty cockle shells

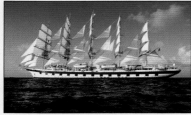

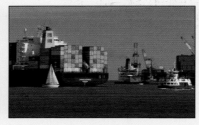

Clipper ships traded goods all over the world in the 19th century.

Modern container ships carry huge amounts of cargo.

Sailing the seas Travelling by sailing ship used to mean months at sea – if disease or pirates didn't get you! – but sailing ships used no fuel and wrecks caused little pollution. Today, ships crossing our oceans are almost all fuelled by oil. Oil pollution is widespread and shipwrecks can destroy wildlife.

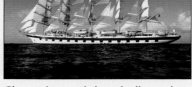

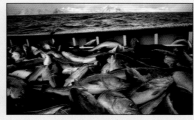

Traditional fishing continues in India.

Modern ships allow fishing far out to sea in deep water.

Hook, line, and sinker Over the past two centuries, fishing methods have changed dramatically. Fishing communities used to catch enough fish to supply their families and local markets. Without fridges the catch could not be sent very far. Today frozen and canned fish can be sent anywhere.

given way to large-scale **commercial** fishing. However, fishing **communities** in some parts of the world still live in *harmony* with the sea, taking only enough for their own needs. Where this **balance** has been lost, the ocean is suffering. Governments are introducing **regulations** to help, such as laws controlling the amount of untreated sewage that can be released into the sea.

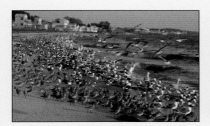
Flocks of gulls and knots are a common sight in estuaries.

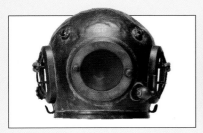
This estuary in Barcelona is now an important Spanish port.

Estuary havens Estuaries – the tidal parts of a river – have always provided shelter and food for wading birds, ducks, and geese. Their rich muddy shores are full of juicy worms and shellfish, and migrating birds use them like motorway service stations. Now many large estuaries have developed into industrial ports.

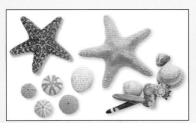
Drying and preserving seashore animals was a popular Victorian pastime.

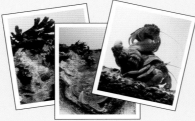
Cameras capture the beauty of the seashore without damage.

Learning from the seashore Seashores provide wonderful outdoor classrooms for the study of marine life. In the 1800s, naturalists wrote about the wonders of the seashore. Many people were inspired to visit the coast, but popular sites were damaged. Now students mostly take photographs.

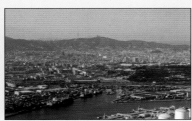
Early divers received air pumped down a tube from the surface.

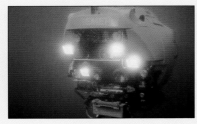
The French Nautile submersible can reach depths of 6,000 m (20,000 ft).

Ocean exploration It has always been difficult to explore under the ocean. Early diving suits were heavy and clumsy and scientific study of the oceans has lagged far behind that on land. Modern submersibles and ROVs (Remotely Operated Vehicles) can explore and film the deep ocean.

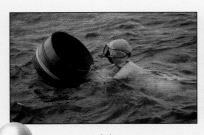
Few pearl divers remain, as pearl oysters are now farmed.

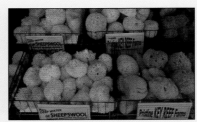
Natural bath sponges are still harvested but today they are rare.

Riches from the sea Pearls and sponges have been harvested from the sea for centuries. Pearl divers could reach amazing depths with no air supply. Use of modern diving gear has resulted in over-collection of valuable corals and sponges.

Natural sponge

coastal ecosystem

The coastal environment is an ever-changing place where the land meets the ocean. Coasts and shores are formed by ocean waves and the geology of the area. Hard granite cliffs can resist the sea and remain unchanged for hundreds of years. However, softer rocks, sand, and mud are easily worn away. Coastal plant communities, such as saltmarshes, help protect the coast by shielding it from the impact of waves and weather.

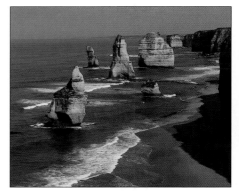

Battering waves carve dramatic rocky stacks and headlands from coastal cliffs. Here, soft limestone cliffs off southeast Australia have worn away to form twelve tall islands called the Apostles.

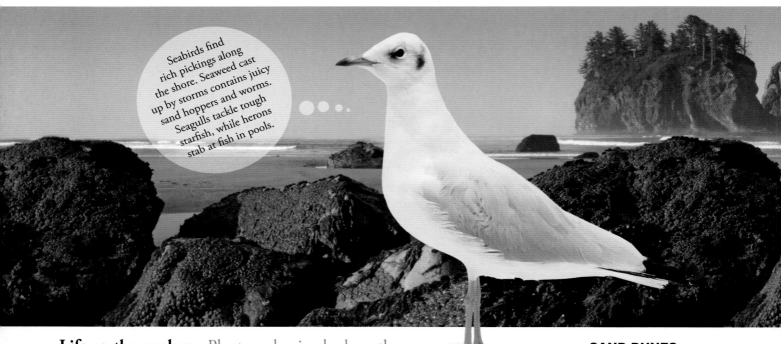

Seabirds find rich pickings along the shore. Seaweed cast up by storms contains juicy sand hoppers and worms. Seagulls tackle tough starfish, while herons stab at fish in pools.

Life on the seashore Plants and animals along the water's edge are mainly those that can tolerate salt spray and occasional submergence in the sea. Those further inland are marine (sea) plants and animals that have adapted to living out of water for a while.

Black-headed gulls are common in the northern hemisphere. They have white heads in winter.

The sea's edge It's a tough life surviving between land and sea. Every tide washes in a fresh supply of food, but also brings in oil and rubbish. Waves roll pebbles and rocks around crushing animals and plants. Wind and sun dry everything out. Yet shores around the world support an amazing variety of life.

SAND DUNES
Low tides expose vast areas of sand, which the wind whips into small mounds and dips called dunes. Marram grass and other plants bind the dunes so they don't blow away.

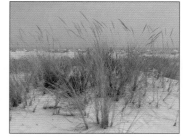

Rockpool oases When the tide is out, rockpools provide a refuge from baking sunshine or freezing cold. Young fish shelter there safe from large predators, but rain can dilute the pools and sunshine can cause them to evaporate.

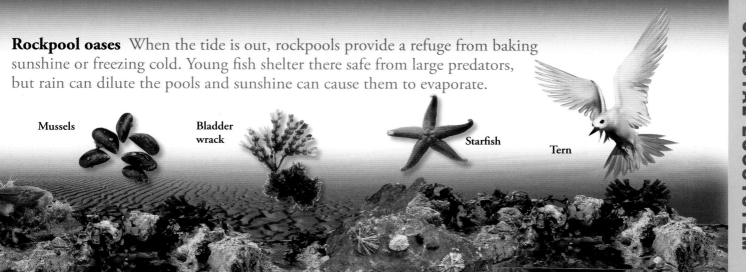

Mussels

Bladder wrack

Starfish

Tern

SHELLFISH
Mussels and oysters can survive pounding waves by fixing themselves to rocks using strong threads (byssus) or special glue.

SEAWEED
The slime that makes seaweeds so slippery stops them from drying out and helps them survive out of water.

STARFISH
Hundreds of tiny sucker-feet help starfish to climb over rocks. Starfish also use them to pull apart and eat shellfish.

SEABIRDS
Terns catch fish by plunging into the sea. Other seabirds patrol the beaches at low tide picking out crabs and worms.

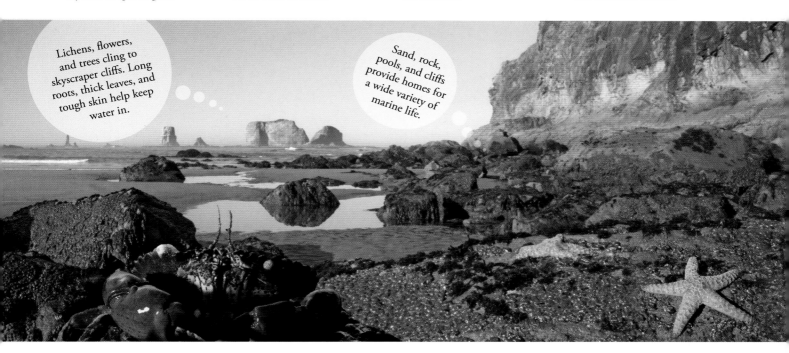

Lichens, flowers, and trees cling to skyscraper cliffs. Long roots, thick leaves, and tough skin help keep water in.

Sand, rock, pools, and cliffs provide homes for a wide variety of marine life.

MANGROVE SWAMPS
Most forests will only grow on dry land. Mangroves however, can tolerate salt and grow along sheltered tropical shores. Their tangled roots stabilize shifting mud and sand.

PEBBLE BEACH
Pebble and shingle beaches and spits build up as strong waves and currents pull stones from deep water and toss them onto the shore. Storms can remove whole beaches just as quickly.

CLIFF LIFE
Steep rocky cliffs provide a home safe from most predators for nesting seabirds, their eggs and young. With little soil or water, a few plants cling on, storing water in their leaves.

NEW COAST
Most coasts form over millions of years, but sometimes a new coastline appears suddenly. Earthquakes push land up or volcanoes pour lava into the sea. Colonization follows swiftly.

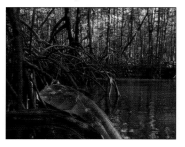

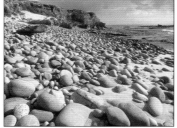

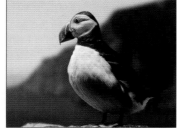

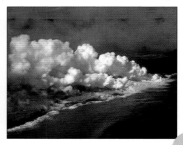

crumbling coast

Stone Age people found plenty of food along the ocean's *shoreline*. Today over **half** the world's population live near the coast. Millions of tourists also visit these areas. All this *activity* damages mangroves, marshes, sand dunes, and coastal coral reefs – natural defences against **erosion** and *flooding*. People living in low-lying coastal areas such as the Maldives and Bangladesh are already suffering the effects of **rising** sea levels.

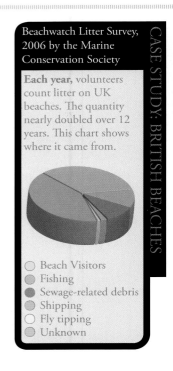

CASE STUDY: BRITISH BEACHES

Beachwatch Litter Survey, 2006 by the Marine Conservation Society

Each year, volunteers count litter on UK beaches. The quantity nearly doubled over 12 years. This chart shows where it came from.

○ Beach Visitors
○ Fishing
○ Sewage-related debris
○ Shipping
○ Fly tipping
○ Unknown

This graph is based on information taken from satellites about sea level increases between 1992 and 2004. It shows what could happen to sea levels over the next hundred years if climate change continues at its current rate.

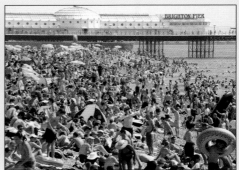

| 1990 | 2000 | 2010 | 2020 | 2030 | 2040 |

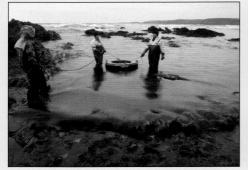

Boating blues Ships and boats from dinghies to oil tankers carry people and goods all over the ocean. Pollution is a risk when ships leak or sink offshore. Oil spills kill seabirds and mammals and smother beaches. Cleaning up the mess is expensive.

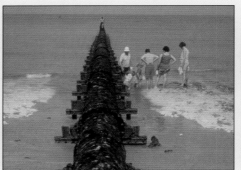

Sewage Raw or poorly treated sewage is pumped into the sea even in developed countries. Out at sea it fertilizes plant plankton, but inshore it is a health hazard to bathers and surfers. Harmful chemicals from factories can also end up on the shore.

People pressure People in cold northern countries go south in search of sunshine for their holidays. Too many seaside hotels, tourist beaches, and golf courses can destroy important wildlife habitats and tourists may trample on and disturb wildlife.

Coastal cities Many of the world's major cities are near the coast where rivers flow into the sea. These places were chosen because the rivers made it easy to get out to sea to trade with other countries. Unfortunately, they also make it easy for storm surges and rising sea levels to flood these cities if they are not protected by barriers.

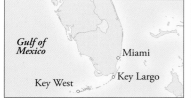

Today

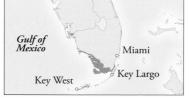

50 years...?

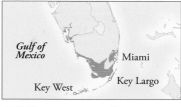

100 years...?

It is very difficult to work out how high the sea level will rise as a result of climate change. Polar ice is melting and adding water to the ocean. As the water itself warms, it expands and takes up more space. The red areas on these maps show which parts of Florida, USA, would be flooded if sea levels rose by 50 cm (1 ft) and 1 m (3 ft).

50 cm (20 in)

40 cm (16 in)

30 cm (12 in)

20 cm (8 in)

10 cm (4 in)

Some of our **cities** might end up under the sea.

050   2060   2070   2080   2090   2100

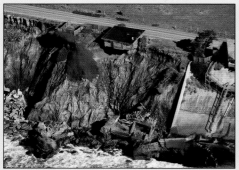

Storm sculpture Over the centuries, coastlines and seashores gradually wear away or build up. This house in California looks set to fall into the Pacific. Violent storms can change a beach overnight, and climate change may bring more intense storms.

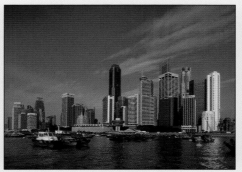

Stealing from the sea To increase their living space, the people of Singapore moved their coastline outwards, reclaiming land from the sea. Some coral reefs have been destroyed and the once clear waters around the island have become murky.

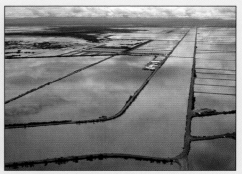

Mangrove farming About half the world's mangrove forests have been destroyed in the last 50 years, mostly to create ponds for prawn and shrimp farms. Villages without mangroves are more likely to be swamped by storms and tsunamis.

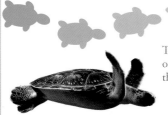

Turtles don't live on beaches, but they visit regularly.

turtle VS

ALL SEVEN SPECIES OF MARINE TURTLE FACE EXTINCTION TODAY. HUMANS POSE THE GREATEST

Although they spend their lives at sea, turtles begin life on land. Take, for example, a green sea turtle in Hawaii. An adult female mates at sea once every two to eight years. She finds the beach where she was born, crawls ashore, and digs a hole

THE CASE FOR TURTLES...

Turtles are already struggling to survive – as few as one in 1,000 babies reaches adulthood. They do not start to breed until they are between 10 and 50 years old, so even with protection it could take many years before numbers start to recover. Turtles need quiet and darkness to lay their eggs. They can't nest when there are people on the beach. The newly hatched babies rely on moonlight reflecting off water to guide them into the ocean so hotel lights send them in the wrong direction. Tourists are bad news for turtles.

In some countries it is now illegal to catch turtles for their meat or to collect turtle eggs, yet both are still being caught and eaten in some parts of the world.

Goods made of turtle shell may not be brought into the UK and US, but poachers still catch and kill turtles to make souvenirs for tourists. Hundreds of turtle shell ashtrays, hairclips, ornaments, and musical instruments have been seized by UK and US customs.

Some fisherman fit hatches called TEDs (turtle exclusion devices) to their fishing nets so turtles can escape.

Take all your litter home after a visit to the beach, particularly plastic bags that turtles might mistake for food.

Divers and snorkellers can frighten turtles by holding onto them under water.

tourist

Tourists love to visit beaches, but sometimes they don't make very good guests.

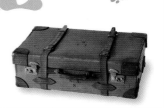

THREAT, AND ALSO OFFER THE BEST CHANCE OF SURVIVAL TO THESE CREATURES.

in the sand where she lays around 100 eggs. She leaves, but may return several times to lay more eggs. Later the eggs hatch. The baby turtles scrabble out of the nest and dash to the sea. They swim off quickly to avoid being eaten by crabs, fish, and birds.

THE CASE FOR TOURISTS...

Tourists are becoming interested in, and concerned for, the wildlife of the places they visit. Local people who once collected turtle eggs to sell as food now guide tourists who wish to see nesting turtles. Tourist centres buy eggs from local collectors and then hatch and rear them, eventually releasing them into the wild. Watching their release is becoming a great tourist attraction. Tourists also help local police return turtles rescued from poachers to the sea. Turtle farms have a part to play in conservation. They are a tourist attraction and they provide meat for local markets. Tourism might be just the thing that saves turtles.

Tourists bring much-needed money to many beautiful but poor parts of the world. The beaches of Bali and Mexico, for example, if properly looked after, can sustain wildlife while also providing a good living to local people through tourism.

Some beaches ask tourists to stay away at night to avoid disturbing nesting turtles.

TURTLE FACTS

🐾 The Hawksbill turtle is the source of the traditional "tortoise shell". Its carapace (shell) is marbled with amber, yellow, or brown.

🐾 The Leatherback turtle is one of the largest living reptiles. The biggest ever recorded was nearly 3 m (10 ft) from nose to tail and weighed 916 kg (2,020 lbs).

🐾 Kemp's Ridley turtles are the most endangered of all. They nest in broad daylight along only one small stretch of coastline in the Gulf of Mexico.

🐾 The temperature of a turtle's nest determines the sex of the young. Turtles are thought to dig their nests to different depths to affect the temperature.

seabed ecosystem

The ocean seabed varies from hard rock to soft sediment. At the edges of the land, it is a patchwork of rock, sand, and mud where vast numbers of sea creatures live. It is here that most of the world's fishing is done. Water current, water temperature, the depth, and type of seabed – these all affect what plants and animals live where.

Volcanic springs, called hydrothermal vents, erupt from the ocean floor. Chemicals in the water nourish bacteria, which are themselves eaten by creatures living on the ocean floor.

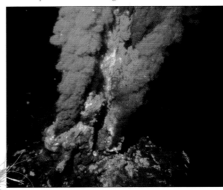

Shrimps and prawns crawl over the seabed.

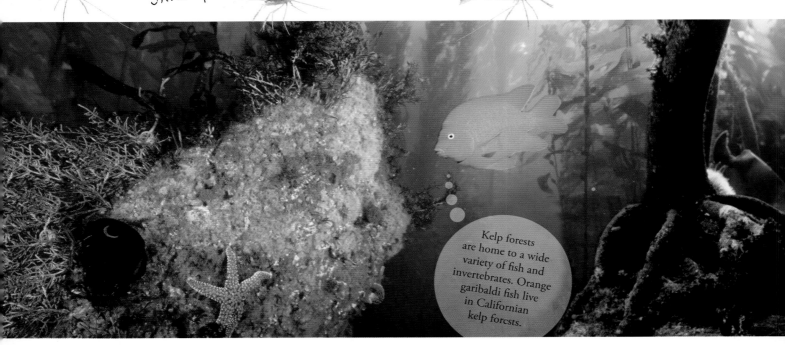

Kelp forests are home to a wide variety of fish and invertebrates. Orange garibaldi fish live in Californian kelp forests.

SHALLOW SEDIMENTS
Much shallow seabed is covered in mud and sand. Valuable scallops lie in shallow depressions hiding from starfish. Buried shellfish take in water using siphons like drinking straws.

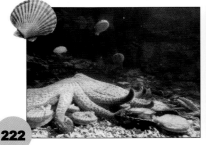

NO PLACE LIKE HOME
Sponges, sea squirts, and similar animals form underwater jungles on rocky seabeds. They do not need to move to find food. Ocean currents bring drifting plankton to them.

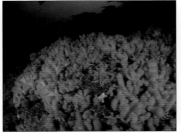

NEW BEGINNINGS
Fixed animals such as sponges cannot move to find a mate, so they produce tiny larvae that drift and then settle on bare rocks. This shipwreck has become covered in marine life.

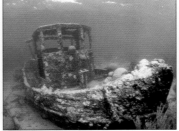

STEALTHY PREDATORS
Colourful sea slugs and other mobile predators graze the kelp forests in the same way that limpets and sea urchins graze seaweeds. Their bright colours warn of their horrid taste.

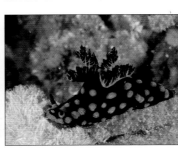

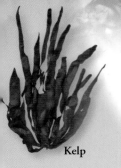

Kelp uses This family of seaweeds has many uses and is harvested from the wild on a commercial scale. Although the holdfast (base of the plant) is left behind to re-grow, some animals lose their home and supply of food when the seaweed is cut.

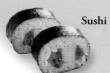

Kelp

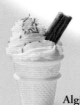

Sushi

Alginates in ice-cream

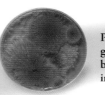

Shampoo

Petri dish growing bacteria in agar

Kelp tablets

SUSHI
Sushi is a Japanese food of rice and raw fish often rolled up in sheets of *nori* (laver), a valuable red seaweed grown in ocean farms.

ALGINATES
If you like ice cream then you like eating seaweed! Kelp and seaweeds contain sticky alginates and gums, which are used in its manufacture.

COSMETICS
Seaweed extracts have been used in cosmetics since Roman times and today are found in shampoo, shaving cream, and skin lotions.

AGAR
Agar is made from harvested red seaweeds. It is a valuable jelly-like substance that is used to grow bacteria in medicine and research.

SUPPLEMENTS
Seaweeds contain many minerals and vitamins and can be taken in tablets to promote health. Seaweed is also widely eaten as food by people and animals.

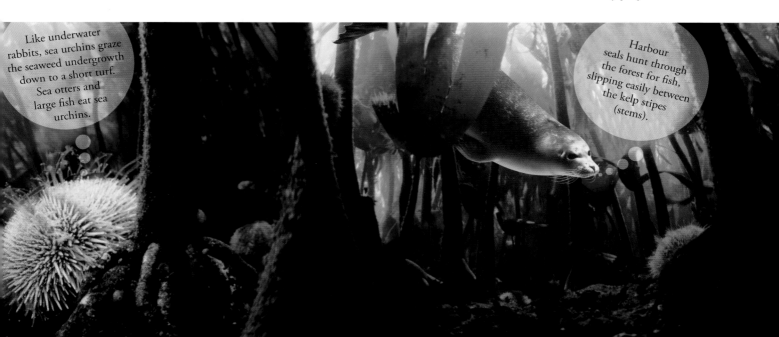

Like underwater rabbits, sea urchins graze the seaweed undergrowth down to a short turf. Sea otters and large fish eat sea urchins.

Harbour seals hunt through the forest for fish, slipping easily between the kelp stipes (stems).

BLUE HOLES
In some places the ocean extends under the land. Dry cave systems in the Bahamas flooded when the sea level rose thousands of years ago. They are now home to rare animals.

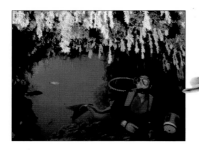

Flattened rays blend in with the seabed.

Kelp forests
These cover the rocky seabed in shallow water around temperate and cold coasts. Off Pacific North America these giant brown seaweeds grow to 50 m (165 ft). Smaller ones grow around Europe and in the Arctic Circle.

seabed destruction

Fishing boats around the world **drag** heavy nets across the seabed to catch fish, shellfish, and shrimps. They **plough up** the seabed and also catch a lot of *unwanted* animals. Fishermen use special **nets** and try to avoid fish-breeding areas to minimize the **damage**, but trawling is still very *destructive*. In the North Sea, the seabed is *scoured* many times every year. This **heavy-duty** fishing damages the homes of the **animals** the fish feed on, resulting in *fewer* fish.

Trawling is incredibly destructive...

... but the extent of the damage is largely hidden from view.

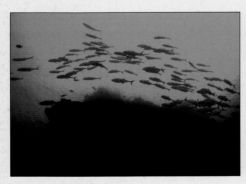

Mountain fisheries Huge shoals of fish and squid circle the tops of seamounts – extinct volcanoes rising thousands of metres from the seabed. Fishing fleets are destroying these unique and remote places. We need to protect them now!

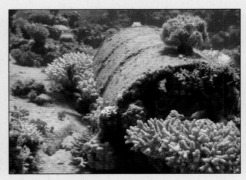

Deepsea dumping The shallow ocean seabed has been used as a dumping ground for many centuries. However, a recent proposal to dump an old oil rig in the deep ocean caused a public outcry. In the depths things only decay very slowly.

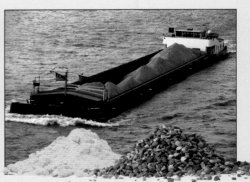

Mining the oceans Each year, thousands of tonnes of sand and gravel seabed are removed for use in the building industry. Areas must be chosen carefully because it takes at least ten years of protection for a mined area to get back to normal.

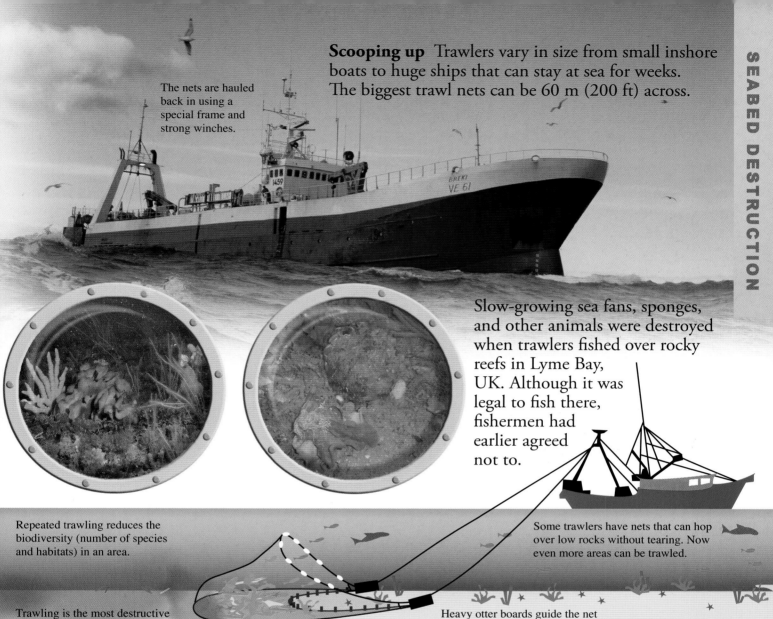

Scooping up Trawlers vary in size from small inshore boats to huge ships that can stay at sea for weeks. The biggest trawl nets can be 60 m (200 ft) across.

The nets are hauled back in using a special frame and strong winches.

Slow-growing sea fans, sponges, and other animals were destroyed when trawlers fished over rocky reefs in Lyme Bay, UK. Although it was legal to fish there, fishermen had earlier agreed not to.

Repeated trawling reduces the biodiversity (number of species and habitats) in an area.

Some trawlers have nets that can hop over low rocks without tearing. Now even more areas can be trawled.

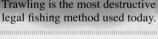

Trawling is the most destructive legal fishing method used today.

Heavy otter boards guide the net over the seabed and keep it open.

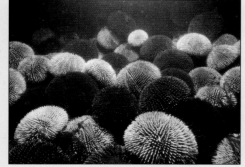

Urchin plagues Plagues of sea urchins can destroy Californian giant kelp forests by munching through seaweed stems so that the plants break off. There are too many urchins because the large sheephead fish that eat them have been over-fished.

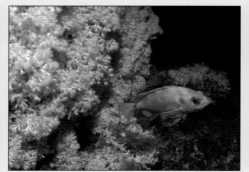

***Lophelia* reef** As shallow fisheries run out of fish, trawlers are targeting deep-water fish. In the North Atlantic, the trawls are destroying delicate reefs of sponges and cold-water corals called *Lophelia*, some of which are thousands of years old.

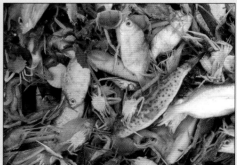

Unsorted catch As a trawl net is hauled in, it comes up with all sorts of unwanted animals as well as the target fish. Most of this by-catch is thrown back overboard. Using different-sized nets can help to prevent this.

coral reef ecosystem

Coral reefs can be found in the warm, clear water of the tropics. Each reef is formed by many different corals growing packed together. Every coral is a colony of tiny animals called polyps, and every polyp builds a hard limestone cup around itself. The polyps divide, adding new polyps with their own cups on top of the old ones, and over time the reef expands. Tiny algae live inside the polyps, sharing the food they make in return for a safe home. Reefs also house clams, sponges, and seaweeds.

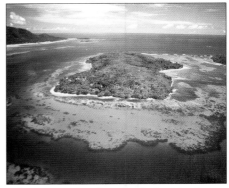

A fringing coral reef surrounds this island with a colourful halo. The corals grow in the shallow water where there is a hard seabed they can fasten onto.

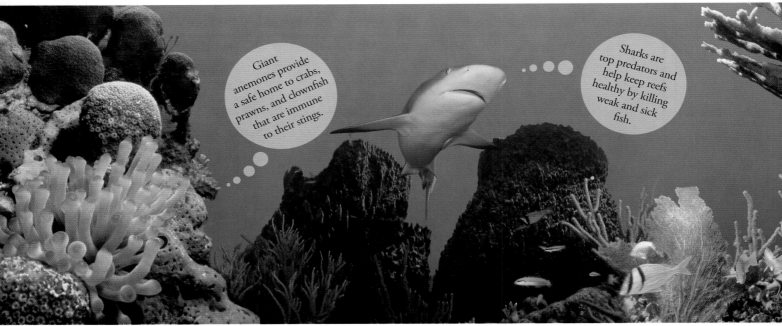

Giant anemones provide a safe home to crabs, prawns, and clownfish that are immune to their stings.

Sharks are top predators and help keep reefs healthy by killing weak and sick fish.

A riot of colour Life is crowded and colourful on a coral reef. Hundreds of species of fish swim around, through, between, and under the coral. In the dense crowds, fish use bright colours and patterns to find a mate, recognize enemies, confuse predators, and camouflage themselves.

Barrel sponges grow large enough to fit a person inside. They grow slowly and live for many years.

CORAL
Corals come in many shapes and sizes. Each colony develops from a tiny larva hatched from a floating egg. The corals grow upwards and outwards, facing towards the Sun.

Underwater rainforest A healthy coral reef bursts with life just as a tropical rainforest does. Hundreds of species of coral provide homes and food for fish, crabs, starfish, sea urchins, and shells. The creatures depend on one another. If one link in this food chain is removed, many other species may also disappear. Destroying the coral is like cutting down forest trees.

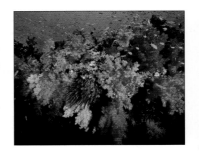

Essential reefs
Local people around the world depend on coral reefs for food and for their living. Reefs also support a huge tourist industry worldwide.

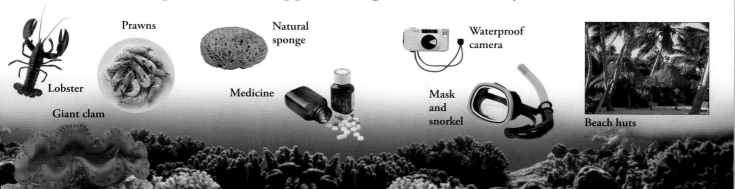

Lobster

Giant clam

Prawns

Natural sponge

Medicine

Waterproof camera

Mask and snorkel

Beach huts

SEAFOOD
Coral reefs provide about 10 per cent of the world harvest of fish and shellfish. That's vital protein for people living near them.

MEDICINES
Scientists are developing the chemicals used by sponges and other reef animals to ward off predators into drugs to treat cancer and arthritis.

TOURISM
Undamaged coral reefs with abundant fish populations attract many tourists. Tourism provides local people with money and jobs.

PROTECTION
Coral reefs form a barrier to waves and protect shorelines from erosion. They can lessen damage to coastal villages from huge waves called tsunamis.

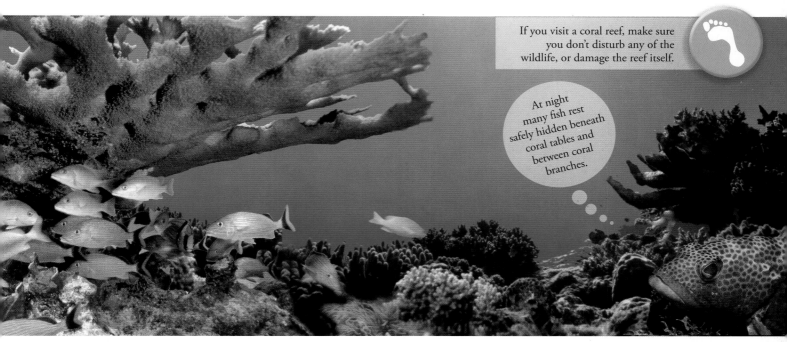

If you visit a coral reef, make sure you don't disturb any of the wildlife, or damage the reef itself.

At night many fish rest safely hidden beneath coral tables and between coral branches.

SPONGES
Many small reef animals find shelter inside hollow sponges, but only turtles and sea slugs relish eating them. The bright colours of sponges warn enemies that they taste dreadful!

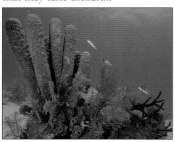

SEA SLUGS
Sharks are not the only predators on the reef. Sea slugs hunt too. They munch holes in anemones, soft corals, sponges, and other fixed animal colonies that cannot escape.

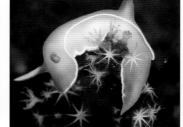

FISH
The reef provides shelter, a place to live, and food for hundreds of fish. Some graze on seaweeds, others eat the coral itself, hunt for worms and crabs in the reef, or stalk other fish.

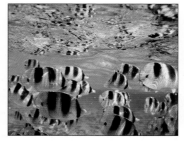

SEAGRASS
Seagrasses grow in shallow sandy areas, often near to coral reefs. Unlike corals, they root themselves in the shifting seabed. Sea cows (dugongs) and turtles graze these lush meadows.

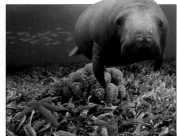

dying coral

Reefs throughout the Indian Ocean were badly **damaged** in 1998 when sea surface temperatures *rose* to the highest recorded levels in 150 years. In some areas, up to 90 per cent of the corals bleached (got rid of the colourful algae that normally live with them) and died. Dead coral is soon smothered in algae and animals and breaks up. The unusual **weather pattern** that caused this is called *El Niño*. It is happening more often, possibly due to global **climate change**. Although the coral is slowly growing back, many reefs will be permanently **destroyed** if regular bleaching takes place.

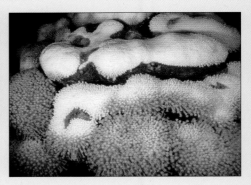

Governments worldwide need to

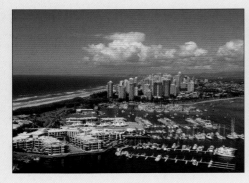

A room with a view Hotels and beach houses built at the edge of the sea cause erosion when trees binding the soil together are cut down. Sewage and silt then drift out and smother reefs. Rising tourist numbers mean more hotels and houses, but careful planning can help.

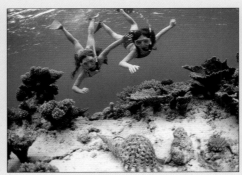

Diver's paradise Coral is easily broken by feet and divers' fins. Some popular reefs in the Red Sea have been nearly destroyed by dive boats dropping their anchors onto them. Permanent mooring buoys are part of the solution, as is raising awareness of the issues among tourists.

White out When corals are stressed – for example, due to an increase in water temperature – they expel the tiny algae that live in their tissues. Without the coloured algae the corals appear white or bleached. The algae return if the stress is taken away but otherwise the corals die.

Disappearing reefs Already at least 11 per cent of the world's coral reefs have been completely destroyed, and a further 16 per cent are badly damaged. Scientists predict that even more will die. Damaged corals will re-grow once the pressure is taken off them, but the variety of coral is often lost.

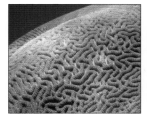

BRAIN
Often, damaged brain corals never recover. They can be several metres across, but take hundreds of years to grow to this size.

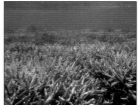

STAGHORN
Thickets of staghorn coral grow in the shallows. They are delicate structures, easily broken by divers' fins and boat anchors.

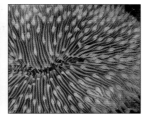

MUSHROOM
Mushroom corals thrive on damaged reefs and can cope with silty water. They can turn themselves the right way up again if upturned.

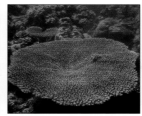

TABLE
Tables of *Acropora* coral are easily broken by storms and the bombs fishermen sometimes use. But they also grow back quickly.

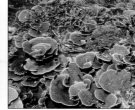

LEAF
Some leafy corals look like crisps, others like cabbages, but all provide important hideaways for small reef animals.

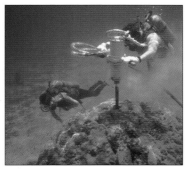

Scientists drill into coral and carefully extract a core.

Like trees, corals have annual growth rings and can live for hundreds of years. They respond to changes in temperature and water clarity by growing at different rates. Scientists can use coral cores to form a record of changing conditions in the ocean.

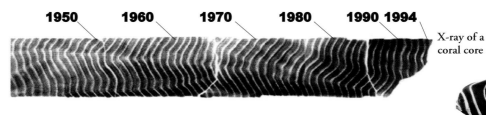

1950 1960 1970 1980 1990 1994

X-ray of a coral core

work together to save our reefs.

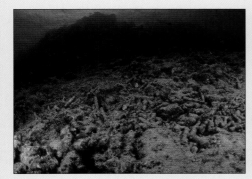

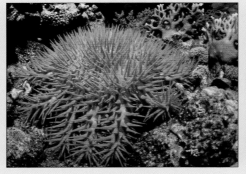

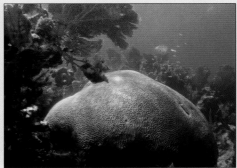

Bombs away In Malaysia, Indonesia, and the Philippines reef fish stocks have declined through over-fishing. Some fishermen have illegally resorted to throwing home-made bombs onto reefs to kill and stun fish. The bombs destroy the reef so fish stocks decline even further.

Coral enemies Crown-of-thorns starfish sit on corals and eat their flesh leaving dead white skeletons. Giant tritons help control starfish numbers by eating them, but because they have beautiful shells, the tritons and other starfish predators are being over-collected to sell to tourists.

Murky waters Coral reefs only grow well in clear water. During land reclamation and forest clearance, silt pours into coastal waters smothering reefs. As the population of small island countries grows, houses, runways, and roads are built and more reefs struggle to survive.

the open

In the open waters of an ocean, there are no solid surfaces. Nothing stays still, so there is nothing for animals to hide behind or under (except maybe one another). They can't pin their prey to the bottom to eat it because the seabed is so far down. Animals either drift with the current or are strong swimmers. Some have bizarre shapes that help them to float, while hunters such as tuna, sharks, and dolphins are streamlined for fast swimming. Some fish, like sardines, live in huge shoals that protect them from predators, but also make them more vulnerable to modern fishing techniques, which can detect and catch whole shoals. Plant plankton floats in the sunlit surface waters. At night, animals rise up to feed on plankton and each other.

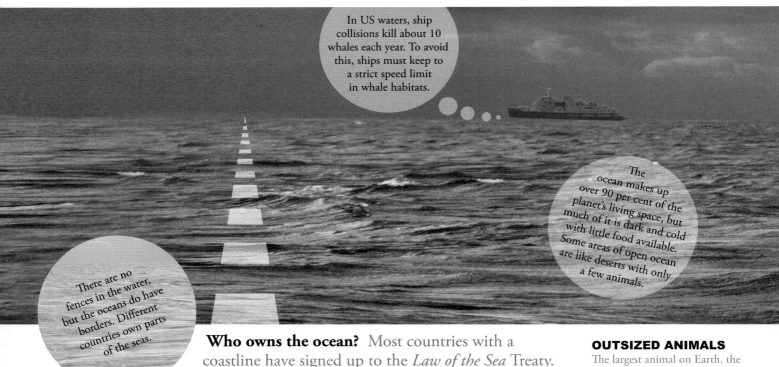

In US waters, ship collisions kill about 10 whales each year. To avoid this, ships must keep to a strict speed limit in whale habitats.

The ocean makes up over 90 per cent of the planet's living space, but much of it is dark and cold with little food available. Some areas of open ocean are like deserts with only a few animals.

There are no fences in the water, but the oceans do have borders. Different countries own parts of the seas.

Who owns the ocean? Most countries with a coastline have signed up to the *Law of the Sea* Treaty. This sets boundaries and gives nations exclusive rights to their waters. Territorial waters extend 12 nautical miles (nm) offshore, and an Exclusive Economic Zone (EEZ) extends 200 nm. Ocean areas beyond EEZs are International.

Roaming free Most open-ocean animals spend their lives in the same general area, but a few are true ocean wanderers. Leatherback turtles travel the oceans in search of jellyfish. Humpback whales migrate each autumn from cold, food-rich waters to the tropics where they breed. International agreements are needed to protect such animals.

OUTSIZED ANIMALS
The largest animal on Earth, the blue whale, roams the open ocean. Whales can grow to huge sizes because salt water is dense and supports their heavy bodies.

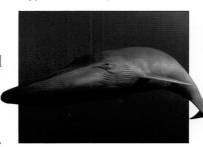

ocean ecosystem

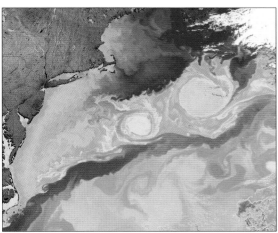

+ Red colour shows warmest water, purple **−** shows coldest.

Walls in the sea Invisible barriers keep floating plankton and fish in their own particular areas and depths. These barriers are ocean fronts and eddies, where water currents of different temperatures and saltiness meet. Here, two warm-water eddies have swirled away into nearby cold water, carrying plankton and fish with them.

Satellites record the surface temperature and amount of plant plankton in ocean water by measuring electromagnetic radiation. Computers convert the data into coloured pictures.

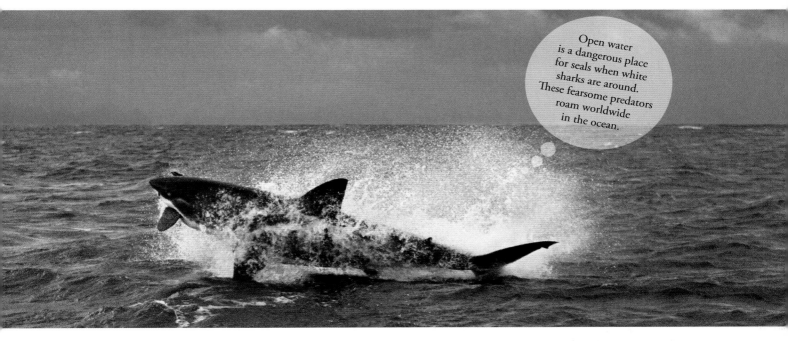

Open water is a dangerous place for seals when white sharks are around. These fearsome predators roam worldwide in the ocean.

LIGHTS ON
Deepsea fish drift in permanent darkness. But many produce their own bioluminescent light. Light patterns help them catch prey, find mates, and avoid enemies.

LIGHTS OUT
The rainbow colours of light, especially reds, disappear a short distance below the surface. This deep-sea red jellyfish always looks black so it is hidden in dim light.

HUGE SHOALS
Out in the open ocean there is nowhere to hide. Living in huge shoals helps protect fish like these sardines from predators, but makes it easier for fishing boats to catch them.

DIVING DEEP
Elephant seals can hold their breath for up to two hours and dive to 1,500 m (5,000 ft) to search for food. Humans need special pressure-proof submersibles to dive this deep.

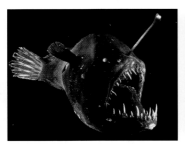

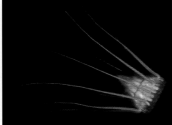

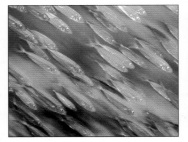

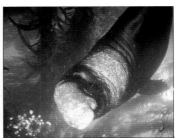

threatened ocean

Out at sea, far away from land, the human impact on the ocean can still be felt. Many of the **threats** are invisible, like changes in water *quality* and chemistry. Even the normal flow of ocean currents may be changing as water *temperatures* increase through global warming. Other effects are more obvious. Great drifts of **litter** collect where ocean **currents** meet. Wandering leatherback turtles die out at sea after eating plastic bags or "balloon race" balloons. As they rest, flocks of seabirds drift into *oily washings* from ships' fuel tanks.

Some of the greatest and most damaging

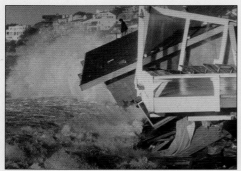

El Niño Every few years, the cold current flowing north along the west coast of South America is diverted by a strong easterly flow of warm water from the central Pacific Ocean. The new balance between warm and cold currents, called *El Niño* alters the weather, affecting fishing. Climate change may bring more *El Niños*.

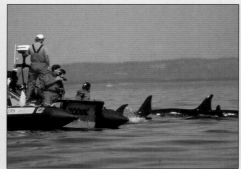

Tourist troubles Watching or snorkelling with whales and whale sharks can be an amazing experience. These animals' value to tourism is a good reason for conservation. However, too much human contact can disturb migration and feeding patterns, so good tour operators follow accepted codes of conduct.

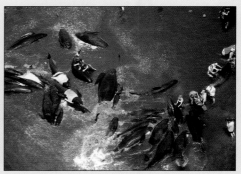

Not so silent ocean Whales and dolphins find their way around underwater by making high pitched noises and then listening for echoes that bounce back, much as bats do on land. Loud noises from earthquake research, naval exercises, and ships can confuse them, and sometimes whole groups get stranded on the shore and die.

The International Whaling Commission (IWC) was set up in 1946 to protect the great whales. The 78 member nations agree how many and which whales can be killed each year.

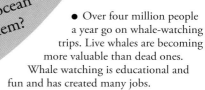

Adopt a whale through a wildlife charity. You'll receive information and photos so you can learn more about whales.

FOR

● Japan catches hundreds of great whales each year, providing vital data for conservation and management of whale stocks. Sending meat to the market helps pay for this research.

● In the Faroe Islands, the annual "grind" – slaughter of pilot whales – is a traditional, and not a commercial, fishing activity carried out by native people.

● Whale stocks have recovered enough to allow some commercial whaling again. The scientific programme should lead to more sustainable whaling in the future.

● All of the Southern Ocean (and part of the Indian Ocean) is a whale sanctuary.

The GREAT WHALE debate...
Is there any reason not to hunt whales for food? Does their intelligence and importance in the ocean ecosystem make it unethical to kill them?

● Over four million people a year go on whale-watching trips. Live whales are becoming more valuable than dead ones. Whale watching is educational and fun and has created many jobs.

● There are few whales left. Their numbers have still not recovered from over-fishing in the 1800s. Many die each year from boat collisions, stranding, and pollution.

AGAINST

● "Scientific whaling" is an excuse to sell whale meat to Japanese supermarkets. There is no need to kill hundreds of whales to collect data. A few would do. Unscrupulous sailors from Korea, Norway and Japan also kill whales illegally and sell the meat.

● Scientists can study living whales. Many can be recognized from photographs of their tail markings, pieces of skin and blubber can be taken for DNA analysis, and movements can be recorded with satellite tags. Together, these supply enough data for management.

● All the products that are, or used to be, made from whales such as oil, soap, glue, leather, and lubricants can now be made synthetically or obtained from other sources.

threats to the ocean are invisible.

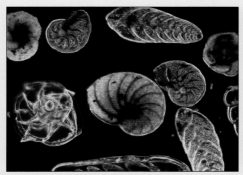

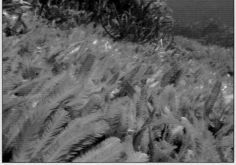

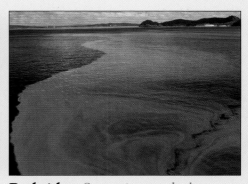

Ocean acidification The ocean absorbs huge amounts of carbon dioxide from the atmosphere. It enables plankton, many bacteria, and seaweed to grow, but burning fossil fuels results in more carbon dioxide entering the ocean making it more acidic. This could dissolve the shells of plant plankton and other animals.

Alien species Animals and plants moved by mistake from one ocean to another can become serious pests. In the Mediterranean, a green seaweed has spread over large areas and is killing seabed animals by smothering them. It probably escaped from an aquarium near Monaco and floated away in ocean currents.

Red tides Sometimes whole areas of ocean turn red when tiny coloured plankton plants called *dinoflagellates* multiply very rapidly. As they grow, they produce poisons that can kill fish and make people ill. Red tides occur naturally but the nutrients from sewage can make them worse.

233

shark finning

SHARKS ARE IMPORTANT TOP PREDATORS IN THE OCEAN. REMOVING THEM IS VERY DAMAGING.

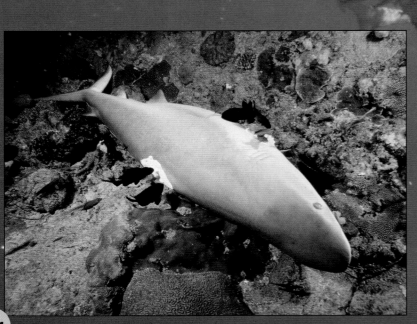

DROWNING SHARK

This Grey Reef shark has been caught, finned, and thrown back onto a reef in Thailand. Sharks grow slowly and give birth to just a few live young after many months of pregnancy. If too many sharks are taken, numbers decline quickly because they cannot breed fast enough to replace those caught.

Don't eat shark-fin soup, and tell your friends and family about shark finning so this harmful practice can be stopped.

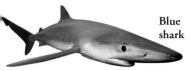

Blue shark

The blue shark is the most heavily fished shark in the world.

In Hong Kong and China, shark-fin soup is traditionally served at weddings and special occasions. As these countries have become richer, demand for the soup has increased.

Shark fins hung out to dry

Shark fins are rather tasteless, so pork and chicken are used to give shark-fin soup flavour. Fibres from the fins make the soup glutinous (gooey).

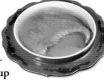

Shark-fin soup

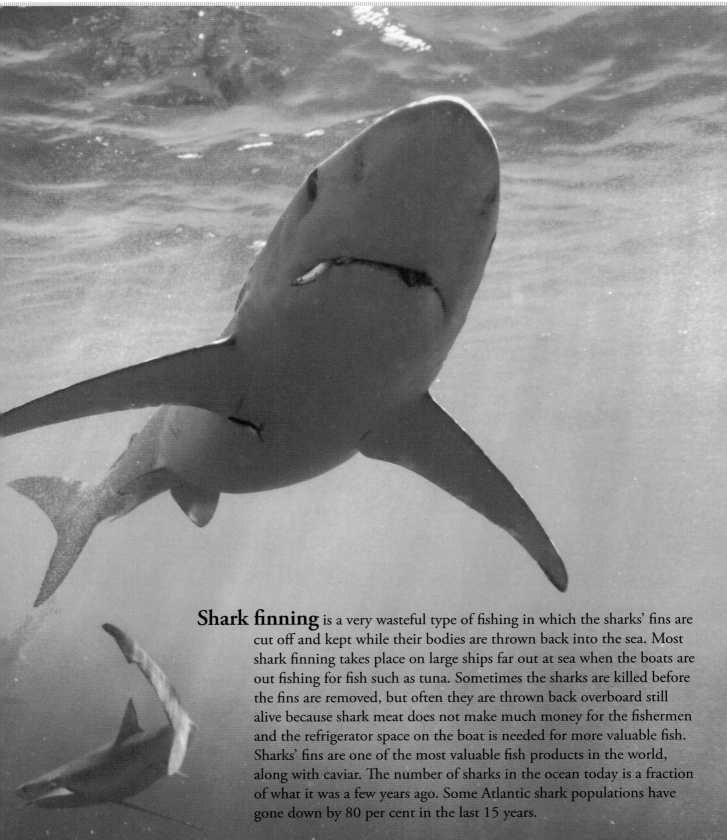

Shark finning is a very wasteful type of fishing in which the sharks' fins are cut off and kept while their bodies are thrown back into the sea. Most shark finning takes place on large ships far out at sea when the boats are out fishing for fish such as tuna. Sometimes the sharks are killed before the fins are removed, but often they are thrown back overboard still alive because shark meat does not make much money for the fishermen and the refrigerator space on the boat is needed for more valuable fish. Sharks' fins are one of the most valuable fish products in the world, along with caviar. The number of sharks in the ocean today is a fraction of what it was a few years ago. Some Atlantic shark populations have gone down by 80 per cent in the last 15 years.

235

Who caught all the fish?

Fishing has undergone a revolution in the last 50 years. Today enormous factory ships roam the seas, equipped with fish-finding sonar and processing systems that include freezing and canning equipment. Dragging enormous nets behind them,

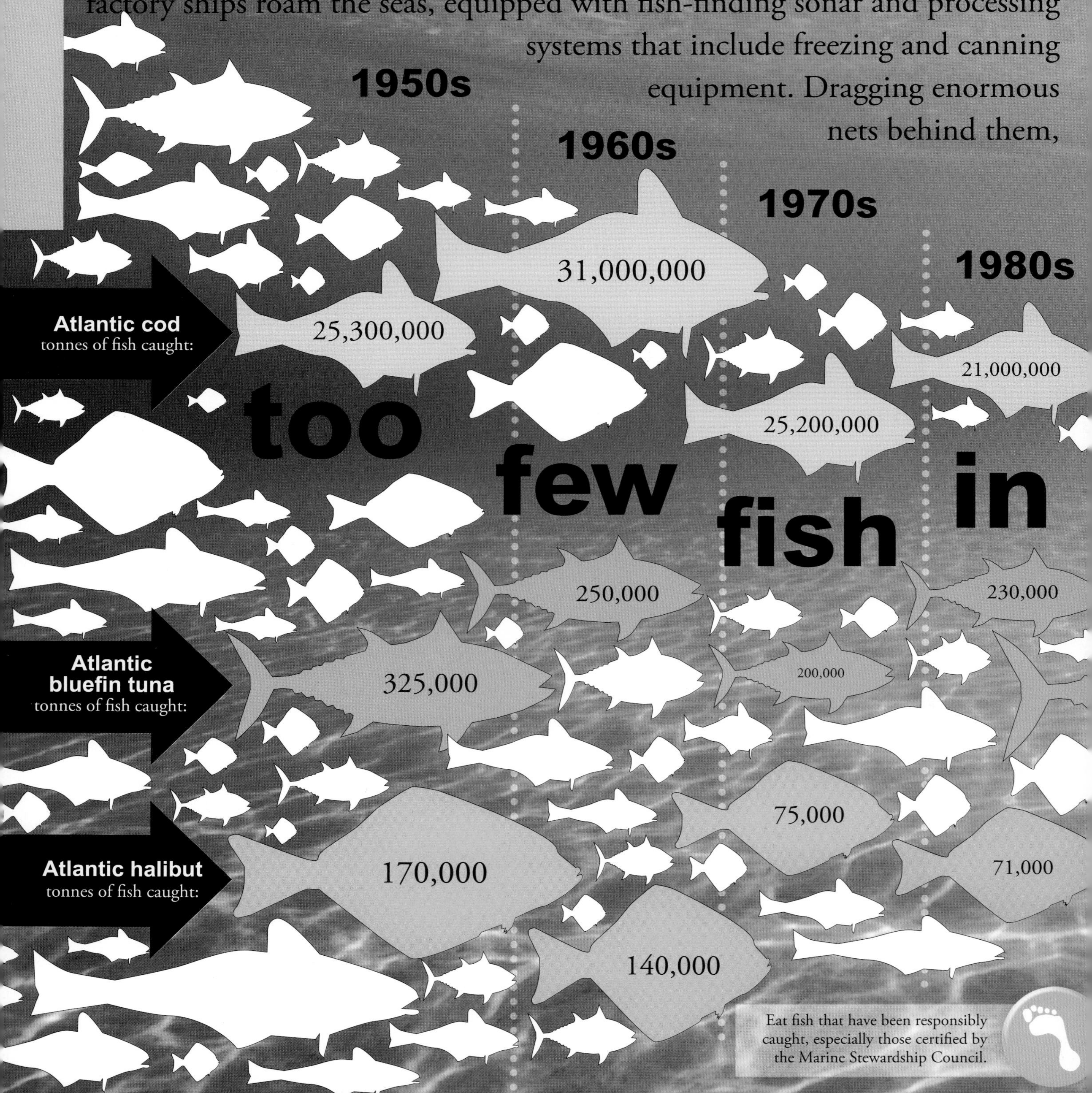

1950s

1960s

1970s

1980s

Atlantic cod
tonnes of fish caught:

25,300,000

31,000,000

25,200,000

21,000,000

too few fish in

Atlantic bluefin tuna
tonnes of fish caught:

325,000

250,000

200,000

230,000

Atlantic halibut
tonnes of fish caught:

170,000

75,000

71,000

140,000

Eat fish that have been responsibly caught, especially those certified by the Marine Stewardship Council.

We did.

they scoop up almost everything in their path, including many unwanted creatures, called by-catch. Most countries regulate fishing, sometimes quite well. But over-fishing means there are already far fewer fish left for us to catch.

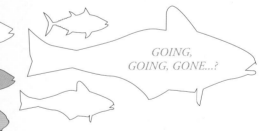

Atlantic cod

THE STORY OF COD

Cod is a wonderful fish. Nutritious and tasty, it is enjoyed by people throughout the northern hemisphere. Cod live in great shoals and one large female can lay several million eggs each year. Early European explorers claimed that there were so many cod, they could catch them by dropping baskets into the water. Everyone thought the supply would never run out. But modern fishing is so efficient that cod stocks are now collapsing.

Cod used to be one of the most abundant fish in the North Atlantic and has always been the favourite fish in "fish and chips". Now, in the North Sea, cod stocks are so low that for the last five years experts have recommended a total cod-fishing ban. But still the fishing goes on.

1990s

12,700,000

2000s
till now

5,400,000

the sea

2010s?

400,000

216,000

30,000

50,000

2020s?

GOING, GOING, GONE...?

"Dolphin-friendly" tuna come from boats that use very long fishing lines with baited hooks. This saves dolphins from being caught in tuna nets. But the bait also attracts albatrosses, and thousands are pulled underwater and drown.

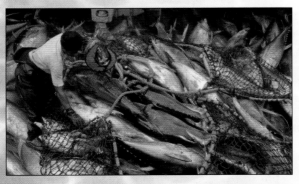

HALIBUT AND TUNA

The amount of halibut caught has been going down since the 1960s as their numbers have dwindled. Blue-fin tuna catches have gone up since the 1970s but in the past two years the catch has plummeted. This is because continuous over-fishing has removed too many adult breeding fish so now too few young are produced.

MAKING A DIFFERENCE

Look out for shark egg cases

Scientists want help to find out more about sharks. Don't worry, there's no danger involved!

Shark egg case

Simply visit your local beach and if you find any egg cases pick them up and take them home. Check out the website below for more info.

www.eggcase.org

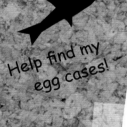

Help find my egg cases!

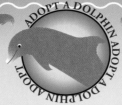

DOLPHIN ADOPTION

This is to certify that

Charlie Duffy
....
(Name here)

is recognised by the Dolphin adoption agency as an official protector of

Smiley the Dolphin
....
(Name here)

what you can do

Adopt a dolphin! With this scheme, you get a cuddly dolphin, certificate, and updates on the dolphin's progress: www.donation4charity.org wwf-adopt-a-dolphin php

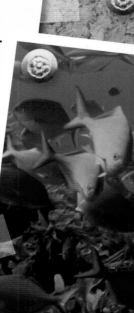

Dear Prime Minister

Please can the government create more marine nature reserves in the UK? These provide an important safe haven for fish, birds, and other seaside creatures from activities that are damaging – like trawling the sea floor or building on coastal land. Even dog-walking can upset nesting birds.

If the reserves include visitor's centres, people could go and learn about the sea and its ecology. The more people value what is beneath the waves, the more life there will flourish.

I look forward to hear

what you can do

Don't buy marine curios (shells, starfish, sponges, even dried out puffer fish). If there is no market, the fish won't be killed.

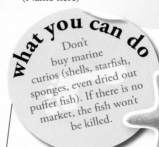

THE PRIME MINISTER
10 DOWNING STREET
LONDON
SW1A 2AA

---

8 THE DAILY NEWS   20th February 2007

HARNESSING THE OCEAN'S POWER

SCOTLAND TO GET MASSIVE "WAVE FARM"

The world's biggest wave energy farm is to be created off the coast of Orkney in Scotland. The Pelamis device has been tested at the European Marine Energy Centre (Emec) on Orkney by Leith-based company Ocean Power Delivery. Scottish Power wants to commission four more at the same site. Deputy First Minister Nicol Stephen announced a £13m funding package that will also allow a number of other marine energy devices to be tested. Ocean Power Delivery has already exported the Pelamis for use in a commercial wave farm. Now Scottish Power is planning a venture which it believes could create enough power for 2,000 homes.

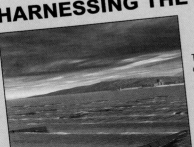

Storms surges battered the coast of England

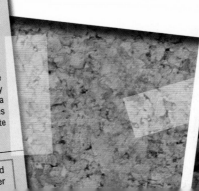

If you love the sea, you can learn more about the creatures living in and near it, and what you can do to help protect them.

PLASTIKI IN THE PACIFIC

David de Rothschild is setting sail in his plastic boat, the *Plastiki*, for the Great Pacific Garbage Patch – to "document an ocean of trash, on a boat made of trash".

This area of the Pacific is a mass of floating plastic pieces caught in a swirling current. It is the size of Texas and 90 m (300 ft) deep, weighing an estimated 3 million tonnes.

Most plastic doesn't biodegrade, it just turns into smaller and smaller pieces until it is the size of dust. Fish and birds mistake the plastic debris for food, and filter-feeders such as jellyfish ingest the tiny particles. The area is a death-trap for marine life.

Plastic is cheap. We use it briefly and then throw it away. But it doesn't really go away. Lots of it ends up in the sea...

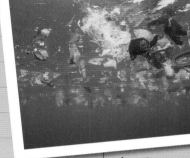

Rubbish floating in the sea

what you can do
Talk "rubbish" with friends and family and spread the word about the Garbage Patch. Pick up litter at the beach, and recycle plastic.

White Island, New Zealand

See this website to find out more:
http://science.
howstuffworks.com/great-
pacific-garbage-patch.htm

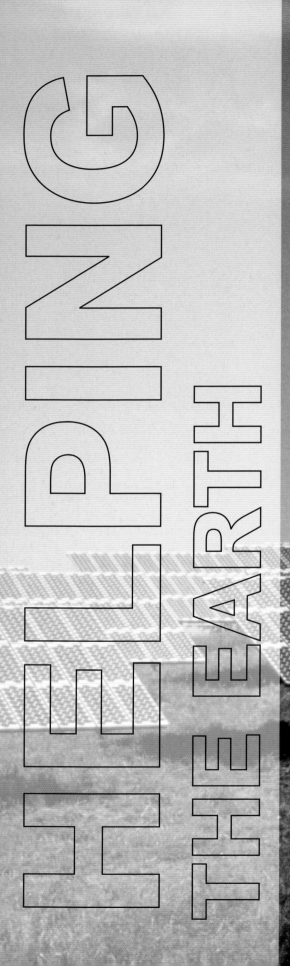

HELPING THE EARTH

The Earth is one huge ecosystem in which everything is **connected** under one atmosphere. How we live in our **small patch** of the planet affects everything, everywhere.

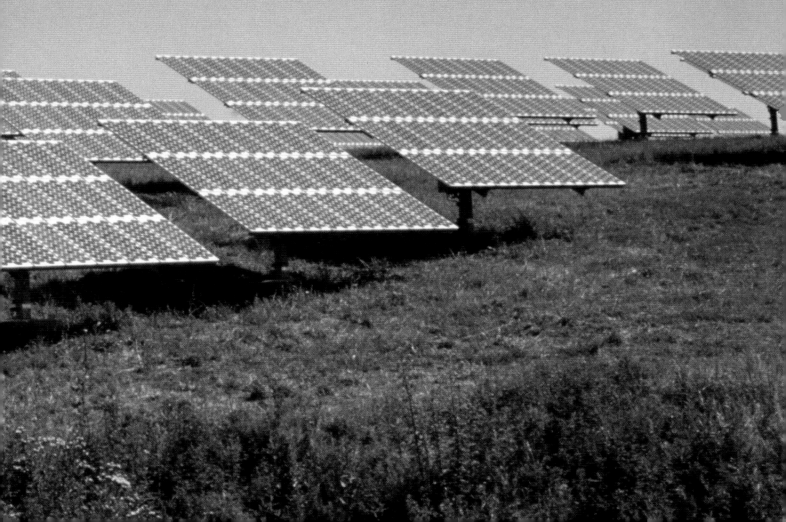

HELPING THE EARTH

living with change

Records show that the world has been getting warmer for the last 100 years. People need to adapt to the changing climate, to **heavier** storms, or in some places, much *less* rain.

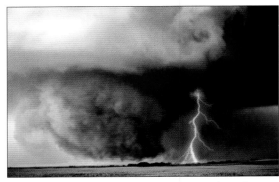
A tornado and lightning hit a field in the USA's Midwest.

The weather is becoming more extreme.

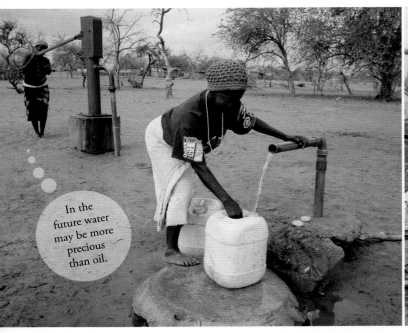

In the future water may be more precious than oil.

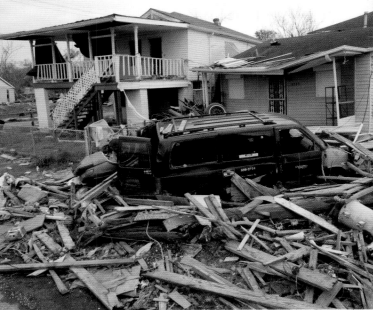

Drought Sub-Saharan Africa, already a poor area, is likely to suffer even worse droughts as a result of climate change. An international agreement called the Kyoto Protocol means that poor countries like those in Africa can get money from rich countries by selling "carbon credits". Carbon credits can be earned by planting trees, or using renewable energy.

Desertification is creating millions of eco-refugees.

Hurricanes Warmer seas are already leading to stronger tropical storms. Hurricane Katrina, which hit the USA in 2005, was one of the most devastating hurricanes ever recorded. Much of the damage was due to the city's flood defences failing. These are now being rebuilt, stronger and higher than ever, and countries all over the world are reassessing their defences.

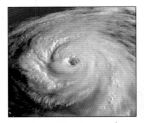
Hurricane Katrina swirling over the coast of Louisiana.

Altering the atmosphere Over the last 600,000 years, the amount of carbon dioxide (CO_2) in the atmosphere has affected the average temperature on Earth. By burning fossil fuels, humans are sending extra CO_2 into the atmosphere and temperatures are rising.

The obvious answer to halting this worrying trend is to reduce emissions of greenhouse gases.

45 YEARS FROM NOW?

NOW

CO_2 concentration measurement

Temperature

600,000 years ago

Present day

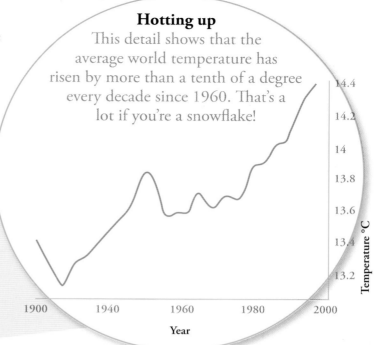

Hotting up
This detail shows that the average world temperature has risen by more than a tenth of a degree every decade since 1960. That's a lot if you're a snowflake!

14.4
14.2
14
13.8
13.6
13.4
13.2

1900 1940 1960 1980 2000

Year

Temperature °C

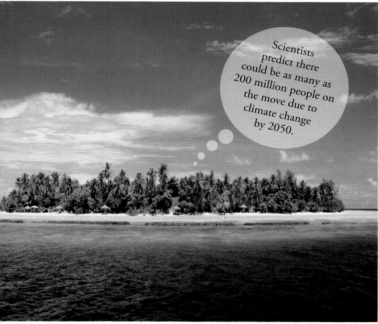

Scientists predict there could be as many as 200 million people on the move due to climate change by 2050.

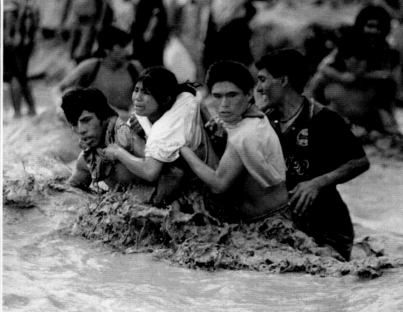

Sinking islands The Maldives consists of 1,200 tiny islands peeping out of the ocean. With sea levels predicted to rise by more than half a metre (2 ft) in the next century, some of the islands could disappear. The

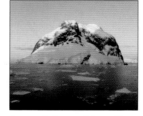

Antarctic ice melting affects sea levels worldwide.

Maldivians are preserving the coral reefs that form a natural barrier against tidal surges, and planting trees to prevent beach erosion. Ultimately, they rely on powerful countries to reduce carbon emissions...

Floods With rising sea levels and heavier rain, floods will be more common in many places. A warm current called *El Niño*, which brings heavy rain to

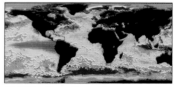

El Niño (in red) moving eastwards along the Equator across the Pacific.

western South America every few years, seems to be happening more often and more strongly. Countries at extra risk of flooding need to bolster their defences, and lay disaster-relief plans. Some may have to prepare for an influx of eco-refugees.

renewable **energy**

Archeologists of the future will look back at our period of human history and call it the Oil Age – when humans relied on *oil* and other **fossil fuels** for almost everything. The Earth provides many other energy sources, which can be harvested indefinitely and will not run out. With a little *technology*, we can make fuel or electricity from wind, water, sunlight, and even the Earth itself.

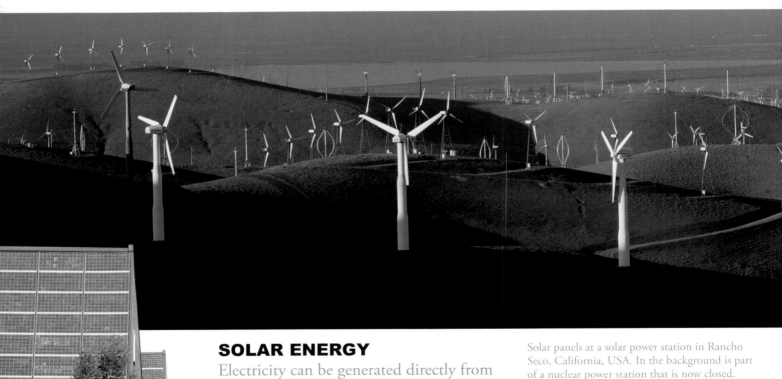

SOLAR ENERGY

Electricity can be generated directly from sunlight, using photovoltaic cells arranged in glass sheets called solar panels. Houses can also use sunlight, instead of a boiler, to heat water by passing it through thin black pipes on a flat surface on the roof. Solar power stations have tens or hundreds of photovoltaic or water-heating solar panels. There is huge potential to generate electricity this way in the world's deserts.

Solar panels at a solar power station in Rancho Seco, California, USA. In the background is part of a nuclear power station that is now closed.

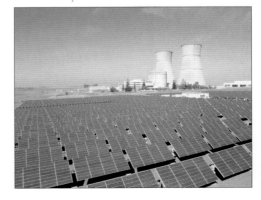

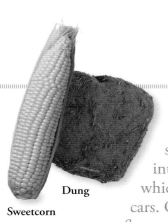

BIOFUELS

Sugary crops like sweetcorn are made into bioethanol, which can run petrol cars. Oily crops like soya or sunflower are made into biodiesel. Food crops aren't the only thing you can use, though. It's possible to make fuel from grass, wood chips, and even wastes such as shredded paper, sawdust, and dung.

Dung

Sweetcorn

Hydroelectricity uses the movement of water as it gushes through a dam.

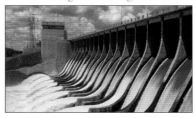

WATER POWER

When you dam a large river, energy builds up behind the dam in a reservoir. Open a gate and water rushes through fast enough to drive a turbine. Worldwide, the amount of energy generated this way has more than doubled since the 1970s.

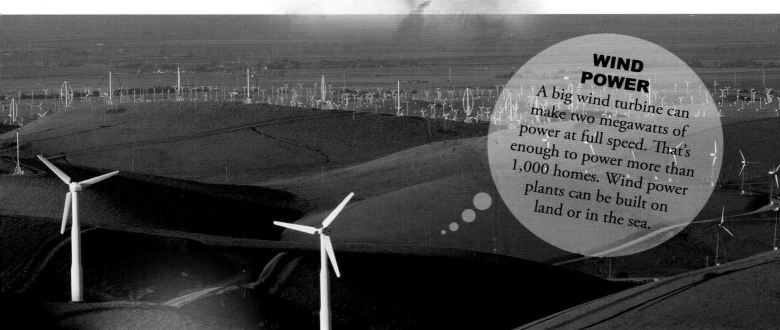

WIND POWER

A big wind turbine can make two megawatts of power at full speed. That's enough to power more than 1,000 homes. Wind power plants can be built on land or in the sea.

Energy from the Earth

GEOTHERMAL ENERGY

"Geo" means Earth, "thermal" means heat. It is warmer underground, especially in geologically active areas where hot rocks create hot springs. The heat can be used to warm water or generate electricity. In Iceland, most houses are heated geothermally, by piping heat out of the ground. Five per cent of California's electricity is generated from underground heat. Even in places without hot springs, it's possible to heat buildings during winter this way, because even when the air gets cold, the ground stays a great deal warmer.

245

using energy well

Energy-efficient housing Experts say it would be possible to cut world greenhouse gas emissions in half by 2020, just by saving energy and doing things more efficiently. Houses of the future will be less wasteful and make better use of the power of nature.

MATERIALS
Bricks and concrete take lots of heat energy to make. Building with other materials, such as these recycled shipping containers, is better for the environment.

INSULATION
Insulation, usually fibreglass or wool, goes between the walls and under the floors and roofs. It stops heat from escaping, or getting in, so you use less energy heating or cooling your inside space.

ENERGY EFFICIENT LIGHT BULBS
These fluorescent bulbs use one-fifth of the power that ordinary bulbs use to shine the same light. They last much longer too.

UNDERFLOOR HEATING
Heat rises, so the most efficient way to heat rooms is from underneath.

REED-BED FILTRATION
Dirty water can be cleaned by running it through reed beds in the garden.

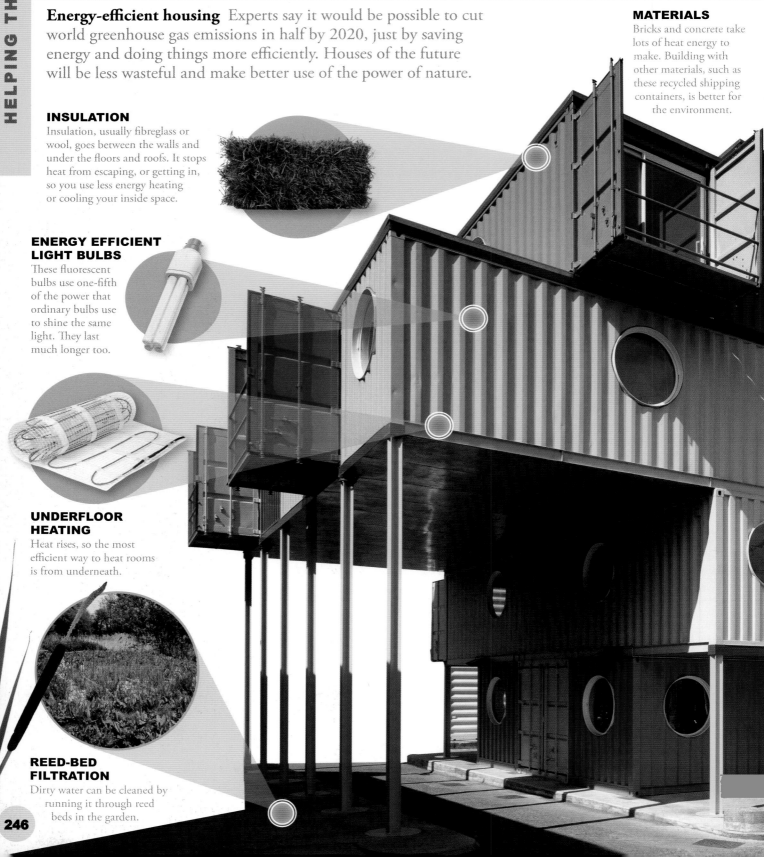

We can reduce *pollution* by using less energy or energy from renewable sources. Helping the Earth starts at home...

SOLAR PANELS

Solar panels can generate electricity or heat water even when it is cloudy. More than half of all the world's solar electricity is generated in Germany, where overcast weather is more common than sunshine.

PASSIVE SOLAR HEATING

Sunlight streaming through a window heats up the inside space. With careful design, this heat can be gathered in the winter, when the Sun is low in the sky, and avoided in the summer.

Imagine living here...

New technology can help in many ways

Here are some new ideas to save energy, pollute less, or cope in the face of climate change.

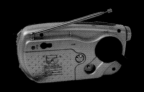

WIND-UP RADIO

Electricity can be generated just by turning a handle. Wind-up power can run radios, torches, and mobile phones.

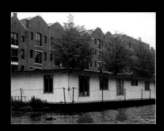

FLOATING HOUSES

Plenty of towns and cities will flood more with climate change. In the Netherlands people have begun building aluminium houses that float. These houses can be linked by walkways, so whole communities can live on the sea.

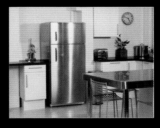

DYNAMIC DEMAND

Fridges run all the time. But they can be programmed to turn off temporarily without losing their cooling function when lots of power is being used elsewhere. If all fridges did this, national electricity grids would work more efficiently.

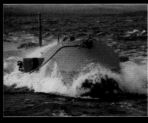

WAVE FARMS

The heave of the ocean waves can be used to make electricity. As seawater fills and empties a chamber, air forced in and out can drive a turbine. Wave energy is not used much yet, but could provide a huge power source.

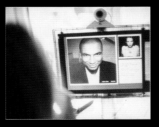

VIDEO CONFERENCING

Modern telecommunications make it possible for people in different parts of the world to have meetings where all the participants can see and hear each other on screen. This saves a lot of air travel.

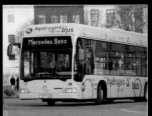

RENEWABLE VEHICLES

Cars and buses can run on renewable energy. This bus is powered by hydrogen. As long as the hydrogen is extracted from water using renewable electricity, there is little damage to the environment.

MAKING A DIFFERENCE

Better habits at home

how to use less energy:

Wash clothes at a lower temperature. Try a lower setting on your washing machine. Your clothes will still come out clean.

Hang your laundry out to dry. Dryers are very energy-hungry so let the wind dry your clothes when it's warm outside.

Reuse your bath water. The dirty water can water your garden in the summer.

Take showers instead of baths. But keep your shower short, otherwise you may use just as much water and energy.

Don't leave appliances on standby. TVs, phone chargers, and other appliances waste a lot of energy when not in use, so switch them off properly.

Switch off lights when you leave a room. And swap all your bulbs for low-energy ones. Get a wind-up torch too.

Don't overfill the kettle. Kettles use a lot of energy. Only boil as much water as you are actually going to use.

Seal the gaps. Use draught excluders under doors and skirting boards. Newspaper, wood, or sealant will also do the job.

Lower your heating by one degree. It won't feel much colder and it will save energy and money.

Adjust your clothing. If you're cold, put on a sweater or vest, rather than turning on a heater. If you're too hot, shut the blinds.

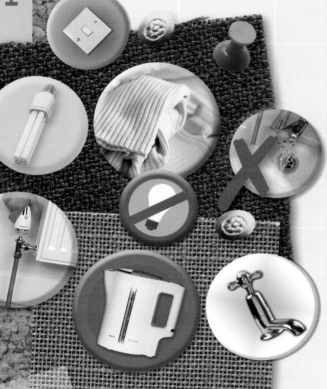

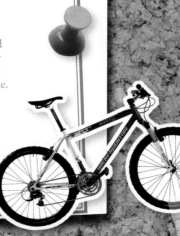

shopping for food

Try to buy food with less packaging You will produce less rubbish, and as packaging adds to the cost of your food, you might even end up saving money.

Buy local and seasonal food Local food doesn't have to travel miles by road or air to reach you. Seasonal food hasn't had to grow in an expensively heated greenhouse. It's probably fresher and healthier too.

Grow your own! Not only is the food you grow yourself very fresh (you just pick, cook, and eat), but gardening is also good exercise and fun.

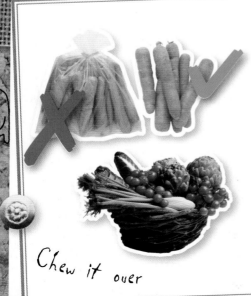

Chew it over

Remember to reduce, re-use, and recycle, and you'll save energy, money, and the Earth!

reusing and recycling

Don't throw out old clothes
Give them a new lease of life by customising them or donate them to charity. Those that are too worn can be cut up and used as dusters and cloths for cleaning.

Donate old eyeglasses to charity Some charities collect glasses and sort them for reuse by people in the developing world.

If you love shopping Start browsing in second-hand shops. You can find treasure and it's often very cheap too!

Collect tins and bottles for recycling There's no reason for these to go to landfill when they can be collected and re-used.

Take trainers for recycling Some companies take trainers apart and recycle them, making soles into playground floors for example.

Make birthday cards yourself Use magazines, packaging, and your imagination. It's fun, and guaranteed to look cool.

take it to the next level

Walk or cycle In heavy traffic, trips of less than 1.5 km (1 mile) can be faster on foot or by bike.

Holiday without flying Travel by car, boat, or train and make the journey part of the holiday.

Buy ethical gifts Buy a practical gift (through a charity) like a donkey for someone who needs it.

Say no to plastic bags Carry a re-usable bag and you won't need to accept yet another plastic bag.

Write to politicians Political change can achieve more than you can on your own, so tell them what you think!

What about the rest of the world?

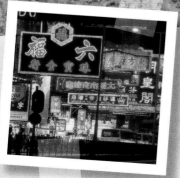

More than a third of the world's population lives in China and India. In both countries, especially in the cities, people are becoming rich: they live in bigger houses, own cars, and use many electrical appliances. But unless they use sustainable forms of energy, this new wealth could have a serious impact on the world's environment.

China is the world's fastest growing economy. It builds a new power station every week. Most are coal-fired, but the Chinese government also encourages large-scale renewable energy too.

India has an entire government department dedicated to encouraging renewable energy like solar power and wind power. Like China, it is worried about the rising price of oil, and would rather produce its own energy.

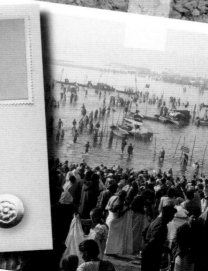

249

INDEX

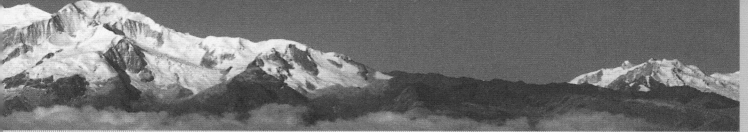

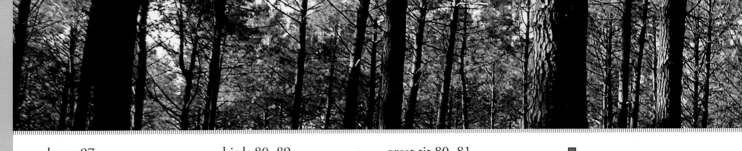

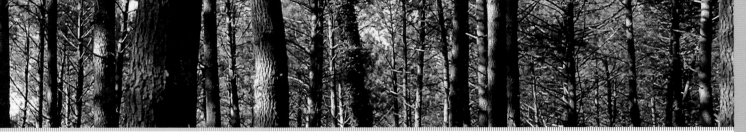

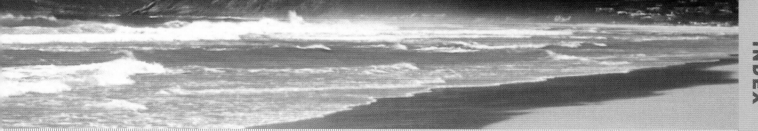

Acknowledgements

Dorling Kindersley would like to thank: Iowerth Watkins for cartography; Ed Merritt for additional cartography; Lee Wilson for proofreading; Chris Bernstein for indexing; and Lucy Claxton, Sarah Crowe, Rose Horridge, Emma Shepherd, and Romaine Werblow at the DK Picture Library.

PICTURE CREDITS

The publisher would like to thank the following for their kind permission to reproduce their photographs:
(Key: a-above; b-below/bottom; c-centre; f-far; jkt-inside jacket; l-left; r-right; t-top)

4Corners Images: Atlantide Phototravel 189t; Atlantide Phototravel/Stefano Amantino 179clb; **Alamy Images**: 121br; Ace Stock Ltd. 99bc; Peter Adams 103c, 108bl; Aerial Archives 219bl; AfriPics.com 109bc; Agripicture Images 122-123; AGStockUSA, Inc. 130cr, 131cr, 135t; Ambient Images Inc 178c (background); Arco Images 43br, 70tl, 92ca, 96c, 167cra, 170-171; Jon Arnold 195br; David Ball 34-35b, 42l; Robert E. Barber 217fbr; Ricardo Beliel 145bl; Blickwinkel 99bl, 155crb, 156bl, 169l, 197l; Steve Bloom Images 116b; Bobo 32t; Mark Boulton 82-83, 132r, 247tr; G P Bowater 59l; Bryan & Cherry Alexander Photography 46bl, 46br, 47bl, 47br, 52bc; Bruce Coleman Inc 167bc; Andrew Darrington 81tl; Carlos Davila 88br; George S de Blonsky 70r; Danita Delimont 103bc, 175bl; Olivier Digoit 233c; Michael Dwyer 32br, 232r; Eduardo Pucheta Photo 156br; Graham Ella 197bl; Elvele Images 60-61, 195tr; Elvele Images/ CGE 92cb; f1online 124b; Paul Felix Photography 201tl; David Fleetham 230br; John T Fowler 69clb; Clint Garnham 224br; Chris Gomersall 96cra, 97tr; Jane Gould 222cr; David Gowans 174r; Peter Haigh 116c, 118tl, 119ca; Andrew Harrington 118tr; Grady Harrison 135ca; Jennie Hart 28-29c; Martin Harvey 217tr; Gavin Hellier 98l; Carole Hewer 247cra; Jack Hobhouse 78bl; Andrew Holt 176-177; Holt Studios International Ltd 81tc; Hornbil Images 157bc; imagebroker 180r, 194bc, 194br; Images and Stories 21b, 94t; J L Images 178t; Jacques Jangoux 131bc; Jon Arnold Images / Gavin Hellier 182bl; Peter Jordan 145bc; Juniors Bildarchiv 171tr, 217br; Wolfgang Kaehler 28br; Steven J. Kazlowski 43tr; KLJ Photographic 35clb; Art Kowalsky 179r; Raghunandan Kulkarni/ephotocorp 155tc; Mark Lewis 225br; Lou Linwei 110-111; LOOK Die Bildagentur der Fotografen GmbH 100-101c, 166-167c, jkt; John E Marriott 179cl; Jenny Matthews 133bl;

Philip Mugridge 179bl; NASA Images 13b; David Noble 107t; David Norton 182br; Michael Patrick O'Neill 229bl; Papilio 195bc; Edward Parker 140clb, 144bl, 155l; Photofusion Picture Library 132c; Robert Preston 168l; qaphotos.com 242cl; Seb Rogers 5bl, 162-163, jkt; Galen Rowell/ Mountain Light 57tr; Joern Sackermann 181bl; Robbie Shone 187br; Stephen Frink Collection 204-205; Keren Su / China Span 86-87; tbkmedia.de 201bl; Mike Tercek 178b; Dave Thompson 166cc; David Tipling 70c; Penny Tweedie 174c, 174l; vario images GmbH & Co KG 135bc; Visual & Written SL 224bl; Visual&Written Sl/Mike Nolan/ VWPics 44crb; David Wall 98br; Lee Warren 194-195c; Dave Watts 189cr; We Shoot 120l; Kim Westerskov 239b; Terry Whittaker 156bc; Wildlife GmbH 37cr, 167bl; Marcus Wilson-Smith 105tr; Worldwide Picture Library 144r, 190r; **Ardea**: Kurt Amsler 226t; Bill Coster 216-217c, 216-217ca; John Daniels 103br; Bob Gibbons 57bc; M. Watson 44br, 61tr, 127r; Andrey Zvoznikov 45bl; **www. atacamaphoto.com**: 95c, 95tl; Adam Broomberg and Oliver Chanarin: 6tl; **Bryan and Cherry Alexander Photography**: 45fbr, 47bc, 52br, 53bc, 53br, 167tr; **Niall Corbet**: 173tl; **Corbis**: 21tl; Peter Adams 102c; Arctic-Images 245b; Yann Arthus-Bertrand 4tr, 90-91, 99t, 188t, 202t, jkt; Atlantide Phototravel 66bl, 84clb, 84-85c; Bjorn Backe/Papilio 101cr; Gary Bell / zefa 239t; Nathan Benn 201c; Niall Benvie 189br; Hal Beral 212ca, 227cra; Tobias Bernhard/zefa 231bc; Andrew Brown 53bl, 143bl; David Butow 107br; Brandon D Cole 222cl; Dean Conger 54-55; Ashley Cooper 214cra; Pablo Corral Vega 175t; C Devan/zefa 212-213c; EPA 144c, 150bl, 203bl, 242cr, 243cr; ER Productions 88bl; Rig Ergenbright 215bl; Kevin Fleming 71bl, 203t, 205tr; Jose Fuste Raga 215tr, 243cl; Raymond Gehman 101bl, 215br; Walter Geiersperger 175bc, 181t; T Gerson 232l; Farrell Grehan 214cla; Clinch Gryniewicz 218l; H et M/photocuisine 30bl; Tony Hamblin 197bc; Timothy Hearsum 32-33c; Chris Hellier 159tr; Jeremy Horner 190c; Hulton Archive 214tl; Zen Icknow 237b; JAI / John Coletti 151br; Peter Johnson 53c, 59r; Steve Kaufman 151bl; Kit Kittle 213c; Bob Krist 66t, 71t; T. Kruesselmann / Zefa 247br; Frank Lane Picture Agency 143cr; Jacques Langevin 102br; Frans Lanting 155bc; Frans Lemmens 96br; George D Lepp 17bl; W. Wayne Lockwood, M.D. 84br; Benedict Luxmoore 246-247c; Arthur Morris 51br; NASA 58l; Naturfoto Honal 78br; Baard Ness / Handout/epa 45bc; John Noble 84t, 85ca; Kazuyoshi Nomachi 95br, 98bc; Michael & Patricia Fogden 149br, 151bc; Paul A. Souders 16-17, 125cra; Smiley N. Pool / Dallas Morning News-15733990 191c; James Randklev 186cl; Walter Rawlings / Robert Harding World Imagery 245tr; Jeffrey L Rotman 225bl; Galen Rowell 51bl, 73br; Ron Sanford 50cra, 50tl, 50-51c, 51bc, 51ca, 74-75; Kevin Schafer 215tl; Gregor Schuster 37cl; Joseph Sohm / Visions of America 244-245c; Hans Strand 50cla; Keren Su 104-105c; Sygma 192bl, 192-193; Roger Tidman 68bl, 230c; Onne van der Wal 214tr; Brian A Vikander 151bl, 151br; Stuart Westmorland 222bc, 232c; Nik Wheeler 200tr; Ralph White 215crb; Witness/Corbis

Sygma 57tl; Lawson Wood 227cr; Tim Wright 219br; Xinhua Press 190l; Robert Yin 222br; **DK Images**: Australian Postal Corporation: stamp 9tr; Julian Baum 14crb; Malcolm Coulson 88tl; Philip Dowell 112cl; Rose Horridge 89bl; Judith Miller 221tr; Lindsey Stock 248cc; **David Doubilet**: 5tr, 208-209; **Ecoscene**: Paul Ferraby 218c; **Kate Edey**: 225ca; **Mario Farinato**: 181br; **Flickr.com**: cocoleroc 123tr; Linda de Volder 173tr; Mark Eadie 154cr, 203bc; Nathan Eagle 177tr; Manuel Haag 1, 2-3t, 14-15 (background); Jeanie's Pics 119br, Stuart Oikawa 119tl; Luca Patriccioli 203br; Mike Peters 203fbr; Doris Rapp 119fbr; Rodrigo Sala 173cla; Jacob Shamberg 125ca; Jeremy Stone 109bl; Tut99 (Roger) 119bc, Dinesh Valke 155cra; Melanie Yare 195bl; **FLPA**: Jim Brandenburg / Minden 92b; Nigel Cattlin 133t; Tui De Roy/Minden Pictures 56-57c; Danny Ellinger/Foto Natura 103cr; Derek Hall 121bl; David Hosking 120c; S Jonasson 225tc; Francoise Merlet 66b, 85cla, 85cr; Mark Moffett / Minden 73bc; Mark Newman 118cl, 118-119c, 119c; Flip Nicklin/Minden Pictures 56br; Terry Whittaker 183bl; Konrad Wothe 97c; **Getty Images**: Pete Atkinson 221b; W Banagan 37tr; Ira Block 106-107t; Larry Broder 48-49; China Photos 109bc; Ed Darack 71b; Peter David 212bl; Reinhard Dirscherl 227br; Georgette Douwma 223cl, 223cr; Michael Dunning 218r; Bob Elsdale 5c, 184-185, jkt; First Flight 214crb; Raymond Gehman 78-79c; Guillermo Gonzalez 73bl; Ken Graham 52bl; Darrell Gulin 72br; Jeff Harbers/Science Faction 62; Hulton Archive 165bl; Arnulf Husmo 214br; The Image Bank/Joseph Van Os 4bl, 40-41; Chris Johns 217bl; Johnny Johnson 50crb; Tim Laman 5tl, 138-139, 226br, jkt; Frans Lemmens 148-149c; Roine Magnusson 198-199; Ray Massey 213br; Joe McDonald 149bc; Eric Meola 189bl; Kevin Miller 228bl; Minden Pictures/Gerry Ellis 143br; Minden Pictures/Norbert Wu 57fbr; Darlyne A Murawski 213fbl; Paul Nicklen 75l; Rei Ohara 227fbr; Oxford Scientific Films / Photolibrary 158-159; Pete Oxford 149cr; Andrew Parkinson 154bl; Michael & Patricia Fogden 140bl, 148cl, 148t, 152-153, 153tl, 154bc; Terje Rakke 245tc; Robert Harding World Imagery / James Hager 51fbr; Andy Rouse 148br; Kelly Ryerson 214bl; David Sanger 214clb; Joel Sartore 138cb; Mike Severns 227bl; Anup Shah 146-147; Peter Sherrard 150bc; Marco Simoni 29bl; Brian J. Skerry 212cb, 227fbl; Moritz Steiger 96-97c; Maria Stenzel 62bl, 143bc; Tom Stoddart 157t; Nobuaki Sumida 4c, 64-65; Superstudio 79bl; Darryl Torckler 228bc; James Warwick 65l; Art Wolfe 227bc; Konrad Wothe 50cb, 68-69c; **Clare Harris**: 66ca, 76-77t; **Image Quest 3-D**: Southampton Oceanography Centre 231fbl; **The Irish Image Collection**: Tim Hannan 213bl; **Johns Hopkins University Applied Physics Laboratory/Southwest Research Institute**: 1997 by the Ocean Remote Sensing Group 231tl; **Lonely Planet Images**: Mark Webster 229bc; **Thomas Marent**: 142bl; **Mike Markey**: Mike Markey 225cla; **Walter Muma**: 69br; **NASA**: Johnson Space Center 24b; Goddard Space Flight Center Scientific Visualization Studio 109t; GRIN 14-15, 23tl, 27t; GSFC / Reto Stoeckli, Nazmi El Saleous &

Marit Jentoft-Nilsen 2-3b; LANDSAT/ University of Maryland Global Land Cover Facility 197tl; **naturepl.com**: Karl Ammann 127c; Peter Blackwell 129tr; Cindy Buxton 57bl; Bruce Davidson 149bl; Sue Flood 57br; Graham Hatherley 97bc; Tony Heald 125bl; Dietmar Hill 125fbr; Paul Hobson 173br; Rhonda Klevansky 172-173c; Neil Lucas 125br; Pete Oxford 149fbr; Peter Oxford 172cl, 172tr; Staffan Widstrand 44-45c; **NOAA**: David Burdick 229ftl, 229tl, 229tr; George E Marshall Album 121t; Dr Dwayne Meadowsreef 229tc; OAR/National Undersea Research Program (NURP) 222tr; **OSF**: Paul Franklin 167br; Rodger Jackman 222fbl; Satoshi Kuribayashi 199tr; Mary Plage 161c; Tui De Roy 45br, 189clb; Survival Anglia 157bl; **PA Photos**: AP Photo 108c, 207br; **Pelamis Wave Power Ltd.**: 238bl; Pelamis Wave Power 247crb; **Photolibrary**: ER Degginger 154cl, 155tr; **Photoshot/NHPA**: A.N.T. Photo Library 169c; Pete Atkinson 233r; Nigel J Dennis 125bc; Martin Harvey 124cl, 125c; Adrian Hepworth 150br; Daniel Heulin 97bl; T Kitchin and V Hurst 69bc; Yves Lanceau 102cl; Haroldo Palo Jr 56ca; Andy Rouse 168r; John Shaw 49tr; Mirko Stelzner 103fbr; **Pro Natura Zentrum Aletsch**: Laudo Albrecht 181bc; **PunchStock**: Digital Vision 220; Photographer's Choice 66cb, 72c (background), 73c (b/g); Stockbyte/ Tom Brakefield 68br; **SaharaMet**: R. Pelisson 17br; **Science Photo Library**: Michael Abbey 16bl; NASA 25bl; Mike Agliolo 242t; Steve Allen 243bl; Nick Bergkessel 79bc; Martin Bond 133bc, 244bl, 244br, 247fbr; Dr John Brackenbury 76clb; Massimo Brega 135bc; British Antarctic Survey 59c; Robert Brook 35cr; Tony Craddock 240-241, 242bl; Christian Darkin 12c; Georgette Douwma 85br; Michael Dunning 18cl; European Space Agency 14ca; P G Adam, Publiphoto Diffusion 39; Bob Gibbons 200b; Andy Harmer 198bc, 198bl, 198br; Jan Hinsch 233l; Manfred Kage 58c; LEPUS 213bc; Dr Ken Macdonald 17bc; NASA/ESA/Stsci/R. schaller 4tl, 10-11; NASA/Goddard Space Flight Center Scientific Visualization Studio 58r; NOAA 210bl, 242br, 243br; Merlin D Tuttle 101tc; Detlev van Ravenswaay 13c, 15t, 24t; M I Walker 19cl; Jason Ware 12t; **Michael Scott**: 155br, 157br, 161t, 179cla; **SeaPics.com**: 229ftr; Clay Bryce 228br; Bob Cranston 231br; Steve Drogin 235tl; Richard Herrmann 234-235, jkt; Espen Rekdal 222bl, 231bl, jkt; Dennis Sabo 223bl; Mark Strickland 234clb; Ron and Valerie Taylor 235tc; Masa Ushioda 227cl, 229br, 235tr; Marli Wakeling 226bl; James D Watt 226c; **Mark W Skinner @ USDA-NRCS PLANTS Database**: 169r; **stevebloom.com**: 231c; Steve Bloom 4br, 114-115, 128-129, jkt; **Still Pictures**: Gil Moti 113bc; Jorgen Schytte 196r; Silke Wedler 112-113bc; **Sublette County Historical Society**: 193tr; **SuperStock**: age fotostock 8, 97br; **TrekEarth**: Tsetsegee Sumiya 103bl; **UNEP**: 106b; **US Geological Survey**: 229cl; **USDA Forest Service** (www.forestryimages.org): Darren Blackford 70bl; **www.UWPhoto.no**: Erling Svenson 225bc

All other images © Dorling Kindersley
For further information see:
www.dkimages.com